Subthalamic and Thalamic Stereotactic Recordings and Stimulations in Patients with Intractable Epilepsy

ISBN : 978-2-7420-0618-2

Éditions John Libbey Eurotext
127, avenue de la République
92120 Montrouge, France
Tél. : 01 46 73 06 60
E-mail : contact@jle.com
Site Internet : http ://www.jle.com

John Libbey Eurotext
42-46 High Street
Esher, Surrey
KT10 9KY
United Kingdom

© John Libbey Eurotext, Paris, 2008
It is prohibited to reproduce this work or any part of it without the authorisation of the publisher or of the Centre français d'Exploitation du Droit de Copie, 20, rue des Grands-Augustins, 75010 Paris, France.

Subthalamic and Thalamic Stereotactic Recordings and Stimulations in Patients with Intractable Epilepsy

Heinz Gregor Wieser and Dominik Zumsteg

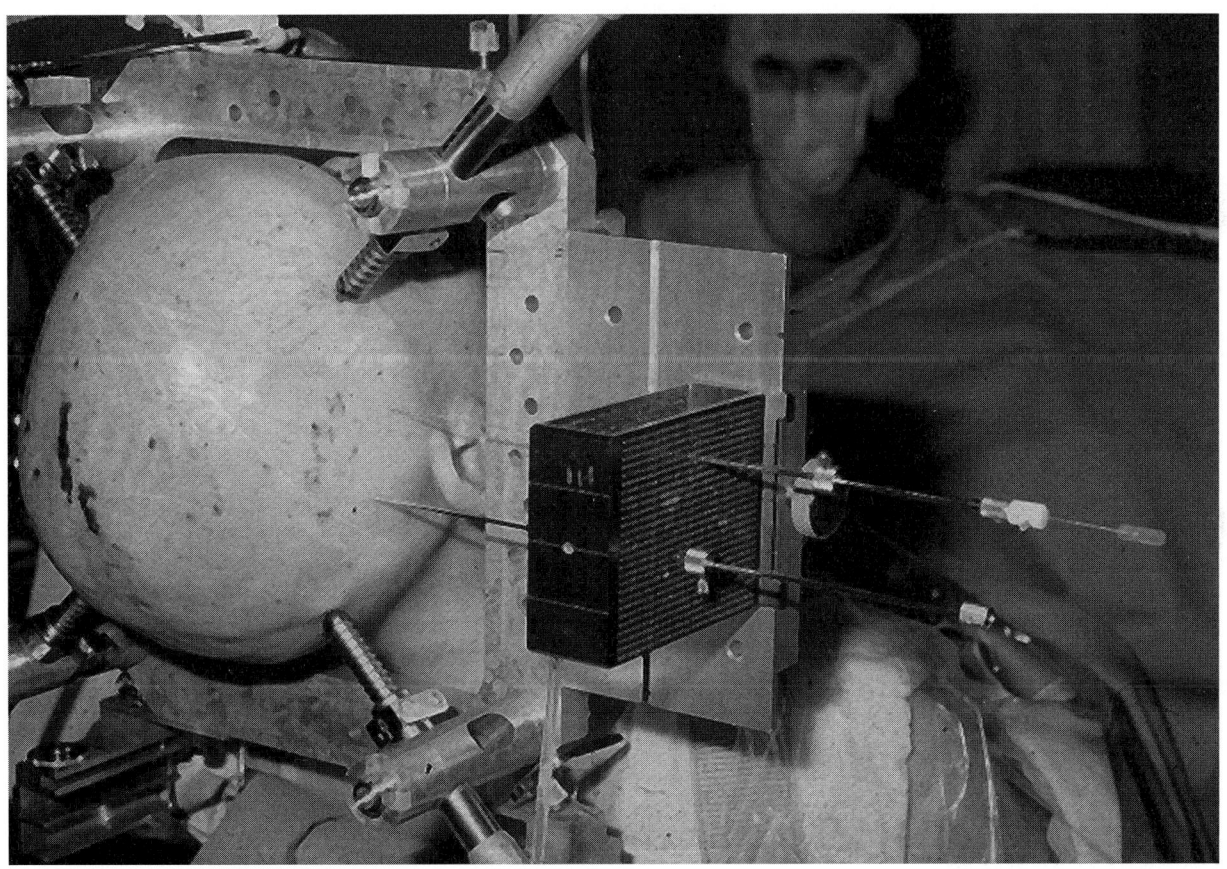

Prof. Dr. med. Heinz Gregor Wieser
Department of Neurology
University Hospital Zürich
Frauenklinikstrasse 26
8091 Zürich
Switzerland

Phone: +41 44 255 55 30 or 31
Fax: +41 44 255 44 29
Email: hgw@usz.ch

PD Dr. med. Dominik Zumsteg
Department of Neurology
University Hospital Zürich
Frauenklinikstrasse 26
8091 Zürich
Switzerland

Email: dominik.zumsteg@usz.ch

Dedication to

Christoph Bernoulli
Former Head of the Stereo-EEG Unit,
Institute of Electroencephalography,
University Hospital Zürich

Klaus Hess
Professor Emeritus, University Zürich,
Former Director of the Neurology Department,
University Hospital Zürich

Rudolf Max Hess [†]
Professor Emeritus, University Zürich,
Former Director of the Institute of Electroencephalography,
University Hospital Zürich

Jean Siegfried
Professor Emeritus, University Zürich,
Former Director of the Stereotaxy Unit,
Department Neurosurgery,
University Hospital Zürich

Gazi Yasargil
Professor Emeritus, University Zürich,
Former Director of the Neurosurgery Department,
University Hospital Zürich

Yasuhiro Yonekawa
Professor Emeritus, University Zürich,
Former Director of the Neurosurgery Department,
University Hospital Zürich

with grateful thanks

Preface

More than thirty years since I have joined the presurgical evaluation and epilepsy surgery program of the University Hospital Zurich (the former Kantonsspital Zurich), and at the end of my professional career, I revisited the stereo-EEG archives to look after some recordings and stimulation data we had performed in deep brain nuclei during these pioneering days of epilepsy surgery. Our archive still contains the complete printouts and magnetic tapes of more than 130 patients who had undergone prolonged video-EEG monitoring with stereotactically implanted depth electrodes. I remembered that we had explored several patients with depth recordings from subthalamic and thalamic sites, as well as from the periaqueductal gray matter. At that time thalamic lesions were made in selected patients with medically intractable epilepsy not amenable to ablative epilepsy surgery. The subthalamic sites, in particular the Forel H fields, were studied in five patients with the goal to learn more about this area with a view towards Jinnai's Forel H-tomy. However, our limited experience with thalamic stereotactic lesions in epilepsy led us to abandon these procedures, and Forel H-tomy was never practiced in Zurich as a treatment modality for epilepsy. Nevertheless, with the renewed interest in deep brain stimulation for patients with intractable epilepsy, I decided to document those case studies that had electrodes in the Forel H fields or the thalamus.

Heinz Gregor Wieser

"Unter den Ameisen findet man Weber, Schlächter, Tierzüchter, Maurer, Kartonfabrikanten, Bäcker, Pilzzüchter, Gärtner, Krieger und Pazifisten, Sklavenjäger, Diebe, Räuber und Parasiten; aber keine Professoren, noch Volksredner, Regenten, Bürokraten und Generale, nicht einmal Korporale, auch keine Kapitalisten und Spekulanten, ebensowenig Schwätzer"

["Among the ants one finds weavers, butchers, animal breeders, masons, cardboard makers, bakers, mushroom growers, gardeners, warriors and pacifists, slave hunters, thieves, robbers, and parasites; but no professors, yet public speakers, rulers, bureaucrats and generals, not even corporals, also no capitalists and speculators, nor gossipers", Translation John Palmer and Marianne Regard]

Auguste Forel (1848-1931),
physician, nature scientist, social reformer
(Exhibition catalog, University of Zurich, 1986, p. 142)

Acknowledgments

Ms. Jeannette Weilenmann and Mr. Sepp Müller helped us with scanning the EEG traces and with some photographs, Mr. Peter Roth with drawing figure 23. Ms. Simone Spring typed parts of the manuscript and helped with the references and permissions. Ms. Vachira Tontrakalpaibul helped with proof reading and checked for completeness of references. Ms. Elsi Urech, former head nurse of the EEG institute, performed an enormous amount of work securing the recording of unparalleled EEGs of the illustrated patients. Mr. Hans Bosshard provided expert technical assistance in the operating theatre and SEEG laboratory. We also thank former fellows, in particular Dr. Stefan Stodieck, Dipl. Ing. Hippolyt Meles and Ing. Sandro Moser. Several authors, editors and publishers gave us generous permission to use previously published material. We would like to express our gratitude to the publishing group of John Libbey Eurotext. Special thanks go to UCB Switzerland for financial support, in particular to Ms. Marianne Tschudi.

Contents

Preface	VI
Abbreviations	X
Introduction	1
Purpose and General Aims of this Book	2
Basic Principles of the Stereo-EEG Technique	3
Direct Current (DC) Recording and Stimulation	14
Neurotransmitter Studies using Push Pull Cannulae	20
Anatomical and Physiological Basis for Stereotactic Exploration of Subcortical Structures in Patients with Epilepsy	29
The Subthalamic Area	30
The Forel H Field	30
The Thalamic Nuclei	41
The Pulvinar	53
The Periaqueductal Gray Matter	54
The Reticular Formation	56
Case Studies	59
Case 1	60
Case 2	66
Case 3	74
Case 4	79
Case 5	82
Case 6	87
Case 7	99
Case 8	103
Case 9	110
Case 10	114
Case 11	119
Case 12	123
Cases 13 to 17	125
Discussion	133
Old and New Treatment Options for Intractable Epilepsies	134
Potential Targets for Deep Brain Stimulation in Epilepsy	136
Conclusions and Outlook	151
References	155
Index	173
Appendix: Historical Note on Auguste Forel	191

Abbreviations

AC	Alternating current
AD	Afterdischarge
AED	Antiepileptic drug
AHE	Amygdalohippocampectomy
ALA	Alanine
AN	Anterior nucleus of the thalamus
ARAS	Ascending reticular activation system
ASN	Asparagine
ASP	Aspartate
BA	Brodmann area
CA	Cornu Ammonis
CD	Cervical dystonia
CJD	Creutzfeldt-Jakob Disease
CLC	Central lateral complex of the thalamus
CM	Centromedian nucleus of the thalamus
CSA	Compressed spectral array
DBS	Deep brain stimulation
DC	Direct current
DM	Dorsomedial nucleus of the thalamus
ECG	Electrocardiography
EDA	Electrodermal activity
EEG	Electroencephalography
EMG	Electromyographic recording
EOG	Electrooculography
EP	Evoked potentials
ER	Evoked response
EPC	Epilepsia partialis continua
FDA	US food and drug administration
FO	Foramen ovale
GABA	Gamma-aminobutyric acid
GLU	Glutamate
GLY	Glycine
GP	Globus pallidus
GPe	Globus pallidus, pars externa
GPi	Globus pallidus, pars interna
GSR	Galvanic skin response
HPLC	High pressure liquid chromatography
ICP	Intercommissural plane
IED	Interictal epileptiform discharges
L.po.	Nucleus lateropolaris
LD	Lateral dorsal nucleus of the thalamus
LHA	Lateral hypothalamic neurons
LORETA	Low resolution electromagnetic tomography
LP	Lateral posterior nucleus of the thalamus
MB	Mamillary body, Corpus mamillare
MCP	Midcommissural plane
MFB	Medial forebrain bundle
MTLE	Mesial temporal lobe epilepsy
MTT	Mamillothalamic tract
NINDS	National Institute of Neurological Disorders and Stroke
NR	Nucleus ruber

NRM	Nuclei raphe magnus
NRP	Nuclei raphe pallidus
OPA	o-pthalaldehyde
PAG	Periaqueductal gray
PC	Posterior commissure
PD	Parkinson's disease
PGM	Periaqueductal gray matter
PGO	Ponto-geniculo-occipital waves
PPN	Pedunculopontine nucleus
PSWC	Periodic sharp wave complexes
PTZ	Pentylenetretrazol
PVP	Posteroventral pallidotomy
rTh	Reticular nucleus of the thalamus
rTMS	Repetitive transcranial magnetic stimulation
sAHE	Selective amygdalohippocampectomy
SEEG	Stereo-electroencephalography
SEF	Spectral edge frequency
SEP	Somatosensory evoked potential
SER	Serotonin
SGI	Stratum griseum intermedium
SNPM	Statistical nonparametric mapping
SNr	Substantia nigra, pars reticulata
SSMA	Supplementary sensorymotor area
STN	Subthalamic nucleus
SWS	Slow wave sleep
tDCS	Transcranial direct current stimulation
TL	Temporal lobe
TLE	Temporal lobe epilepsy
TMN	Tuberomamillary neurons
TMS	Transcranial magnetic stimulation
V.c.a.	Nucleus ventrocaudalis anterior
V.c.p.	Nucleus ventrocaudalis posterior
V.c.pc.e	Nucleus ventrocaudalis parvocellularis externus
V.c.pc.i	Nucleus ventrocaudalis parvocellularis internus
V.im.e.	Nucleus ventrointermedius externus
V.im.i.	Nucleus ventrointermedius internus
V.o.	Nucleus ventro-oralis
V.o.a.	Nucleus ventro-oralis anterior
V.o.i.	Nucleus ventro-oralis internus
V.o.p.	Nucleus ventro-oralis posterior
VA	Nucleus ventralis anterior
Vca	Anterior vertical line perpendicular to the AC-PC line
Vcp	Posterior vertical line perpendicular to AC-PC line
VEP	Visual evoked potential
VI	Ventral intermedial nucleus of the thalamus
VIP	Vasoactive intestinal peptide
VL	Ventral lateral nucleus of the thalamus
VNS	Vagus nerve stimulation
VP	Ventral posterior nucleus of the thalamus
VPL	Ventral posterolateral nucleus of the thalamus
VPM	Ventral posteromedial nucleus of the thalamus
WGA-HRP	Wheat germ-agglutinin-conjugated horseradish peroxidase

Introduction

Purpose and General Aims of this Book

Brain stimulation for seizure control has succeeded the era of lesioning deep relay nuclei. The successful history of cochlear implants (US Food and Drug Administration (FDA) approval in 1985) followed by deep brain stimulation (DBS) for tremor (1997), vagal nerve stimulation for epilepsy (VNS, 1997), DBS for Parkinson's disease (2002) and primary dystonia (2003) are ample evidence that interaction of science and clinical work has benefited both groups. The *National Institute of Neurological Disorder and Stroke (NINDS)* is presently supporting investigations using electrical recording and electrical stimulation and local drug delivery in the central nervous system at demand.

Cerebellar stimulation, VNS, repetitive transcranial magnetic stimulation (rTMS), DBS either targeting the subthalamic nucleus (STN), the anterior thalamic nucleus (AN) or the hippocampal formation have been used in the management of epilepsy patients who are medically intractable and not amenable to classical resective epilepsy surgery. However, with respect to the role of DBS in epilepsy, data are still very limited and much has to be done in order to answer the questions as to the efficacy of DBS. The Grenoble experience includes five patients with high frequency STN stimulation [Benabid et al., 2004], and the Cleveland experience four patients [Neme et al., 2004]. Patient selection criteria (focal vs. generalized), stimulation modality (constant vs. cycling, open loop vs. closed loop), stimulation parameters, stimulation target nuclei vs. fiber tracts have to be studied before the effectiveness of this treatment modality can be assessed. At present DBS is an experimental procedure that warrants further studies.

On the background of this exciting and ongoing discussion on the role of thalamic and subthalamic nuclei in epilepsies and given the potential therapeutic role of DBS of thalamic and subthalamic nuclei on the other, we present 11 patients who underwent stereo-EEG (SEEG) explorations with a view towards epilepsy surgery at the Zurich University Hospital. These patients had electrodes in Forel H (patients 1 to 5), in thalamic nuclei (patients 6 to 10) or in the brainstem (patient 11). We also illustrate one patient with Creutzfeldt-Jakob Disease (CJD) with simultaneous thalamic and cortical recordings (patient 12). Furthermore, we summarize our limited experience with recordings and stimulations in the periaqueductal gray matter (PGM, patients 13 to 17), with DC recording and DC polarization, as well as with biochemical measurements of excitatory and inhibitory transmitters and transmitter candidates released in the primary epileptogenic area during spontaneous and electrically induced epileptic discharges. All patients are illustrated with their most relevant findings in order to elucidate the following basic questions.

(1) Do cortical seizure discharges spread to the above mentioned deep brain structures, and with which characteristics?
(2) Do interictal epileptiform graphoelements originate in or spread to these deep brain structures?
(3) What is the effect of cortical and subcortical electrical stimulation, with regard to (a) deep brain nuclei, (b) interictal and ictal epileptiform EEG potentials, and (c) biochemical measurements?
(4) Which components of SEP and cognitive potentials can be recorded in these deep brain structures?
(5) Finally, what is the clinical efficacy of lesions in thalamic sites in those patients with therapeutic stereotactic lesions?

Some of the patients in this book in part have been presented in previous publications. Two patients (Nos. 7 and 8, Fig. 6) with bihemispheric SEEG exploration through two symmetric thalamic electrodes and two patients (Nos. 9 and 10) with unilateral exploration of the suspected primary epileptogenic area and simultaneous recording from the ipsilateral thalamus have been previously presented in a book chapter by Wieser and Siegel [1993]. We have also summarized findings in patients with severe pain syndromes, recorded from electrodes targeted to the PGM. These electrodes allowed for simultaneous recordings from the PGM and the posterior thalamus and were correlated to recordings from scalp electrodes [Wieser and Siegfried, 1979a, b]. The thalamic and cortical recordings of patient 12 with CJD have been recently illustrated [Wieser et al., 2004, 2006].

We are fully aware of the descriptive nature of this volume and understand it as an intermediate between an atlas and a series of well-illustrated case studies undertaken with a view towards possible epilepsy surgery at a time when modern diagnostic tools were not available. Since exhaustive invasive presurgical evaluation is diminishing because of the today's availability of modern non-invasive imaging techniques, the findings of these patients might help to better understand the role of the explored deep brain structures in various types of epilepsy.

Basic Principles of the Stereo-EEG Technique

The first intracerebral recording from man was made by Berger [1931] and later by Foerster and Altenburger [1935] using insulated needles. The first multi-target depth electrode studies in humans date back to 1953 [Ribstein, 1960], but this technique was not based on precise stereotactic principles. Professor Lars Leksell was one of the first to develop a stereotactic device exclusively for human functional neurosurgery in 1949, following the pioneering work of the American neurosurgeons Ernest A. Spiegel and Henry T. Wycis in 1947. Leksell's stereotactic frame was based on the Horsley-Clarke apparatus developed for animal experimentation by Sir Victor Horsley at University College London in 1908, but instead of using the Cartesian coordinate frame, it used polar coordinates [Leksell, 1949]. In humans, these stereotactic methods were first applied by Spiegel and Wycis to investigate the thalamus and hypothalamus in petit mal epilepsy [Spiegel et al., 1947; Spiegel and Wycis, 1950, 1951, 1952, 1961; Hayne and Meyers, 1950; Riechert and Mundinger, 1955; Talairach et al., 1958]. Using similar techniques, Williams and Parsons Smith [1949], Kirikae and Wada [1951] and Jung et al. [1952] conducted functional investigations towards treatment of seizures within the concept of the so-called "centrencephalic" seizure origin. Yet, the use of simultaneous functional stereotactic exploration of many cortical and subcortical structures had to await the publication of atlases providing their spatial coordinates [Talairach et al., 1957, 1967]. The simultaneous recording from many stereotactically inserted electrodes together with scalp EEG was pioneered in St. Anne, Paris, and became known as stereo-electroencephalography [Talairach et al., 1952; Bancaud, 1959]. The term stereo-electroencephalography (stereo-EEG; SEEG) simply denotes that this method is based on stereotactic principles, and that it aims at measuring the EEG in a 3-dimensional way. The combination of stereotactic depth electrodes and scalp EEG recordings minimizes the spatial sampling problem, which is inherent in depth EEG recordings. In this fashion, the shortcomings of each method are compensated by each other: The extremely sharp but relatively "tunneled vision" of depth electrode recordings is balanced by the distorted and "blurred vision" of scalp EEG recordings.

Studies of intracerebral activity in the epileptic patient have contributed enormously to our understanding of the origin and spread of seizure discharges. In 1987 we have published the proceedings of a scientific meeting on "Presurgical Evaluation of Epileptics" taking place in Zurich in 1985, outlining the value of stereo-EEG [Wieser, 1987a; Wieser and Elger, 1987]. At that time, SEEG was considered a *step II* procedure, that is, it was generally performed after establishment of hypotheses about the seizure origin in candidates for epilepsy surgery. As an invasive method, SEEG was performed with the explicit aim of (a) improving inconclusive or insufficient data of the non-invasive *step I* diagnosis in order to allow firm judgments whether surgical treatment can be offered, and (b) of resolving discrepancies of non-invasive investigations which otherwise would have precluded surgical treatment.

The Implantation of SEEG Electrodes

Although most stereotactic techniques allow the electrodes to be implanted from any angle, most centers prefer to use the orthogonal approach in their routine work. The Yale group has advocated depth probes inserted through occipital guide pins and coursing through the long axes of both hippocampi. The most commonly explored targets are the medial temporal lobe structures including the amygdala, the pes hippocampi and the parahippocampal gyrus, mostly by using anterior, middle and posterior electrode placements. Orbital and mesial frontal cortical (supplementary sensorymotor area, SSMA) as well as anterior and posterior cingulate cortical areas have also been targeted in a large number of patients in Paris and Zurich (Fig. 1). Although most of the extratemporal structures in principle can be explored stereotactically, there is now a tendency to use either subdural strips/grids instead of stereotactic depth electrodes, or to combine the two methods in patients with extratemporal epilepsy [Wieser et al., 1985a].

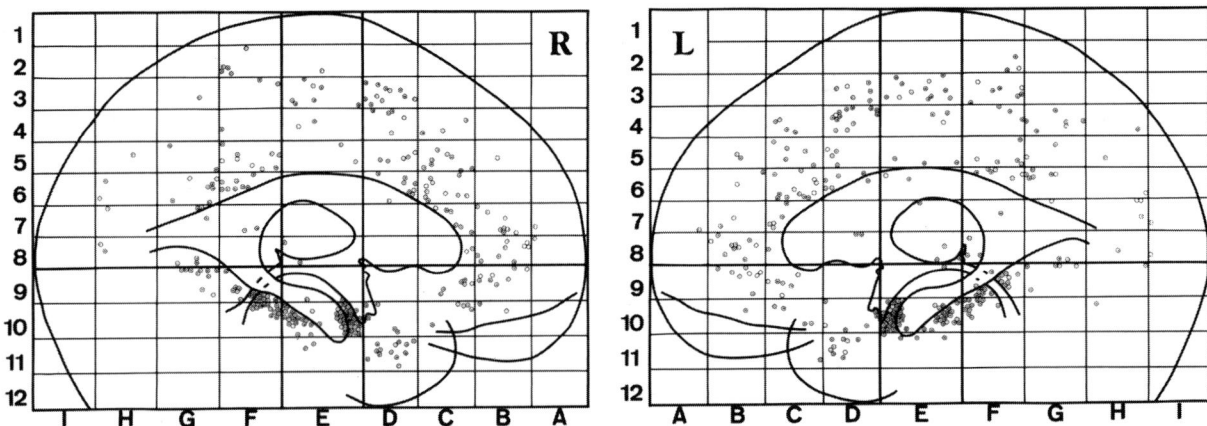

Figure 1. Superposition of the targets for the SEEG electrodes in 60 patients shown in the normalized Talairach system based on the anterior and posterior commissures and their verticals.

Modified from: Siegfried J, Wieser HG. The actual role of stereotactic operations on deep brain structures in the treatment of medically refractory epilepsies. In: Broggi G ed. The Rational Basis of the Surgical Treatment of Epilepsies. London: Libbey 1988: 113-119.

Prior to implantation, the brain and its vessels had to be known in the stereotactic reference system, which was achieved by performing a so-called "repérage". This neuroradiological examination under stereotactic conditions was a necessary precondition not only for the calculation of the targets but also for minimizing the risks of electrode insertion. Before the MRI era, the "repérage" consisted of mounting the stereotactic Talairach frame, performing a pneumencephalography and, if necessary, ventriculography with contrast medium. Finally, the vessels were visualized angiographically by carotid, and if necessary, vertebral angiography (Figs. 2 and 3). The "repérage" and the insertion of the depth electrodes was usually a two-step procedure with an interval of about 6 weeks, which allowed for the calculation of the depth electrodes position outside the operating theatre, leading to shorter general anesthesia time and, presumably, to a lower risk. However, in certain instances the "repérage" and the insertion of depth electrodes were performed in one session. Burr holes of a diameter of 3 mm were placed following a small skin incision using a special drill with a stopper (Fig. 2c). The dura was then penetrated with a special coagulation electrode and the depth electrodes were inserted using an in-house modified Talairach system (Figs. 2b and 5).

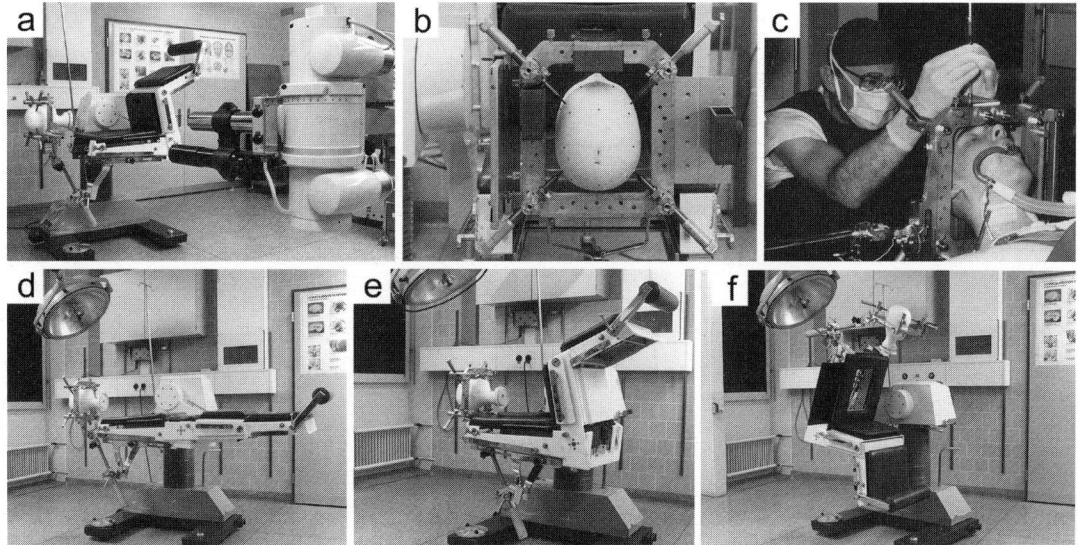

Figure 2. a, teleradiography; **b**, Talairach frame; **c**, a 3 mm diameter burr-hole is placed using a special drill; **d, e, f**, the table of Alexander in various positions (in order to prevent distortion of the object due to magnification, the x-rays (a) should be paralleled, which is approximatively achieved by keeping a source-object distance of greater 4.75 m).

See also: Talairach J, Szikla G, Tournoux P, Prossalentis A, Bordas-Ferrer M, Covello L, Jacob M, Mempel E, Buser P, Bancaud J. *Atlas d'anatomie stéréotaxique du télencéphale.* Paris: Masson 1967.

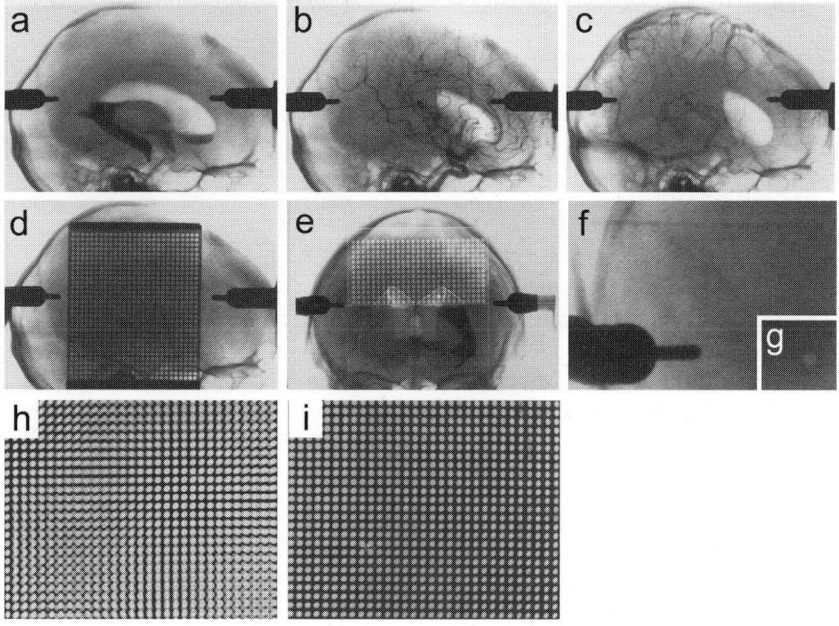

Figure 3. Illustration of the neuroradiological examination under stereotactic conditions, the so-called "repérage". **a**, lateral x-ray with ventriculography with air and positive contrast medium; arterial **(b)** and venous **(c)** phase after carotid angiography; **d**, lateral view of the double grid in position; **e**, anterior-posterior x-ray composite with the double grid and ventriculography; **f**, anterior-posterior view of an inserted electrode; **g**, orthogonal view of a burr hole; **h** and **i**, illustration of the teleradiography with an incorrect sighting-line with a too short source-object distance and a correct sighting-line with a sufficient source-object distance (with the use of a good sighting-line, the holes of the double grid display as one circle).

Modified from: Wieser HG. Stereo-Electroencephalography. In: Wieser HG, Elger CE eds. *Presurgical Evaluation of Epileptic Patients.* Berlin Heidelberg: Springer 1987a: 192-204.

Introduction

Today there is a variety of commercially depth electrodes available, but patients illustrated in this work were all implanted with homemade electrodes developed in collaboration with the Straumann Company [Comte et al., 1983]. This so-called hollow core electrode permitted the insertion of the electrode with its guiding stylet inside, minimizing the traumatization of the brain (Fig. 4). Moreover, this electrode could also be used to host other devices in the inner lumen such as a push pull cannula, which in turn allowed for the investigation of extracellular fluid for known and putative transmitters in relation to EEG changes and in particular in relation to epileptiform events [Wieser et al., 1989a; Cuénod et al., 1990; see page 20].

In patient Nos. 6, 7, 10 and 12 of the present compilation (Fig. 6), thalamic recordings were performed by using rigid multicontact depth electrodes, so-called "electrodes de type aigu" [Talairach et al., 1967]. The diameter of the standard depth electrodes was 0.9 mm, with a length and intercontact spacing of 1 mm for each contact, except the longer intercontact spacing between contact 4 and 5. In patient Nos. 8 and 9, a wing electrode ("Seitenelektrode") was used for thalamic recordings and stimulations. Depth electrodes were numbered with numerals (in the illustrated recordings they are indicated with the first large and bold numeral) and their topographical position was indicated in the patient's individual brain map with lateral and anteroposterior views (Fig. 6). As a rule, each depth electrode had 10 contacts (exceptionally only 8), numbered 1 to 10 (or 8, respectively) from inside out. These contacts were indicated with the small numerals following the electrode number in the recordings.

Example: In Fig. 6, the depth electrode 5 in patient No. 1 was targeted to the anterior cingulate gyrus; 5/1-2 therefore indicates that contact 1 against 2 of electrode 5 is recording in a bipolar fashion from the anterior cingulate gyrus, whereas 5/9-10 indicates that the recording was performed from the lateral frontal opercular neocortex (Brodmann area 45).

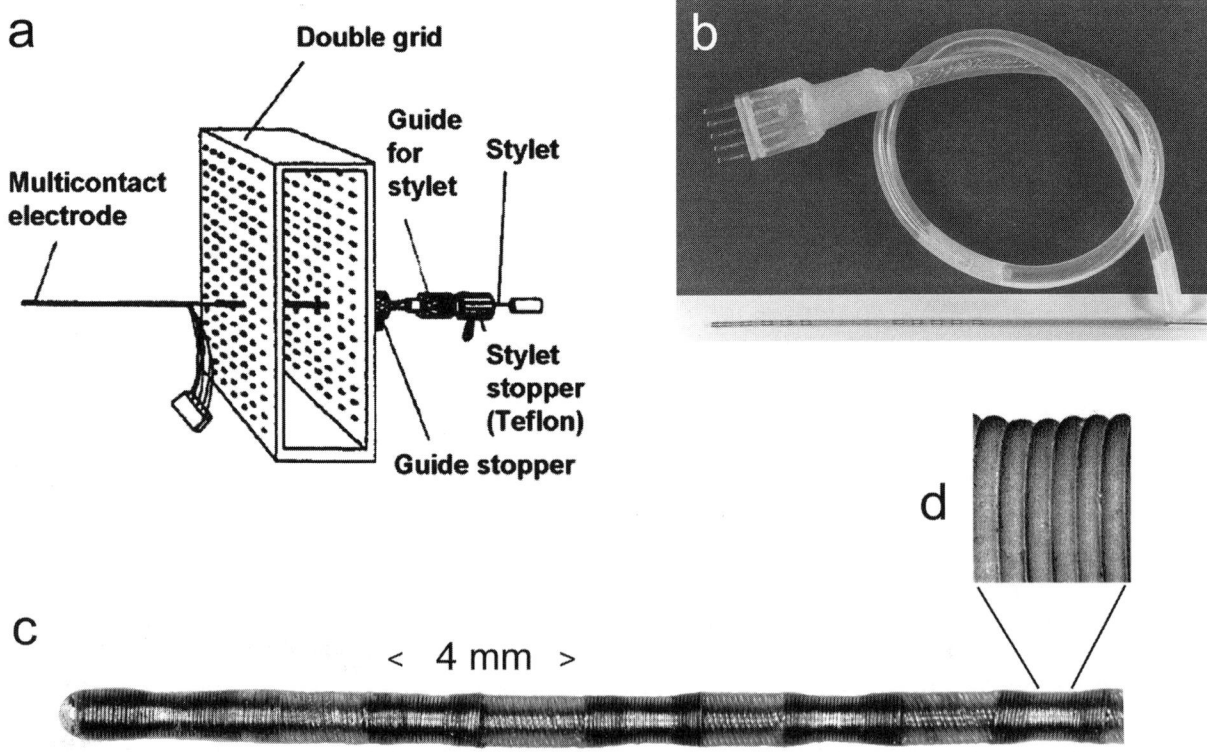

Figure 4. Multicontact hollow core electrode with a 10-pin connector (b) and guiding device mounted on the Talairach grid (a). Details of slightly recessed contacts (c) showing the wiring of the electrode in greater detail (d).

Parts a and d modified from: Comte P, Siegfried J, Wieser HG. Multipolar hollow-core electrode for brain recordings. Appl Neurophysiol 1983; 46: 41-46.

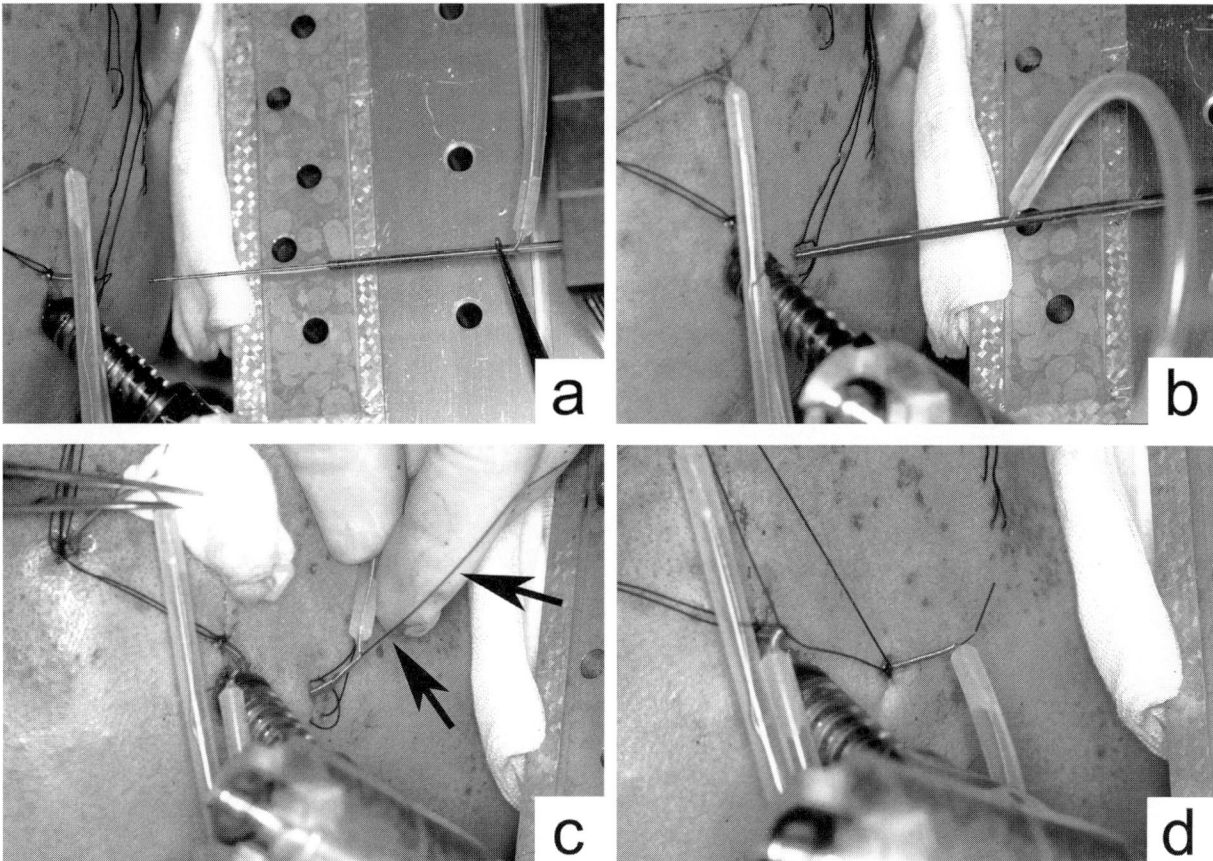

Figure 5. Stereotactic insertion of a multicontact hollow core electrode. **a**, multicontact hollow core and special guiding device mounted on the Talairach grid; **b**, insertion of the guiding device into the small 3 mm burr hole; **c**, insertion of the depth electrode, z-suture and introduction of the plastic wire (black arrows) into the hollow core of the electrode; **d**, tied z-suture, the electrode is in its final position and is fixed to the scalp.

SEEG Recordings

Scalp EEG recordings were carried out using standard scalp electrodes (Ag/AgCl cup-shaped disc electrodes) placed according to the Hess system [Hess, 1969] or the international 10-20 electrode system and referenced to linked earlobes. Depth EEG recordings were usually performed using bipolar derivations of two neighboring contacts of an electrode. Commonly, bipolar recordings were then followed by monopolar recordings using a common average electrode fed by "inactive" contacts situated in the white matter. Continuous 32-channel paper printout of selected scalp and depth EEG derivations was supplemented by polygraphic recordings including electrocardiogram (ECG), oculogram (EOG), respiration, heart rate and galvanic skin response (GSR). All recordings were stored on a 32-channel tape and video-monitoring device (Figs. 7-10). For special recording sessions, EEG traces were subjected to analog 0.3 to 70 Hz bandpass filtering, 200 Hz digitization, and electronic storage. This allowed for quantitative EEG analysis using Stellate® (http://www.stellate), Spectralab® (Bruno Fricker, http://www.spectralab.ch) and in-house purpose-built software. The latter was based on forerunners of the nowadays commercially available MATLAB software package (The MathWorks Inc., Natick, MA, USA). These software packages allowed for plotting *compressed spectral arrays* (CSA) of up to six EEG channels simultaneously with real time EEG recording and display, *spectra and band activity* for up to eight user defined frequency bands, *coherence and phase spectra* measuring the relationships between two channels over time, and the production of *spectral activity maps* displaying topographical representations. *Phase- and coherence analysis* (Stellate®) was used for estimation of phase delays, reflecting propagation of EEG activity. *Long-term trend of band activity* and *spectral edge frequency* (SEF) were used to quantify vigilance in association with *automatic spike detection algorithms* (Figs. 26 and 30). *Amplitude maps* were calculated when appropriate.

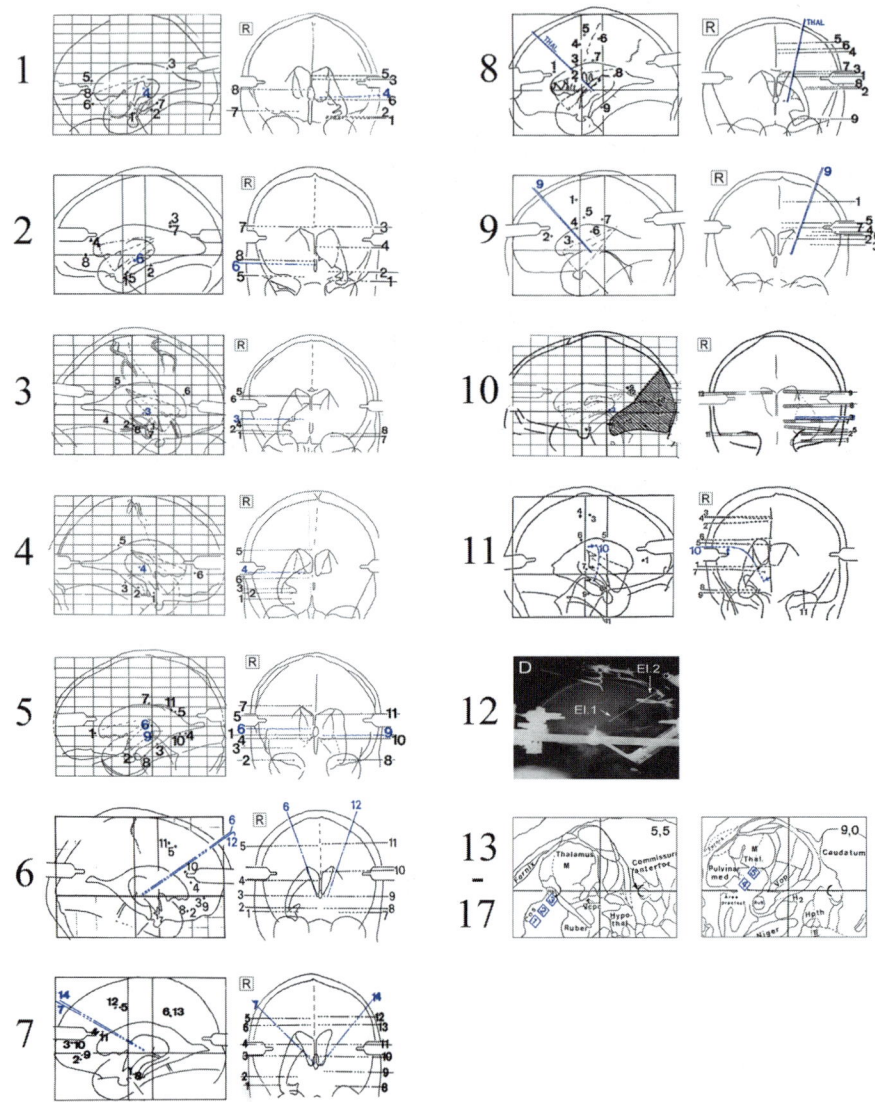

Figure 6. Survey of the presented case studies with depth electrodes located in subthalamic (patient Nos. 1 to 5), thalamic (patient Nos. 6 to 10, and 12) and brainstem sites (patient Nos. 11, and 13 to 17). Case studies 8, 9 and 11 illustrate patients with Rasmussen's encephalitis, case study 12 a patient with CJD, and case studies 13 to 17 pain patients with electrodes in the PGM.

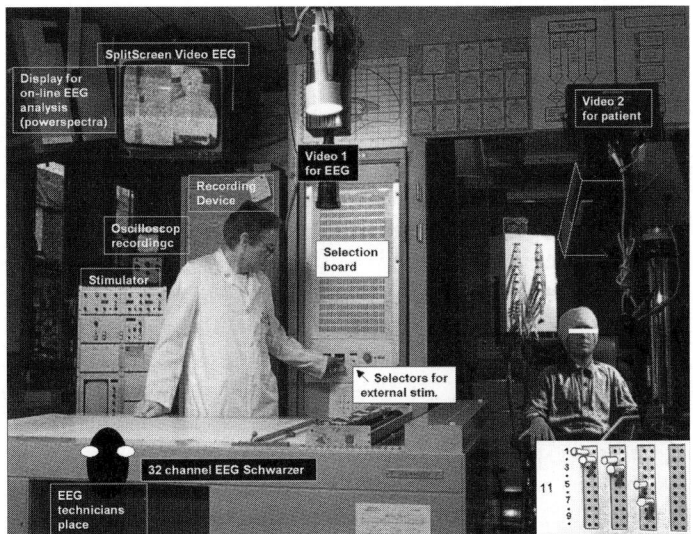

Figure 7. Photograph of the Zurich SEEG laboratory (1980) situated in a Faraday cage, showing the main parts of the recording and stimulation devices.

The selection board used the principle of a "Kreuzschiene", allowing for the selection of every conceivable combination of electrode contacts for recording and stimulation paradigms.

The lower part of the selection board hosted the selectors (the two black rectangles) for external electrical stimulation. There were 32 channels (horizontal) versus 17 × 10 signal entries (vertical). The insert (bottom right) illustrates a detail of the selection board indicating that channel 1 recorded from contacts 1-2 of the depth electrode no. 11, channel 2 from contacts 2-3, etc.

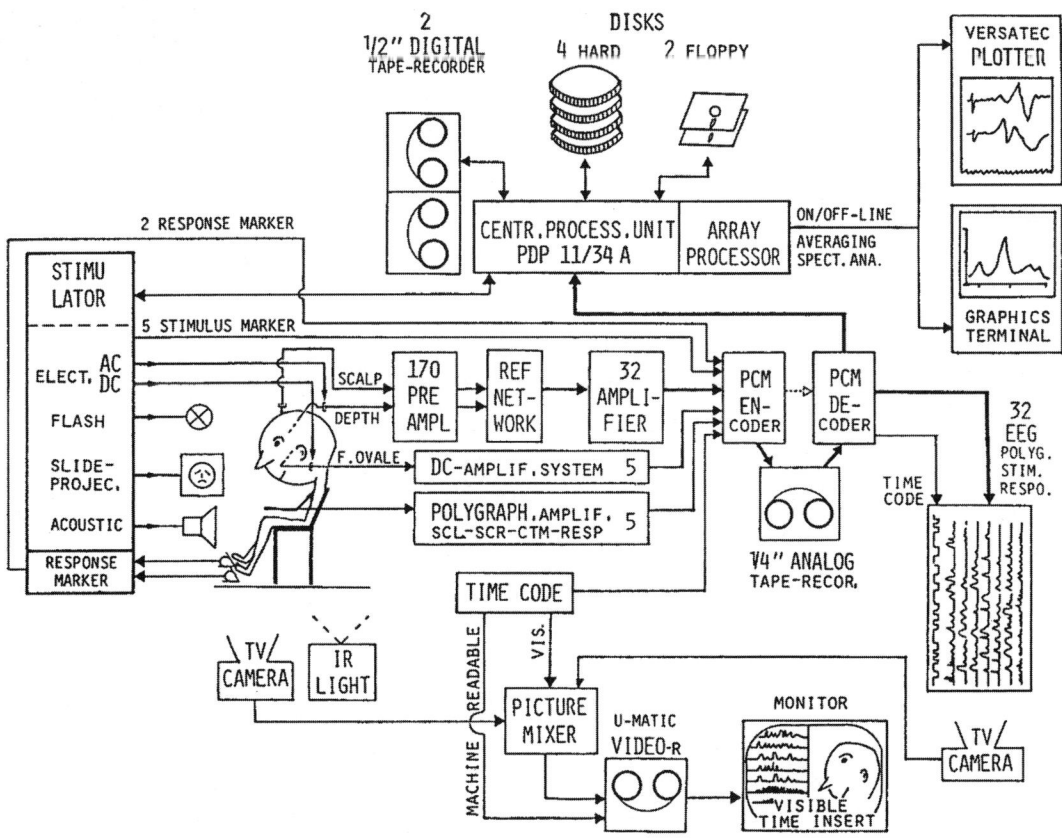

Figure 8. Diagram of the Zurich SEEG laboratory equipment (1980).

Modified from: Wieser HG. Selective amygdalohippocampectomy: Indications, investigative technique and results. In: Symon L, Brihaye J, Guidetti B, Loew F, Niller JD, Nornes H, et al. eds. *Advances and Technical Standards in Neurosurgery.* Vienna, New York: Springer 1986a; 13: 39-133 (Fig. 5).

Introduction

Intracerebral Stimulation

Intracerebral stimulation was usually performed at the end of the SEEG exploration session spanning over two consecutive days. Intracerebral stimulation during night sleep was carried out during the night in between these days of stimulation. In general, repetitive single pulse stimulation (120 pulses delivered at 1 Hz, pulse width of 0.7 ms, voltages from 5 to 10 V) was performed through innermost and outermost neighboring contacts (bipolar short distance) of each depth electrode with simultaneous recording of the remaining depth and scalp derivations. Stimulation was terminated when afterdischarges occurred. Based on the information gained from single pulse stimulation, 50 Hz train stimulation was performed the following day, usually by using a pulse width of 1 ms and voltages from 3 to 10 V, depending on the afterdischarge threshold. The duration of the 50 Hz train was individually adjusted to the afterdischarge threshold and/or clinical symptoms, and was usually between 3 and 5 seconds [Wieser, 1983a]. Fig. 11 depicts a representative example of single-pulse and 50 Hz train stimulation.

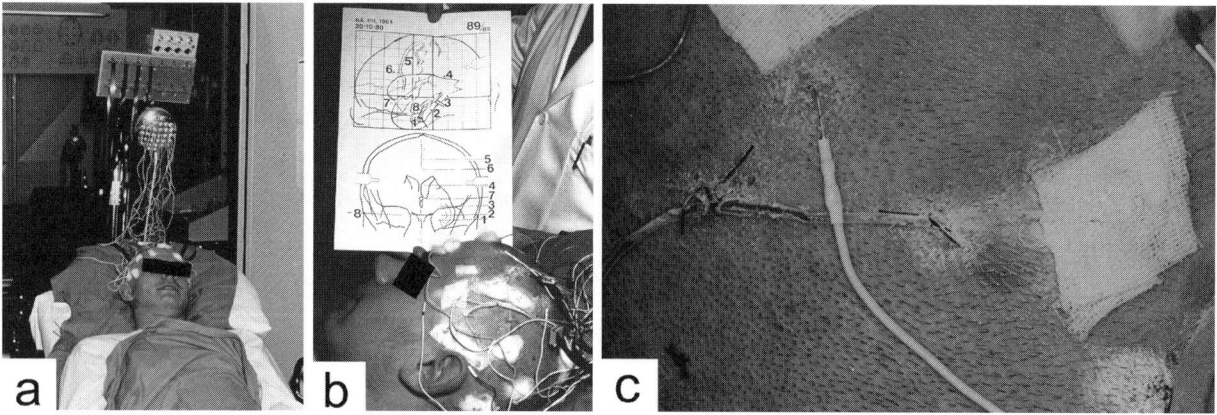

Figure 9. **a**, photograph of the preamplifier connected to the electrodes; **b** and **c**, photographs of the implanted and fixed depth electrodes.

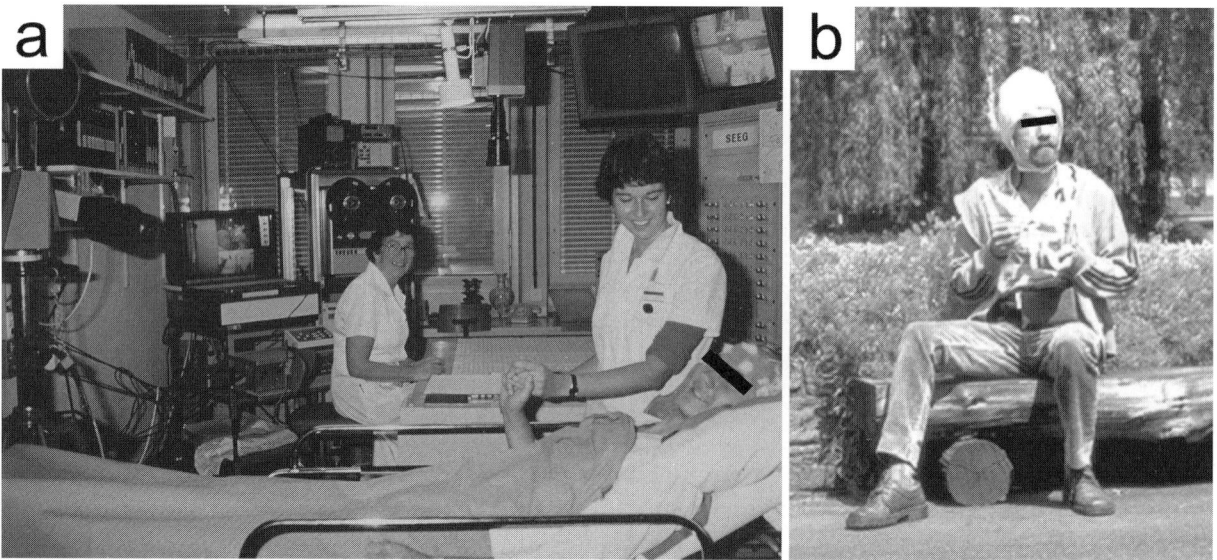

Figure 10. **a**, recording session in the SEEG laboratory; **b**, head dressing for ambulatory cassette depth and scalp EEG monitoring.

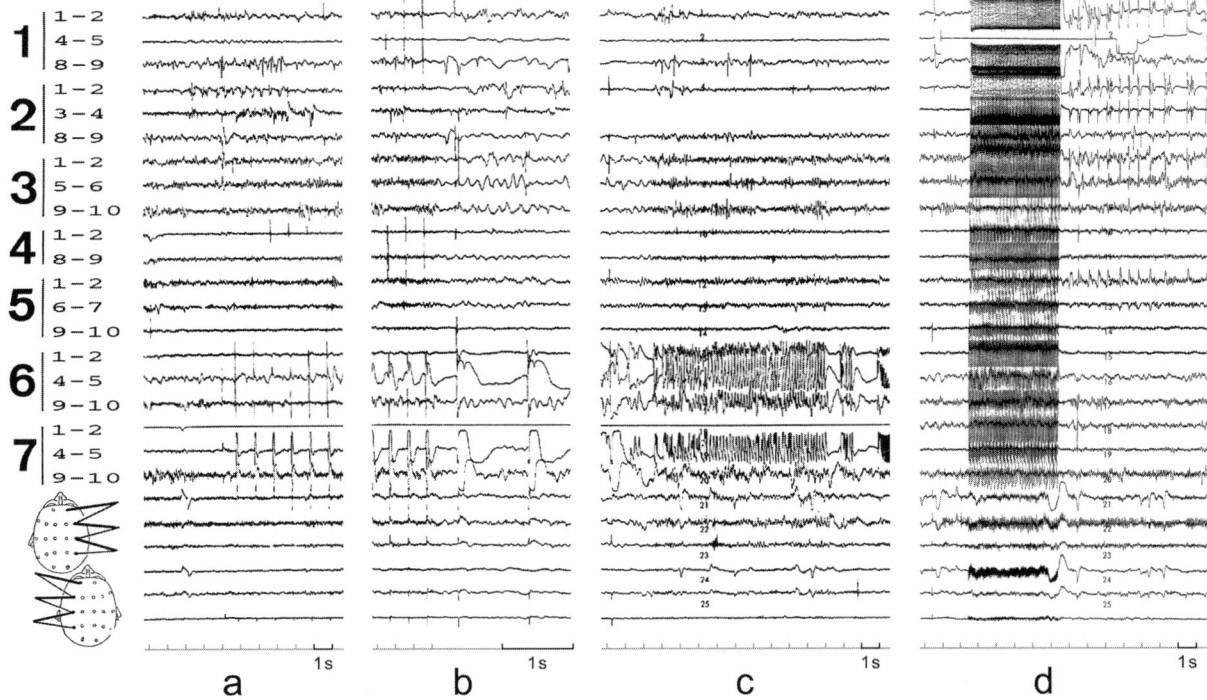

Figure 11. **a**, repetitive 1 Hz single pulse stimulation of the right hippocampus (electrode 7, contacts 1 and 2) with 4 V and 0.1 ms pulse duration; **b**, single pulse stimulation (same parameters) displayed with a paper speed of 60 mm/s; **c**, localized afterdischarge of the right mesial temporal region (6/4-5 and 7/4-5) following single pulse stimulation during 44 seconds; the patient was confused and amnesic during this episode; **d**, 50 Hz train stimulation of the left periamygdalar area (1/4-5) during 5 seconds with 5 V and 0.1 ms pulse duration. Immediately after onset of the train stimulation the patient reported his habitual epigastric aura. Depth electrode targets: **1**, left amygdala; **2**, left anterior hippocampus; **3**, left posterior hippocampus; **4**, left posterior cingulate gyrus; **5**, left anterior cingulate gyrus; **6**, right amygdala; **7**, right middle hippocampus.

Part c modified from: Wieser HG, Valavanis A, Roos A, Isler P, Renella RR. "Selective" and "superselective" temporal lobe memory tests. I. Neuroradiological, neuroanatomical and electrical data. In: *Advances in Epileptology*. New York: Raven Press 1989b; 17: 20-27 (Fig. 5).

Conventional averaging techniques were carried out for the calculation of evoked responses (ER, Fig. 13). Averaged ERs were usually displayed using two different time windows, i.e. – 100 to 236 ms for better visualization of early components, and – 192 to 1,000 ms for the demonstration of later ER components. Stimuli were generally delivered at time 0 ms and the amplitudes of the ERs were indicated by numbers denoting the ratio of the ER amplitude in comparison to the averaged background amplitude, multiplied by factor 10 (Fig. 14).

Paired pulse stimulation was performed to study the "recovery period" of the ERs. The main interest was to see at what time the second pulse would overcome the "inhibitory effects" elicited by the first pulse. The working hypothesis was that the reappearance of the response to the second stimulus would be related to the autochthonous background activity of a certain brain region. Fig. 15 shows an example with paired pulse stimulation of the hippocampus and recording from the ipsilateral amygdala with a preferred background rhythm of about 4 to 5 Hz. In addition to direct electrical stimulation of intracerebral structures as outlined above, we also studied depth recorded visual (VEP), somatosensory (SEP), and cognitive evoked potentials.

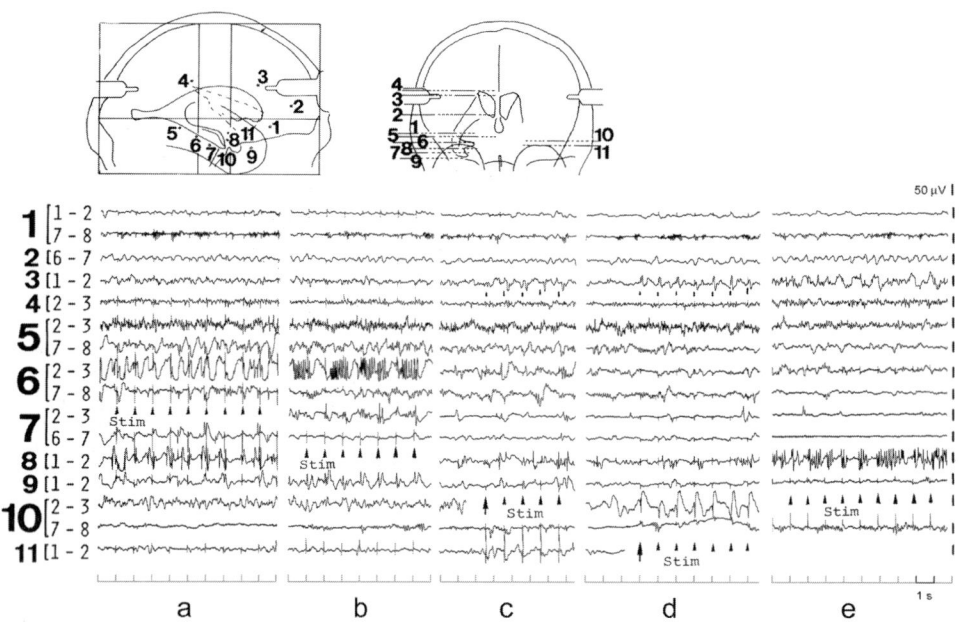

Figure 12. a-e, intracerebral evoked responses (ERs) elicited by 1 Hz single pulse stimulation at various sites (stimulation sites are labeled with black arrows).

Part e modified from: Wieser HG. *Electroclinical Features of the Psychomotor Seizure*. Stuttgart, London: Gustav Fischer-Butterworths 1983a: 127 (Fig. 64).

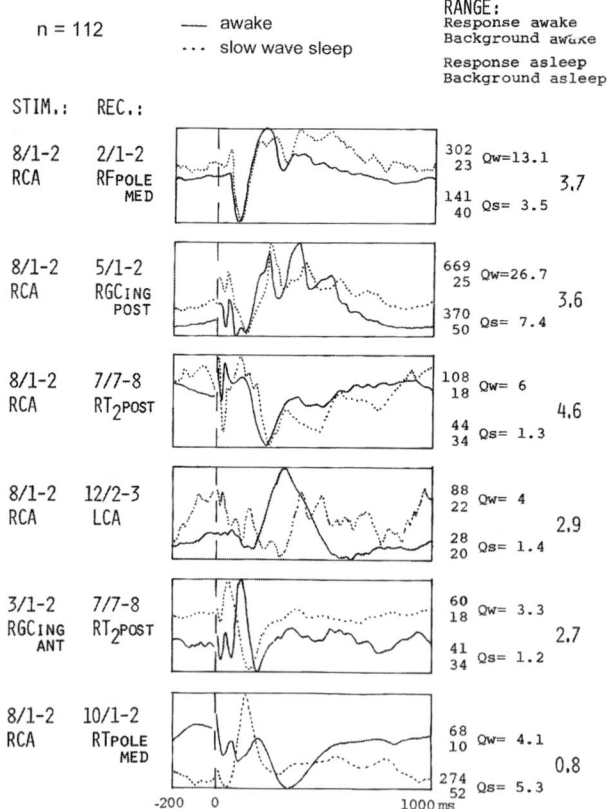

Figure 13. Averaged ERs (n = 112) following 1 Hz single pulse stimulation during the waking state (solid line) and Slow Wave Sleep (SWS, dashed line). Single ERs before averaging of this patient are shown in Fig. 12.

STIM, stimulation site; REC, recording site; ERs are normalized to full scale and expressed as a quotient (Q) against background amplitude. These quotients are calculated during the waking state (Qw) and during SWS (Qs). The numbers at the very right indicate the quotient Qw/Qs.

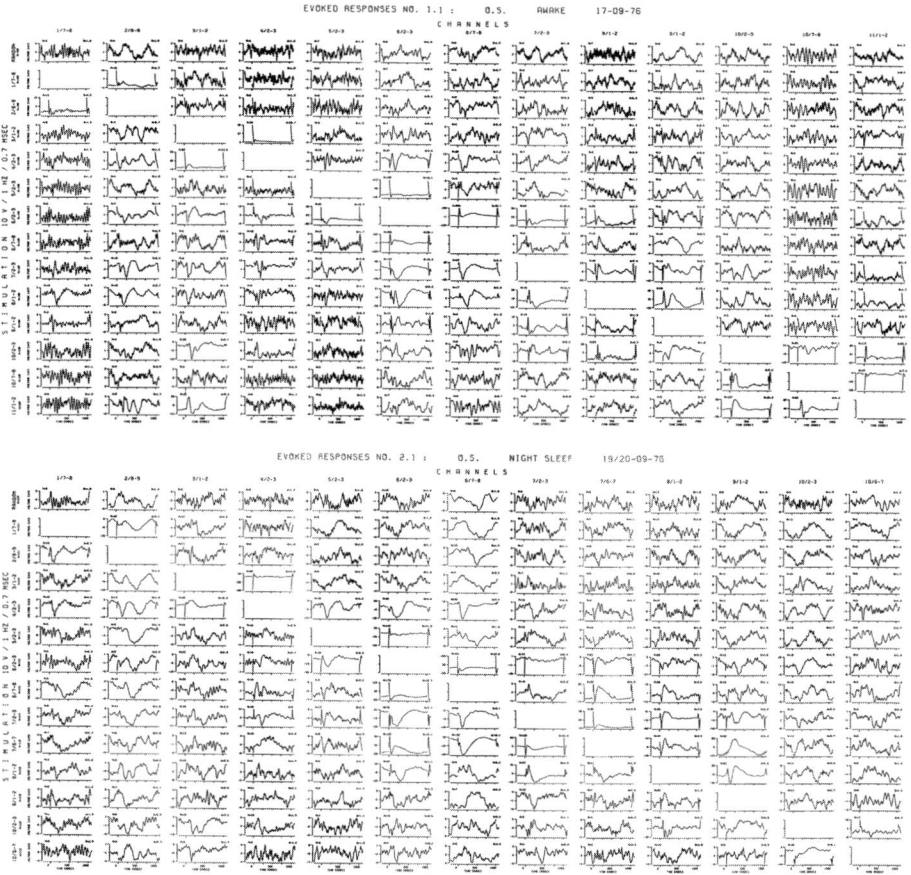

Figure 14. Example of intracerebral ER maps elicited by 1 Hz single pulse stimulation.

The upper part depicts ERs elicited in the waking state, the lower part during night sleep (SWS). The ERs are normalized to full scale and expressed as quotient (Q) against background amplitude.

Modified from: Wieser HG. *Electroclinical Features of the Psychomotor Seizure.* Stuttgart, London: Gustav Fischer - Butterworths 1983a: 130-131 (Figs. 67A & B).

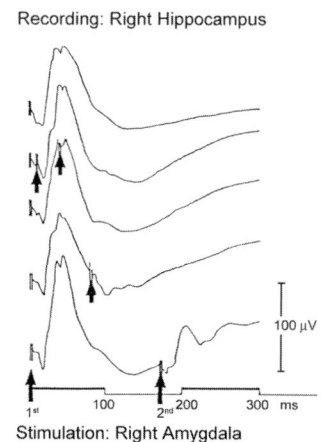

Figure 15. Example of averaged ERs (n = 64) of the amygdala following paired stimulation of the right hippocampus, showing a refractory period of about 100 to 180 ms (a second pulse delivered after an interval of 180 ms elicits a small response). Position of electrodes is as indicated in Fig. 12.

The ER to the second pulse returned to normal with an interval greater than 250 ms in this setting (not shown).

Modified from: Wieser HG. *Electroclinical Features of the Psychomotor Seizure.* Stuttgart, London: Gustav Fischer - Butterworths 1983a: 129 (Fig. 66, part C).

Direct Current (DC) Recording and Stimulation

Since this book was written with a view towards DBS, we include here a short chapter on our experience with DC recording and stimulation. There is evidence from experimental animal studies [Caspers, 1974; Mayanagi and Walker, 1975; Speckmann and Caspers, 1979] and electrophysiological studies in man [Goldring, 1963; Cohn, 1964; Stodieck and Wieser, 1987] that the extracellular potential recorded by DC-coupled amplifiers, the so-called DC potentials, reveal slow fluctuations during epileptic activity and during the sleep-wakefulness cycle. Under normal conditions, there are potential differences in the order of mV between the cortical surface (negative) and the subcortical white matter (positive). In increased cortical activity states, such as epilepsy or afferent stimulation, there is a negative DC shift, whereas an increase of pCO_2 is accompanied by a positive DC shift. The occurrence of an initial negative DC shift during focal or generalized seizures is in keeping with this concept [Ikeda et al., 1999; Vanhatalo et al., 2003].

However, the exact origin of the DC potential is not entirely clear; several mechanisms have been proposed including dendritic potentials [Caspers, 1959], extracellular glia potentials [Cohen, 1976], synaptic depolarization of apical dendrites and pH- and CO_2-dependent barrier potentials between the brain and cerebrospinal fluid [Creutzfeldt, 1983]. It is also pertinent to note that DC potentials are not reliably detected by conventional clinical EEG techniques but require genuine DC-EEG amplifiers and nonpolarizable electrodes (e.g. Ag/AgCl). The practical solution to obtain a DC-stable electrode-skin interface is a challenge (Vanhatalo et al., 2002). We profited from foramen ovale (FO) electrode recorded DC shifts (see technical note to FO electrodes, page 15).

Whether or not a potentially epileptogenic stimulus triggers a seizure depends on the *recruitability*, which is a function of *facilitation* and *availability* (Fig. 16). It is reasonable to assume that anodal and cathodal polarization of neurons may influence the recruitability of neurons and therefore may prevent or facilitate epileptiform spikes and seizures. This has been experimentally put to test with anodal and cathodal polarization of the primary epileptogenic hippocampus (Figs. 17 to 22).

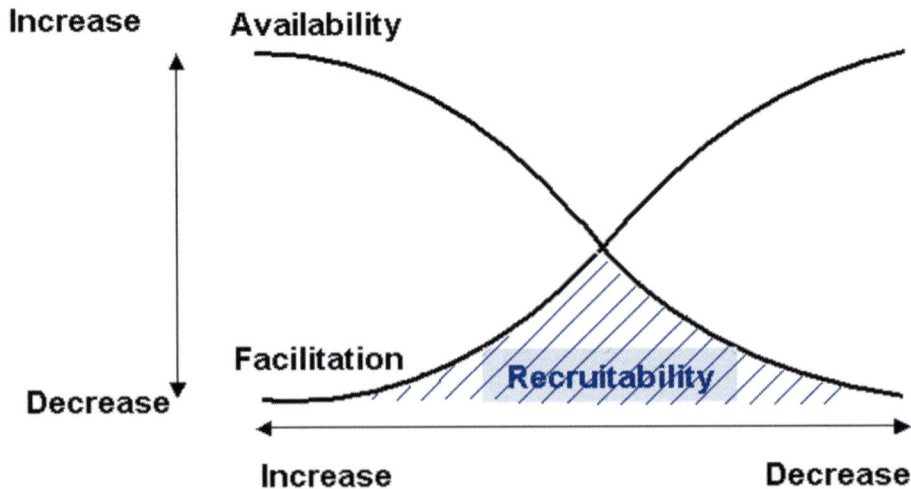

Figure 16. Graph illustrating the concept of the recruitability as a function of facilitation and availability of neurons.

Courtesy of Prof. Dr. E-J Speckmann. Modified from: Speckmann E-J. Experimentelle Epilepsieforschung - Grundlagen, Modelle. Wissenschaftliche Buchgesellschaft, Darmstadt 1986; Konzept und Realisation: AMV AV-Kommunikation und Medizin-Verlag, München. Produktion: Bayerl & Partner Film, München Desitin Videothek, Hamburg 1989.

DC Recording

In some patients, DC recordings were accomplished with newly developed FO electrodes [Wieser *et al.*, 1985a]. DC recordings were referenced to a disc-shaped sintered Ag/AgCl electrode of 12.5 mm diameter (In Vivo Metric Systems, Healdsburg, CA) implanted subgaleally at the vertex (Cz electrode).

Technical note: *Our FO electrode consisted of cylindrical Ag/AgCl pellet (0.4 mm in diameter, 4 mm in length) sintered around the tip of a silver wire of 0.25 mm diameter. The lead wire was teflon-insulated, the Ag/AgCl pellet covered at the top with insulating varnish to achieve a smooth and round tip. The impedance of these FO electrodes (3 to 6 days) was less than 120 Ω at 100 Hz (0.01-2 V AC), less than 150 Ω at 5 Hz (0.01-2 V AC), and less than 210 Ω at 2 V DC (measured in Ringer solution after soaking for 3 min and an approximate distance of 30 mm between to contacts). DC offset voltage (bias potential) was less than 2 mV.*

Spontaneous spikes and focal high frequency seizure discharges (AC recorded) were accompanied by a negative DC values as illustrated in Fig. 17. In generalized seizures the polarity drifted suddenly to positive DC values, indicating that the vertex region with the subgaleal reference electrode exhibited a much stronger negativity than the FO electrode (Fig. 18).

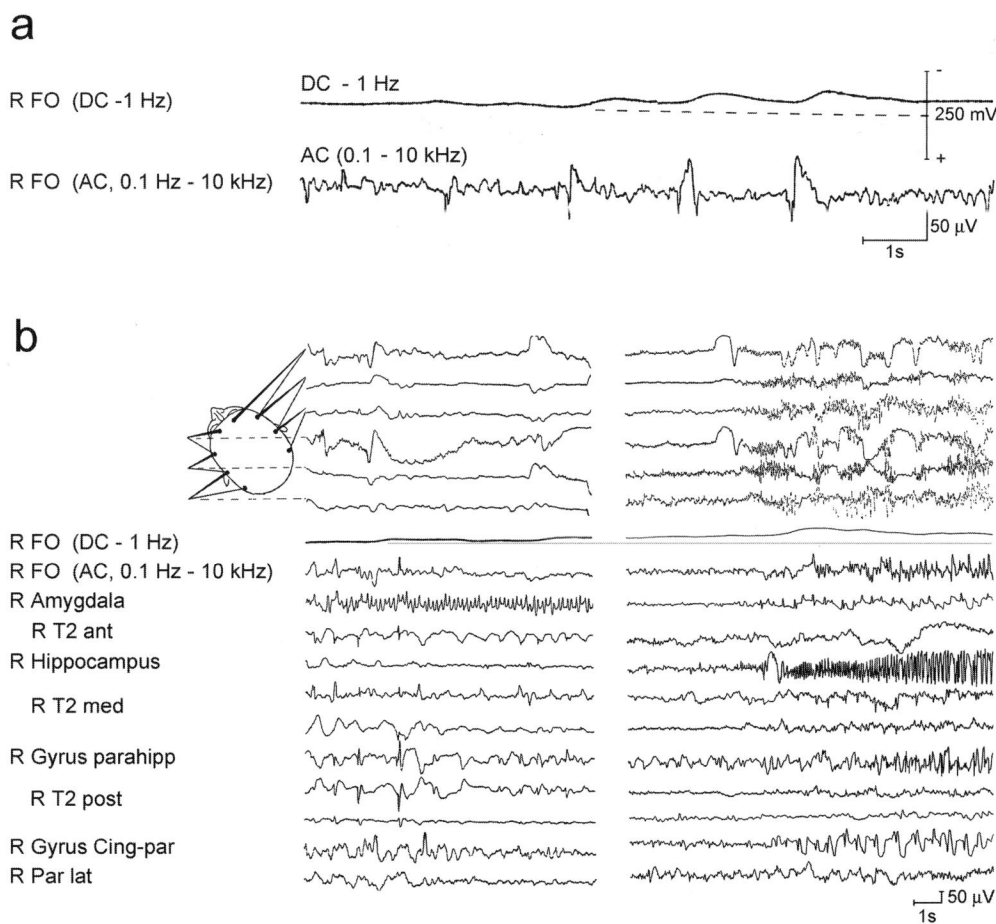

Figure 17. Negative DC values accompanying spontaneously occurring spikes **(a)** and focal high frequency seizure discharges **(b)**.

R, right; **FO**, foramen ovale electrode; **T2**, second temporal gyrus; **ant**, anterior; **med**, medial; **Gyrus parahipp**, parahippocampal gyrus; **post**, posterior; **Gyrus Cing-par**, parietal cingulate gyrus; **Par lat**, parietal neocortex.

Modified from: Wieser HG, Elger CE, Stodieck SRG. The "Foramen Ovale Electrode": A new recording method for the preoperative evaluation of patients suffering from mesio-basal temporal lobe epilepsy. Electroenceph Clin Neurophysiol 1985a; 61: 314-322.

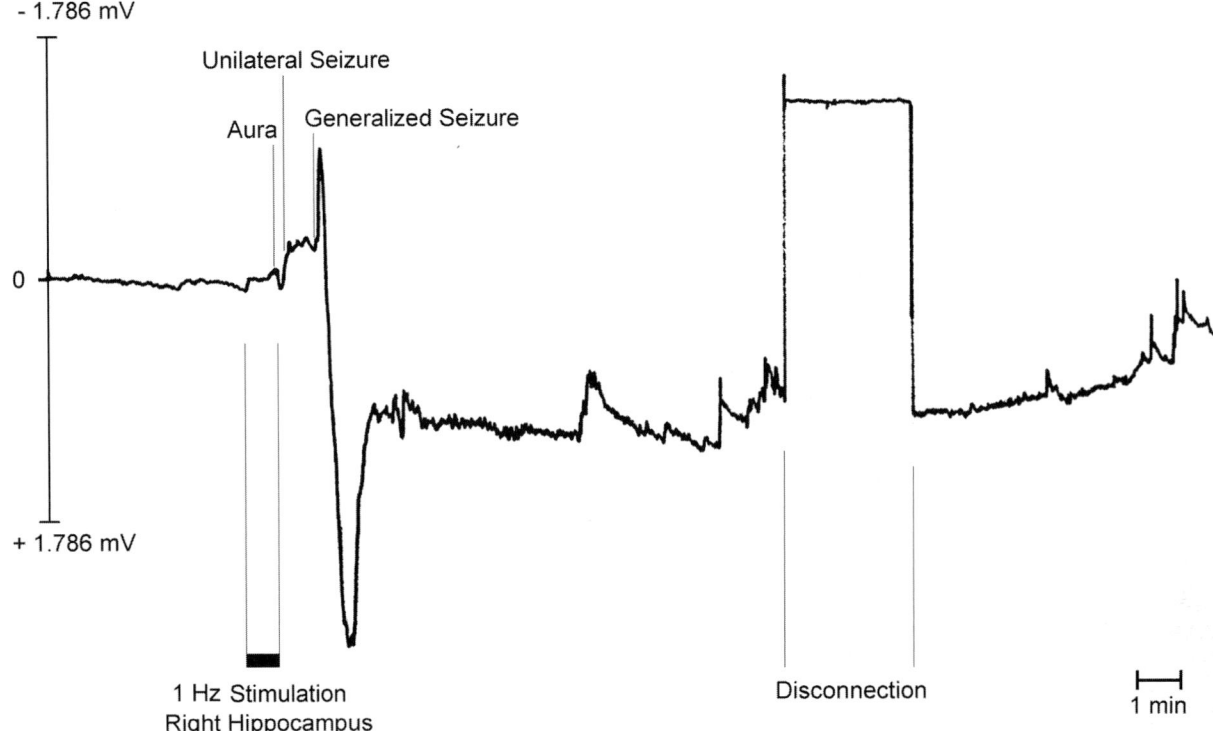

Figure 18. DC recording from the right FO electrode during a secondary generalized seizure, provoked by repetitive 1 Hz single pulse stimulation of the right hippocampus (black bar).

With the onset of the afterdischarge the patient experienced his habitual aura. The electrically induced focal mesial temporal seizure was accompanied by a moderate negative DC shift. With the secondary generalization of the seizure, this DC shift increased and then flipped polarity to positive DC values, indicating that the vertex region with the subgaleal reference electrode exhibited a much stronger negativity than the FO electrode.

Modified from: Wieser HG and Schindler K. Foramen ovale and epidural electrodes in the definition of the seizure onset zone. In: Lüders HO, Najm I. Bingaman W eds. *Textbook of Epilepsy Surgery.* Abingdon UK: Taylor & Francis Group (2007, in press).

DC Stimulation

Transcranial DC electrical polarization of the brain is a technique for modulating brain function that enjoyed periods of clinical and scientific interest as long as two centuries ago [Priori, 2003]. Numerous studies have reported on transcranial direct current stimulation (tDCS) in animals [Bindman et al., 1962; Purpura and McMurtry, 1965]. More recently, transcranial magnetic stimulation (TMS), which allows noninvasive focal manipulation of brain function, was introduced and applied in patients with epilepsy, although without significant beneficial results [Theodore et al., 2002]. However, there is convincing physiological evidence for the effects of DC polarization on cortical neurons from recent experiments using changes in the muscle twitch evoked by TMS to the motor cortex. Human behavioral studies, measurements of cortical evoked potentials in animals [Bindman et al., 1962], and single neuron recording both in vitro [Terzuolo and Bullock, 1956] and in mammalian cortex [Purpura and McMurtry, 1965] showed that cortical DC polarization is polarity-dependent. When the anode is located near the dendrites of an isolated neuron or placed on the scalp or cortex, polarization tends to be activating (both behaviorally and neurophysiologically). When the polarity is reversed and the cathode is near the dendrites or the cortical surface, depression of both cell firing and behavior is assumed. Little is known about the mechanism of these polarity-specific effects. It has been argued that the effects probably rely at least in part on changes in neuronal membranes, rather than on changes at the level of synapses, and that the tDCS technique currently used does not cause resting neurons to fire, but appears to modulate the firing rate of spontaneously active neurons. Hence, transcranial DC brain polarization may not refer to "stimulation" in the way that TMS causes neuronal firing with rapidly changing electrical current. tDCS should certainly be distinguished from conventional transcranial electrical stimulation with brief pulses, electroconvulsive therapy and other forms of transcranial electrotherapy using weak alternating currents known as "cranial electrotherapy stimulation" and "electrosleep".

tDCS presently witnesses a rediscovery due to the work of the Göttingen Group [Nitsche and Paulus, 2000; Paulus, 2004; Antal et al., 2006] and other research groups [Fregni et al., 2005; Iyer et al., 2005]. In the study of Fregni et al. [2006a], 19 patients with refractory epilepsy and malformations of cortical development have been subjected to single sessions of DC polarization (20 min, 1 mA) targeting the epileptogenic focus. tDCS was applied through a saline soaked pair of surface sponge electrodes (35 cm^2): the anode electrode was placed as the "active" electrode over the epileptogenic area and the cathode electrode contralateral over the supraorbital area, or over an epileptologically silent area. The number of interictal epileptiform discharges (IED) in the EEG were measured before (baseline), immediately after, and 15 and 30 days after either sham or active DC polarization. Seizure frequency after the treatment was compared with baseline seizure frequency. The authors found a significant reduction in the number of IED (mean reduction of 64%) with active compared to sham DC polarization, but only a trend for decrease in seizure frequency. The authors found that both anodal and cathodal polarization decreased IED, although cathodal surface stimulation showed a stronger effect. Considering the finding that epileptic seizures are usually accompanied by a negative DC shift it can be suggested that a field with the opposite effect on the epileptogenic area may have beneficial effects. Crucial problems besides strength of the field and polarity are the geometry of neurons in relation to the applied DC field, the local network characteristics with excitatory and inhibitory interneurons and the participation of glia.

Wassermann and Grafman [2005] demonstrated an improvement of working memory with tDCS applied to left prefrontal cortical areas, applying anodal polarization with 40 mA/cm^2. The authors speculate that the observed antidepressant effect was due to neuronal depolarization, in analogy to animal studies suggesting that cathodal tDCS reduces spontaneous firing of cortical neurons by hyperpolarization of the cell body. tDCS applied to specific brain areas has also been shown to alter verbal fluency, motor learning and perceptual thresholds. Recently, the therapeutic usefulness of tDCS has been investigated in various diseases, including migraine [Antal et al., 2006], stroke [Hummel et al., 2005, Fregni and Pascual-Leone, 2006] and major depression [Fregni et al., 2006b].

With a view towards the application of tDCS in epilepsy and the results of the first controlled clinical trials [Fregni et al., 2006c], our early DC polarization studies in three patients are interesting in many ways. Stimulations were carried out before surgical removal of mesial temporal lobe structures. All patients gave informed consent. A large (5 × 5 cm) plate scalp electrode was placed over the ipsilateral fronto-temporal region, and the current was applied using a constant-current device powered by a conventional 9 V battery. The current flow was continuously monitored by an ampere meter in series (Fig. 19). DC currents of 1 to 60 µA (up to 200 µA in one patient) were applied with stepwise increments over a total duration of 2 minutes. First of all, we were able to apply an inhomogeneous field with one electrode situated directly in one subcompartiment of the primary epileptogenic zone, i.e. the amygdala, with the other large scalp electrode placed over the ipsilateral scalp. This fashion, we induced a graded field with a maximum in the epileptogenic zone and found strong polarity-dependent effects, in the sense that anodal polarization of the hippocampus produced a desynchronized (attenuated) nearly spike-free hippocampal EEG, whereas cathodal polarization prompted no or, in one patient, the opposite effect, leading even to a seizure (Fig. 20).

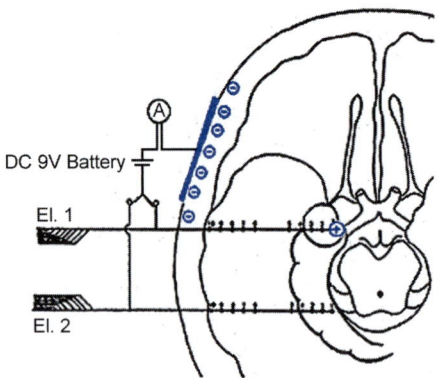

Figure 19. Illustration of the experimental settings during polarization of the mesial temporal lobe structures. **(A)** ampere meter; **El. 1**, depth electrode with its tip in the amygdala; **El. 2**, depth electrode with its tip in the posterior hippocampus.

Modified from: Stodieck SRG, Wieser HG. The effects of polarization on human epileptic foci. In: *Proc. 1st Vienna International Workshop on Functional Electrostimulation*. Thoma H ed., Vienna, 1983 (Abstract see: Artif. Organs 8/3:392, 1984) and Wieser HG, Bjeljac M, Khan N, Müller S, Siegel AM, Yonekawa Y. Interplay of interictal discharges and seizures: some clinical and EEG findings. In: Wolf P ed. *Epileptic Seizures and Syndromes*. London: John Libbey 199: 563-578 (Fig. 4).

During polarization, scalp and depth EEG were continuously recorded. In general, anodal (positive pole) polarization of the primary epileptogenic area resulted in a decrease of interictal spike incidence, whereas cathodal polarization (negative pole) had the opposite effect. In one patient, the latter setting induced a seizure originating in the polarized structures (Fig. 20). The effects on background activity, however, were more variable. Anodal polarization sometimes led to a reduction of the amplitude of the background activity, and, in one patient, both polarities equally activated rhythmic delta waves in the polarized hippocampus.

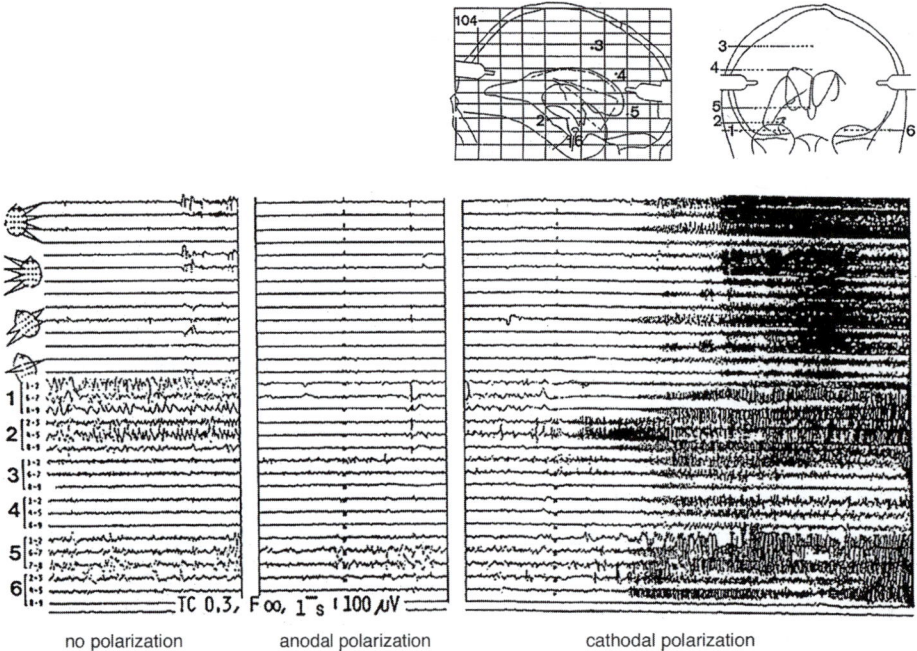

Figure 20. Effects of anodal and cathodal polarization of the mesial temporal lobe structures. Anodal polarization of the right amygdala led to a suppression of interictal epileptiform activity. Cathodal polarization of the right amygdala provoked a seizure discharge.

Modified from: Stodieck SRG, Wieser HG. The effects of polarization on human epileptic foci. In: *Proc. 1st Vienna International Workshop on Functional Electrostimulation*. Thoma H ed., Vienna, 1983 (Abstract see: Artif. Organs 8/3: 392, 1984) and Wieser HG, Bjeljac M, Khan N, Müller S, Siegel AM, Yonekawa Y. Interplay of interictal discharges and seizures: some clinical and EEG findings. In: Wolf P ed. *Epileptic Seizures and Syndromes*. London: John Libbey 1994: 563-578 (Fig. 5).

We also studied the influence of the DC field on ERs following electrical 1 Hz pulse stimulation of the amygdala, while recording from the ipsilateral hippocampus. The experimental setting is depicted in Fig. 21. For each investigation, we started with low initial current flow (1 µA) for 10 seconds and stepwise increased the intensity of the DC current (up to 60 µA, up to 200 µA in one patient) for a duration of up to 2 minutes, while carefully observing electroencephalographic and behavioral changes.

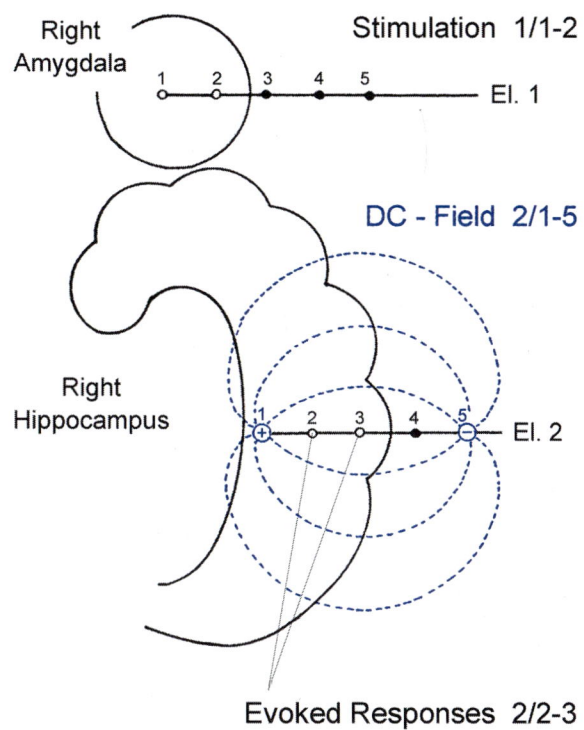

Figure 21. Experimental setting for the investigation of the influence of a DC field on hippocampal ERs to stimulation of the ipsilateral amygdala.
Modified from: Stodieck SRG, Wieser HG. The effects of polarization on human epileptic foci. In: *Proc. 1st Vienna Internatinal Workshop on Functional Electrostimulation.* Thoma H ed., Vienna, 1983 (Abstract see: Artif. Organs 8/3: 392, 1984) and Wieser HG, Bjeljac M, Khan N, Müller S, Siegel AM, Yonekawa Y. Interplay of interictal discharges and seizures: some clinical and EEG findings. In: Wolf P ed. *Epileptic Seizures and Syndromes.* London: John Libbey 1994: 563-578 (Fig. 6).

A weak polarizing DC field across the hippocampus clearly altered the morphology of hippocampal ERs to stimulation of the ipsilateral amygdala. The phase of the main biphasic potential with the opposite polarity to the applied field increased in amplitude and duration (Fig. 22). These effects were reproducible and clearly related to the current intensity of the applied DC field.

This experimental setting induced a seizure in one patient, but otherwise there were no side effects. The patients were generally unable to tell whether they were under the influence of direct current stimulation or not. However, in one patient there was a marked behavioral alteration with psychotic features (the history, SEEG recordings, surgery and outcome of this patient are described on p. 60). For the present, it is enough to note that this 37-year-old gentleman never had suffered any overt psychotic episode, never had consulted a psychiatrist and that there was no psychiatric illness in his family. His acute psychotic episode started about one hour after the polarizing experiment: the patient behaved awkwardly, became extremely agitated and revealed frank paranoid hallucinations. He reported seeing non-existent persons threatening him and he obviously received commands from them. He disappeared from the ward and when he was found (still inside the hospital), he explained that he had to use "another telephone" because the one he had access to on the ward "was controlled by his enemies". Orientation to time and space was always preserved. The scalp EEG during this

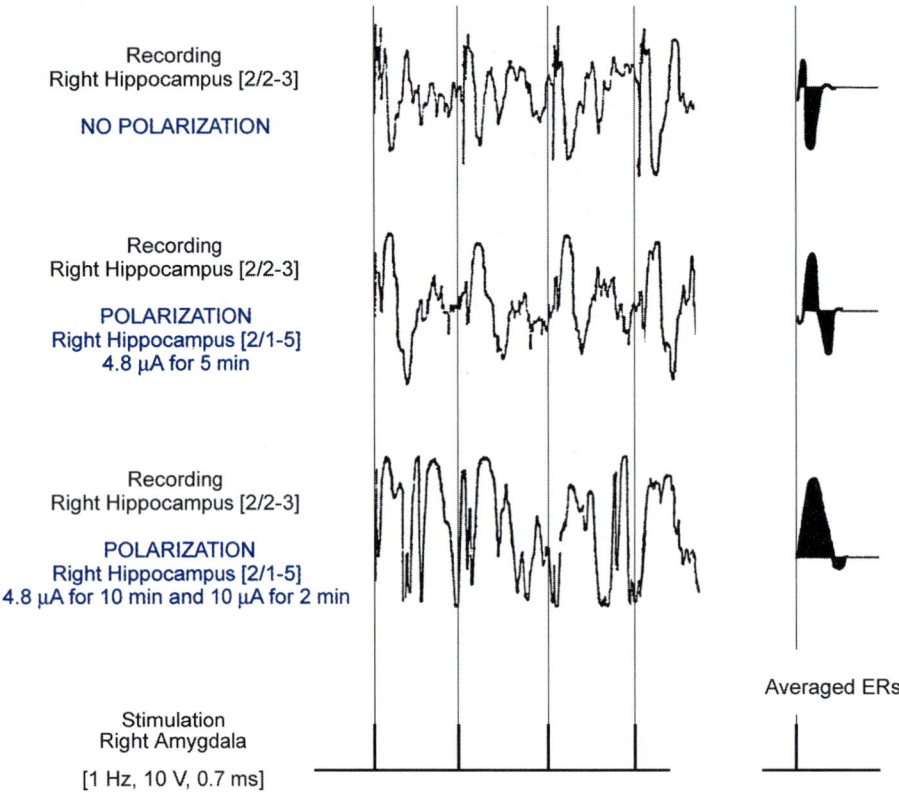

Figure 22. Effect of a polarizing DC field across the hippocampus [2/1-5] on ERs recorded from the hippocampal electrode [2/2-3] following stimulation of the ipsilateral amygdala [1/1-2].
Modified from: Stodieck SRG, Wieser HG. The effects of polarization on human epileptic foci. In: *Proc. 1st Vienna International Workshop on Functional Electrostimulation.* Thoma H ed., Vienna, 1983 (Abstract see: Artif. Organs 8/3: 392, 1984) and Wieser HG, Bjeljac M, Khan N, Müller S, Siegel AM, Yonekawa Y. Interplay of interictal discharges and seizures: some clinical and EEG findings. In: Wolf P ed. *Epileptic Seizures and Syndromes.* London: John Libbey 1994: 563-578 (Fig. 6).

episode showed low amplitude background without epileptiform activity. No epileptic seizures were witnessed during this psychotic episode, despite careful observation. The depth electrodes were removed without any problems. Overall, the acute psychotic symptoms lasted for about six hours and completely resolved within 3 days without the need for any special treatment. It is interesting to note that the patient remained seizure free for a period of about two months. Finally, a palliative left selective amygdalohippocampectomy SAHE was performed, with unfavorable outcome (i.e. persisting seizures).

The psychotic episode obviously occurred in clear relation to a weak direct polarizing current applied to the primary epileptogenic zone. We believe that this patient represents a very interesting case with regard to an experimentally induced "forced normalization" [Wieser, 1998]. The discussion of this observation with many experts in this field nourished the idea to measure potential changes of the extracellular ionic milieu using ion sensitive microelectrodes, but this procedure could not be realized because ion sensitive microelectrodes fitting into the hollow core depth electrodes were not available these days.

Neurotransmitter Studies using Push Pull Cannulae

It has been demonstrated that concentrations of excitatory amino acids, in particular aspartate (ASP), are positively correlated with the spike frequency of the EEG [Cuénod *et al.*, 1990; Do *et al.*, 1991]. Similar studies using microdialysis showed an increase in extracellular glutamate and a decrease in gamma aminobutyric acid concentrations before seizure onset [During, 1991; During and Spencer, 1993; During *et al.*, 1994, 1995]. These findings are of major interest with respect to on demand seizure prevention (time-adjusted pharmacotherapy), providing the development of reliable seizure detection algorithms.

In collaboration with the Zurich Brain Research Institute (Prof. Michel Cuénod and Dr. Kim Q. Do), we performed neurotransmitter studies using push pull cannulae in four patients with depth electrodes, with the aim to investigate the pattern of neurotransmitters or transmitter candidates released in the primary epileptogenic area during spontaneous and electrically induced epileptiform discharges. All patients gave their informed written consent and the study was approved by our local ethical committee. Push pull cannulae were inserted into the lumen of hollow core multicontact hippocampal depth electrodes, a technique that allowed for simultaneous perfusion and EEG recording of epileptic tissue at the tip of the electrode. Sterilized Gey's solution was perfused through the push pull cannula at a flow rate of 20 µl/min, and one minute fractions were collected over a period of one hour in anaesthetized patients (Fig. 23). The perfusate was analyzed by OPA (o-pthalaldehyde) precolumn derivatization high pressure liquid chromatography (HPLC) allowing for the quantification of the putative amino acid transmitters concentrations. Computer assisted analyses of the background depth-EEG activity as well as of spontaneous and electrically induced epileptiform events were performed. These recordings were correlated with the biochemical measurements. In the following, we will present the results of two of four patients investigated at our center.

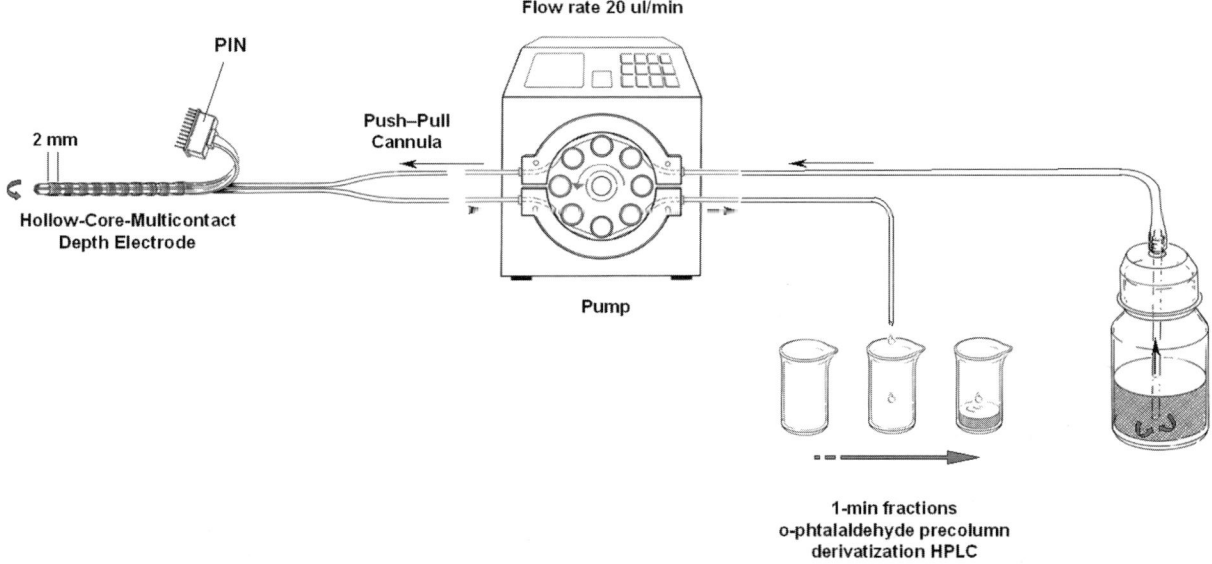

Figure 23. Illustration of the experimental setting: Sterilized Gey's solution was perfused through the push pull cannula at a flow rate of 20 µl/min, and 1 minute fractions were collected over a period of one hour. Perfusates were analyzed by OPA precolumn derivatization HPLC.

Patient A

This 31 year-old man had tonic clonic seizures at regular intervals since age 4. Complex partial seizures, sometimes with secondary generalization, occurred since age 7. The scalp EEG showed a left temporal background abnormality at that time. The seizure frequency steadily increased over the following years, despite polytherapy with antiepileptic drugs (AED) in various combinations. Seizures often occurred in the early morning hours, regularly while coming out of sleep. Non invasive phase I investigation was non conclusive, suggesting either a right frontal or a right temporal seizure onset (a judgment that was mainly based on ictal signs and symptoms). A decision was made to perform a presurgical evaluation with 10 depth electrodes (Fig. 24).

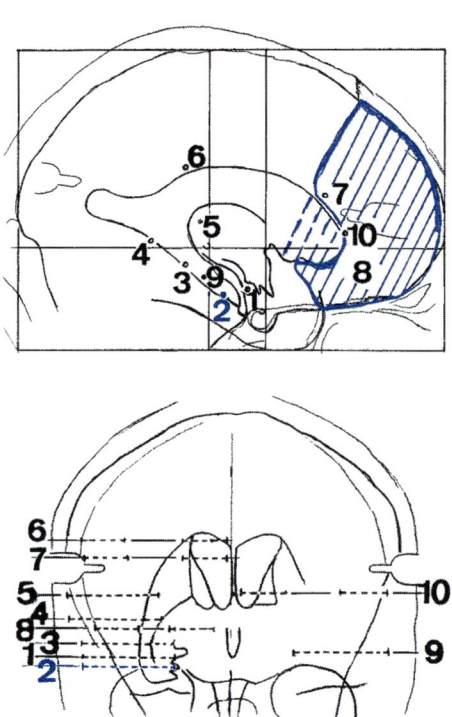

Figure 24. Localization of the depth electrodes in patient A. A push pull cannula was inserted into the lumen of an intrahippocampal standard hollow core multicontact depth electrode placed in the hippocampus (electrode 2, blue). The region shaded in blue indicates the area of resection.

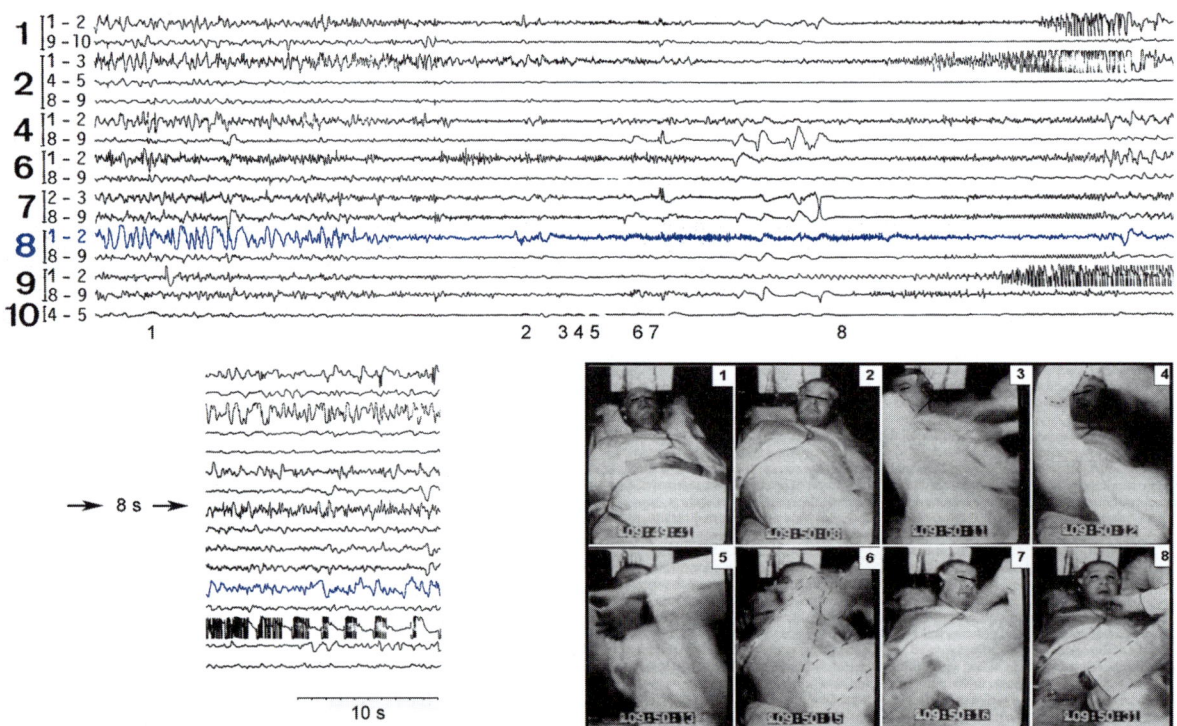

Figure 25. Representative SEEG recorded spontaneous seizure with widespread decrement followed by a low amplitude high frequency discharge in right fronto-orbital [8/1-2] (blue) structures, spreading to both mesial temporal lobes (right hippocampus, [2/1-3]; left hippocampus [9/1-2]).

Note that 8 seconds have been omitted between the top and the bottom section. The numbers below the EEG traces correspond to the video pictures 1-8.

Modified from: Wieser HG, Swartz BE, Delgado-Escueta AV, Bancaud J, Walsh GO, Maldonado H, Saint-Hilaire JM. Differentiating frontal lobe seizures from temporal lobe seizures. *Adv Neurol* 1992; 57: 267-285.

The SEEG recordings revealed a very active interictal spiking focus in the right fronto-orbital region. Thirty-four habitual complex partial seizures were recorded following mild AED tapering during a 6 day investigation. Ictal electroclinical semiology confirmed a right fronto-orbital seizure onset with secondary spreading to both mesial temporal lobes (Figs. 25). A partial right frontal lobe resection was carried out (corresponding to the shaded area in Fig. 24) but seizures continued to occur (Engel outcome class III, follow up of 16 years).

During the 1-hour session with collection of the perfusate through the push pull device inserted into electrode number 2 (with its tip located in the right pes hippocampi) the following electrical stimulations were performed (numbers correspond to samples):

#11 Repetitive single 1 Hz pulses (6 V, 0.7 ms) at [2/1-2] inducing an afterdischarge (AD) in the right amygdala.

#13 Repetitive single 1 Hz pulses (10 V, 0.7 ms) at [2/1-2] with an AD in the right amygdala.

#16 50 Hz train stimulation (4 V, 1 ms) at [2/1-2] without AD.

#20 50 Hz train stimulation (6 V, 1 ms) at [2/1-2] with AD in the right hippocampus and amygdala for a total duration of 11 s.

#21 Sample taken at the end of the AD following sample #20.

#22 50 Hz train stimulation (6 V, 1 ms) at [1/1-2] with an AD in the right hippocampus, amygdala and parahippocampal gyrus as well as in the right temporal neocortical region with propagation to the contralateral, left hippocampus. The AD in the right temporal lobe lasted 25 s, the AD in the left hippocampus 44 s.

#23 Sample taken during the ADs following sample #22.

#30 50 Hz train stimulation (6 V, 1 ms) at [1/1-2] with an AD in the right hippocampus, amygdala and parahippocampal gyrus as well as in the right temporal neocortical sites.

#31 Sample taken exactly at the end of the AD following sample #30.

#35 50 Hz train stimulation (7 V, 1 ms) at [2/1-3] with an AD in the right hippocampus, amygdala and parahippocampal gyrus with slight propagation to [5/1-2] the pontes grisei caudolenticulares, with a total duration of 19 s.

#37 Sample taken during increased spontaneous spiking in the right hippocampus [2/1-2].

#42 50 Hz train stimulation (6 V, 1 ms) at [1/1-2] with an AD in the right hippocampus, amygdala and parahippocampal gyrus as well as in the right temporal neocortical sites (left hippocampus not recorded). This AD lasted 25 s.

Patient B

This 20 years-old man had frequent seizures since age 11 after a traffic accident at age 10 with head trauma. His seizures were characterized by auras with nausea and/or visual symptoms, followed by head version to the right and frequent secondary generalization. Seizure control was not achieved, despite AED polytherapy in various combinations. Presurgical investigation with eight depth electrodes was carried out (Fig. 28). Seizures originated in left posterior temporal neocortical areas and revealed rapid propagation into left mesial temporal structures. The patient passed a selective temporal lobe amytal memory test [Wieser et al., 1997, 2007b; Hajek et al., 1998] and a *palliative* sAHE [Wieser et al., 2003] was performed. During the first two postoperative years, the patient continued to have infrequent simple partial seizures, characterized by flushing and short elevation of the right arm. At age 22, he had four secondary generalized seizures, but was seizure free thereafter (with a follow up of 14 years).

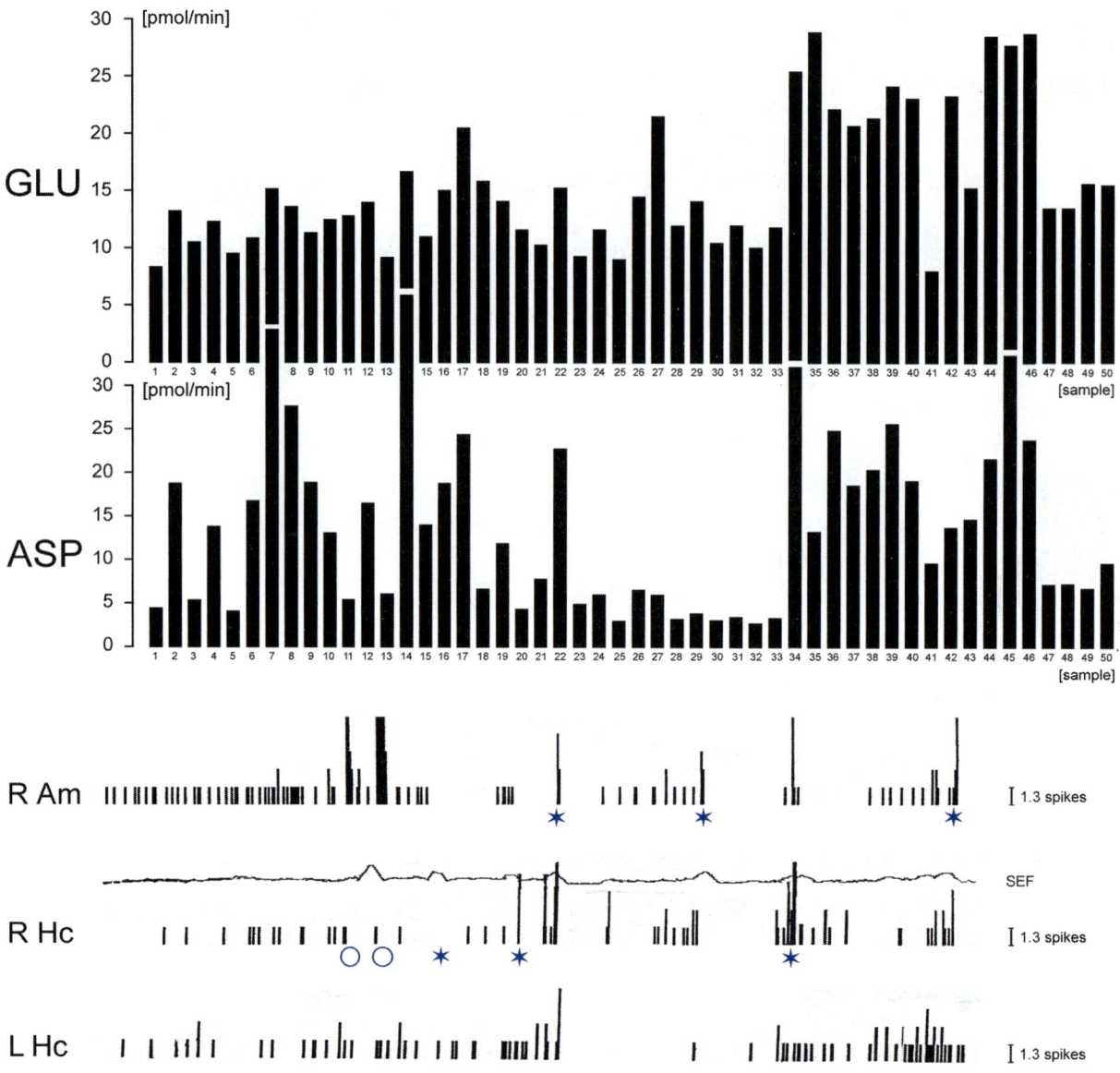

Figure 26. Correlation between the time course of concentrations of the excitatory amino acids glutamate **(GLU)** and aspartate **(ASP)** in the perfusates from the right hippocampus with the EEG of the right hippocampus **(R Hc)**, the right amygdala **(R Am)** and the left hippocampus **(L Hc)**.

The stimulations are indicated by symbols: "circles" for 1 Hz single pulse stimulation and "stars" for 50 Hz train stimulation. Blue symbols represent stimulations that were followed by afterdischarges. The increase of ASP and, to a lesser extent, GLU seemed to correlate with the AD (note that there is a delay of about 90 s of the perfusate samples with regard to the stimulation and the electrical events). The EEG of the interesting brain regions (lower part) was analyzed by using spike detection algorithms of J. Gotmann Stellate® (http://www.stellate) and, occasionally, Bruno Fricker (Fricker Spectralab®, http://www.spectralab.ch), as well as with compressed spectral array (CSA) defining the power in certain frequency bands and plotting the spectral edge frequency (SEF).

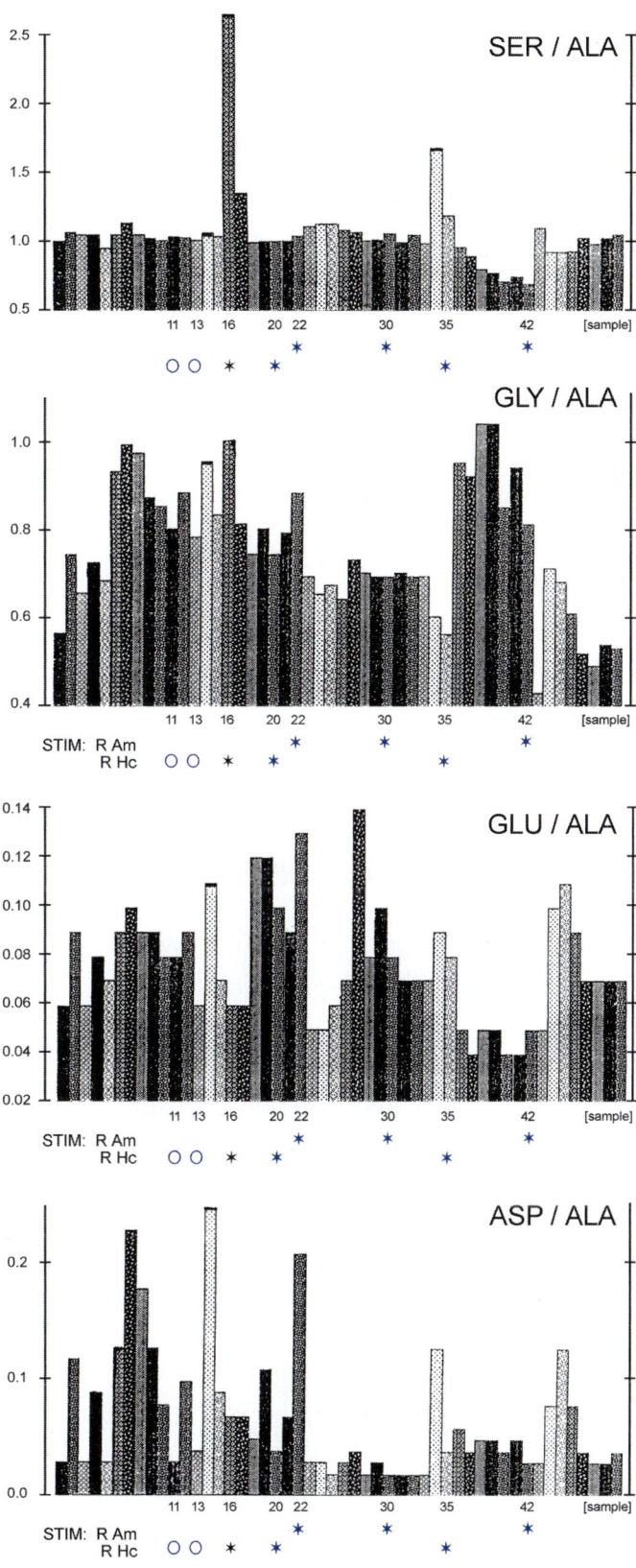

Figure 27. Time course of concentrations of the excitatory amino acids serotonine **(SER)**, glycine **(GLY)**, glutamate **(GLU)** and aspartate **(ASP)** in the perfusates from the right hippocampus expressed as quotients over alanine **(ALA)**.

The stimulations of the right amygdala **(R Am)** or the right hippocampus **(R Hc)** are indicated by symbols, i.e. "circles" for 1 Hz single pulse stimulation and "stars" for 50 Hz train stimulation. Blue symbols represent stimulations that were followed by afterdischarges.

Introduction

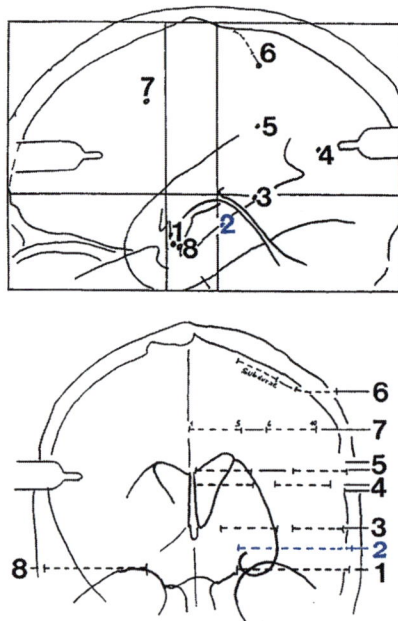

Figure 28. Localization of the depth electrodes in patient B. A push pull cannula was inserted into the lumen of an intrahippocampal standard hollow core multicontact depth electrode placed in the left hippocampus (electrode 2, blue).

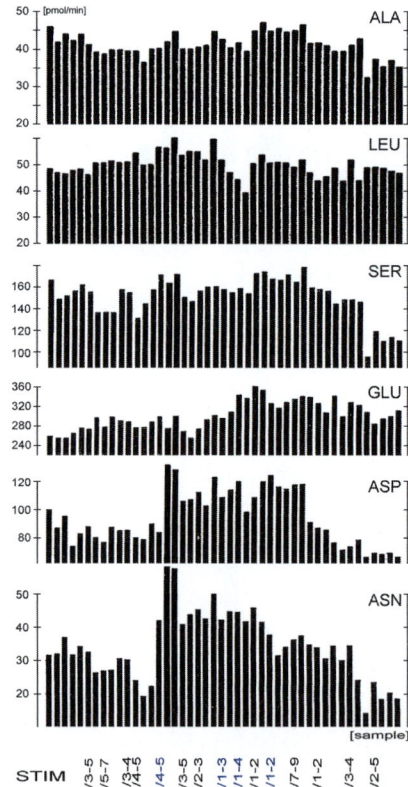

Figure 29. Time course of the concentrations of alanine **(ALA)**, leucine **(LEU)**, serotonine **(SER)**, glutamate **(GLU)**, aspartate **(ASP)** and asparagine **(ASN)** in perfusate samples 6-50 taken from the right hippocampus (electrode 2 in Fig. 28) during spontaneous EEG activity and during electrical stimulation. The sites of stimulation are indicated at the bottom of the figure, blue numbers represent stimulation followed by AD.

The first stimulation [2/4-5] followed by an AD was accompanied by an elevation of the concentrations of ASP and ASN.

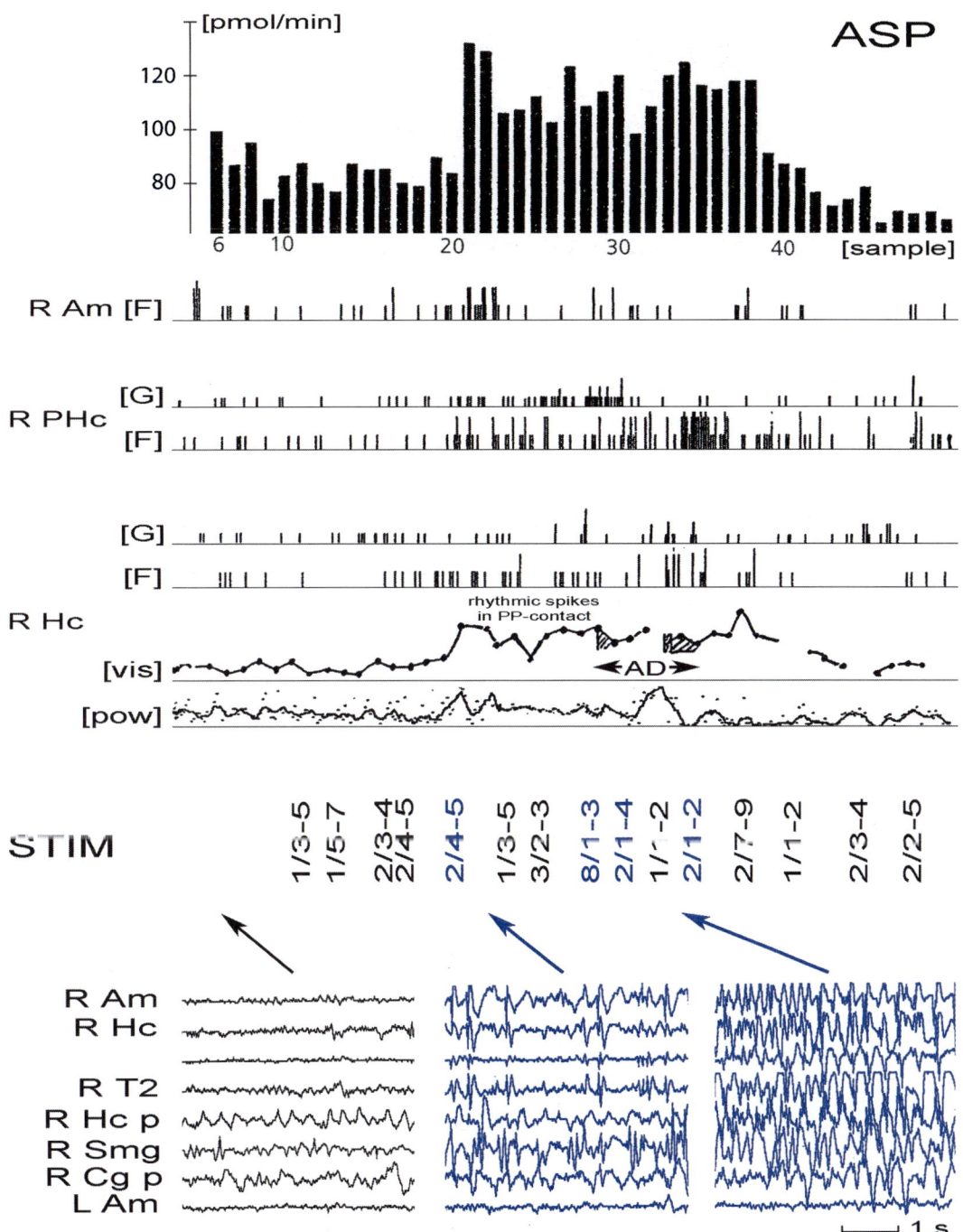

Figure 30. Time course of the aspartate (ASP) concentration in correlation to EEG findings.

The EEG traces recorded in brain regions of interest were analyzed with sharp slow wave detection algorithms developed by B. Fricker **(F)** and J. Gotmann **(G)**, by visual spike counting **(vis)**, and with compressed spectral array (CSA) defining the spectral power **(pow)** in defined frequency bands (8-32 Hz) plotting the spectral edge frequency. The stimulation sites (blue numbers represent those stimulations that were followed by ADs) and three representative EEG samples are shown at the bottom: **left**, relatively spike-free period before stimulation, corresponding to perfusate sample 6; **middle**, with spiking in the right mesial temporal lobe including the right posterior neocortical derivation, corresponding to perfusate sample 23; **right**, with an electrically induced AD involving all channels on the right side but not the contralateral amygdala, corresponding with perfusate sample 34. **R Am**, right amygdala; **R PHc**, right parahippocampal gyrus; **R Hc**, right hippocampus; **R T2**, right middle temporal gyrus; **R Hc p**, right posterior hippocampus; **R Smg**, right supramarginal gyrus; **R Cg p**, right posterior cingulate gyrus; **L Am**, left amygdala.

Modified from: Cuénod M, Audinat E, Do KQ, Gähwiler BH, Grandes P, Herrling P, Knöpfel T, Perschak H, Streit P, Vollenweider F, Wieser HG. Homocysteic acid as transmitter candidate in the mammalian brain and excitatory amino acids in epilepsy. In: Ben-Ari Y ed. *Excitatory Amino Acids and Neuronal Plasticity*. New York: Plenum Press 1990: 57-63, and Wieser HG, Bjeljac M, Khan N, Müller S, Siegel AM, Yonekawa Y. Interplay of interictal discharges and seizures: some clinical and EEG findings. In: Wolf P ed. *Epileptic Seizures and Syndromes*. London: John Libbey 1994: 563-578 (Figs. 8 and 9).

Anatomical and Physiological Basis for Stereotactic Exploration of Subcortical Structures in Patients with Epilepsy

The Subthalamic Area

The pars ventralis diencephali situated caudoventrally to the hypothalamic sulcus may be divided into *hypothalamus* and *subthalamus* on phylogenetic, ontogenetic and functional grounds. The *hypothalamus* includes the structures forming the floor of the third ventricle as far caudally and including the mamillary bodies together with structures embedded in the cranioventral sidewall of the ventricle. The main hypothalamic structures are the nucleus praeopticus medialis, nucleus praeopticus medianus, nucleus suprachiasmaticus, nucleus supraopticus, nucleus anterior hypothalami, nucleus paraventricularis, nucleus dorsomedialis hypothalami, nucleus ventromedialis hypothalami, nucleus arcuatus, mamillary bodies, nucleus posterior hypothalami, the lateral hypothalamic zone and the zona incerta [Künzle, 1994; Haymaker et al., 1969]. The main aggregations of nerve cells in the *subthalamus* are the cranial end of the red nucleus, the cranial end of the substantia nigra, the STN, the nucleus of the prerubral or tegmental field (Forel H field), and the entopeduncular nucleus or nucleus of the ansa lenticularis. Warwick and Williams [1973] also include the zona incerta into the subthalamus.

According to the goals of this book we shall concentrate on the Forel H field and the STN, but will also briefly mention the mamillary bodies and the fornix, since these structures play an important role in the current literature on DBS in patients with epilepsy.

The Forel H field

In 1877, Auguste Forel (see also Appendix) noticed a subthalamic field, which he called H (H refers to Haubenfelder) and was later named after him, the Forel H field [Forel, 1877]. The Forel H field is also known as Corpus Luysii. Anatomically, it comprises a concentration of cortical, pallido-rubro-thalamic, cerebellar and other projection fibers. It was soon recognized as a functionally important structure regarding the pathogenesis of movement disorders, pain syndromes and epilepsy.

Anatomy and Fiber Connections

The fields of Forel are three circumscript myelin rich regions of the subthalamus, namely the H1, H2 and H3 field. The *H1 field* corresponds to the thalamic fasciculus, which is a horizontal fiber stratum at the junction of the subthalamus and the overlying thalamus, comprising uncrossed pallidothalamic and crossed cerebellothalamic fibers (the latter are also known as the brachium conjunctivum). The zona incerta separates the H1 field from the more ventrally placed H2 field. The zona incerta is a flat, obliquely disposed plate of gray matter in the subthalamic region, medially adjacent to the prerubral area and laterally continuous with the reticular nucleus of the thalamus. The zona incerta is a derivative of the ventral thalamus and receives afferents from the precentral motor cortex and the cerebellum. The *field H2* is formed by the lenticular fasciculus, which is composed of pallidal efferent fibers crossing the internal capsule, is insinuated between the subthalamic nucleus and zona incerta, and joins in the formation of the thalamic fasciculus. The *field H3* (or prerubral field) is a large field of intermingling gray and white matter directly rostral to the red nucleus that unites the H1 and H2 fields around the medial margin of the zona incerta. Its gray matter forms the prerubral nucleus.

The human Forel H field is of considerable variability. Iukharev [1976] studied 100 preparations of the diencephalon and midbrain in serial frontal sections made 1 mm from one another, and found that the shape of the Forel H field is very variable, changing from rectangular to triangular shape in pararubral parts, and from oval to semioval shape in prerubral parts. He also found that the size and position of the Forel H field changed in relation to intracerebral reference points, such as the posterior commissure, the medial and intercommissural planes (as used in stereotactic technique). Figs. 31 and 32 depict the basic anatomical structures and fiber tracts of the Forel H field. The stereotactic coordinates of the Forel H field are shown in Figs. 33 and 34.

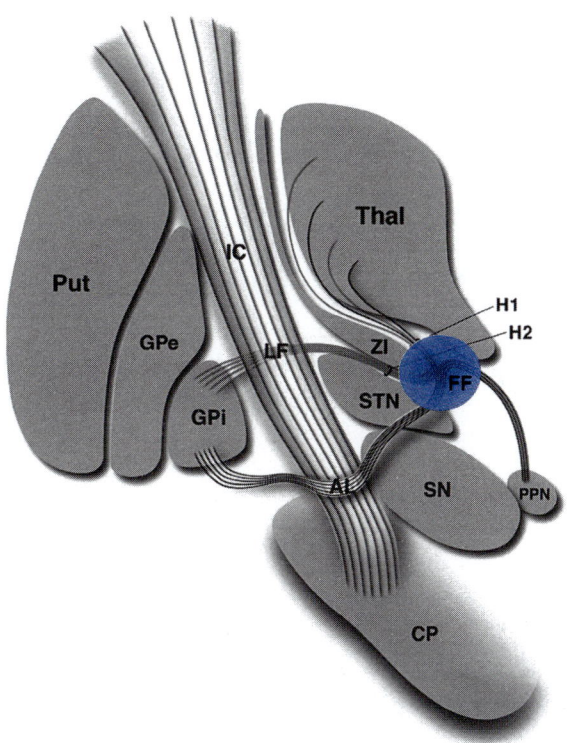

Figure 31. Schematic diagram of the Forel H field and its basic fiber tracts.

FF, Fields of Forel; **STN**, subthalamic nucleus; **ZI**, zona incerta; **SN**, substantia nigra; **PPN**, pedunculopontine nucleus; **Thal**; thalamus; **Put**, putamen; **GPe**, globus pallidus, pars externa; **GPi**, globus pallidus, pars interna; **CP**, cerebral peduncle; **H1**, H1 Field of Forel (thalamic fasciculus); **LF**, lenticular fasciculus (H2); **IC**, internal capsule; **AL**, ansa lenticularis.

Modifed from. Hamani C, Saint Cyr JA, Fraser J, Kaplitt M, Lozano AM. The subthalamic nucleus in the context of movement disorders. *Brain* 2004a; 127: 4-20.

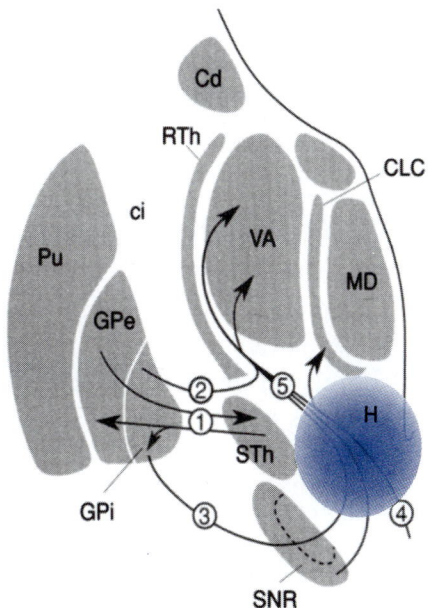

Figure 32. Schematic diagram of the pallido-thalamic and pallido-subthalamic fiber tracts.

H, Forel H field; **STh**, subthalamic nucleus; **SNR**, substantia nigra; **VA**, ventralis-anterior complex of the thalamus; **CLC**, central lateral complex of the thalamus; **MD**, medial dorsal thalamic nucleus; **RTh**, reticular nucleus of the thalamus; **Cd**, caudate nucleus; **Pu**, putamen; **GPe**, globus pallidus, pars externa; **GPi**, globus pallidus, pars interna; **ci**, internal capsule; ①, subthalamic fasciculus; ②, lentiforme fasciculus; ③, ansa lentiformis; ④, cerebellothalamic tract. ②, ③, and ④ converge into the Forel H field and constitute the fasciculus thalamicus ⑤.

Modified from: Künzle H. Aufbau und Verbindungen der Basalganglien. Chapter 16.17. In: Drenckhahn D, Zenker W eds. *Benninghoff Anatomie*, Band 2, 15th revised edition. München, Wien, Baltimore: Urban & Schwarzenberg 1994: 572-582 (Fig. 16.17-4).

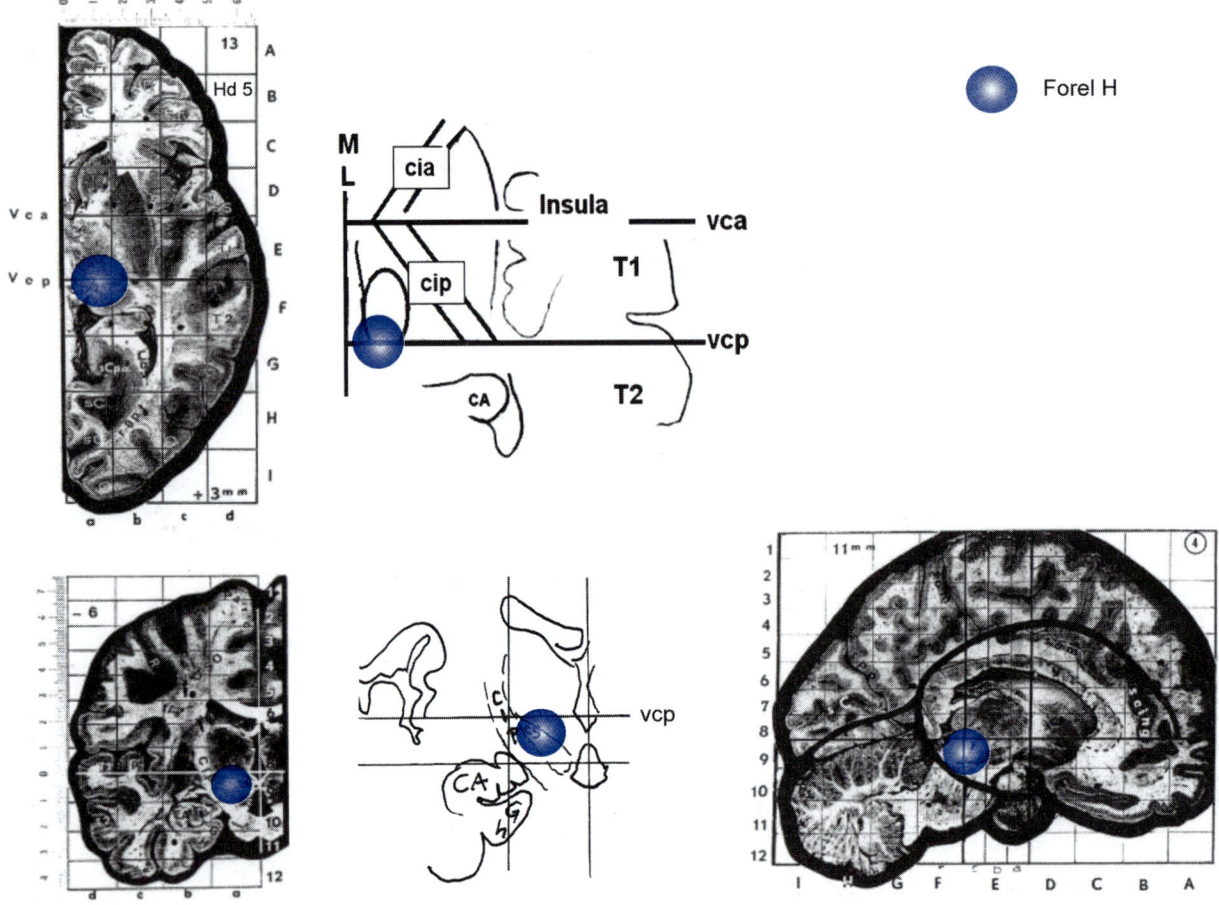

Figure 33. Stereotactic coordinates of the Forel H field, as shown in the atlas of Talairach *et al.* [1967].

cia, internal capsule, anterior limb; **cip**, internal capsule, posterior limb; **T1**, superior temporal gyrus; **T2**, middle temporal gyrus; **vca**, anterior vertical line perpendicular to AC-PC line, at the posterior border of the anterior commissure (AC); **vcp**, posterior vertical line perpendicular to AC-PC line, at the anterior border of the posterior commissure (PC); **ML**, midline (linea mediana cerebri); **CA**, cornu Ammonis.

Modified from: Talairach J, Szikla G, Tournoux P, Prossalentis A, Bordas-Ferrer M, Covello L, Jacob M, Mempel E, Buser P, Bancaud J. *Atlas d'anatomie stéréotaxique du télencéphale*. Paris: Masson 1967 (horizontal sections: Hd 5, planche XCVIII, + 3 mm, section 13, p. 133; vertico-frontal section: VF48; planche LXVII, -6, section 14, p. 101; and sagittal section: S 34D; planche XXXIV, 11 mm, section 4, p. 65).

The knowledge of afferent and efferent fiber connections of the Forel H field is mainly based on experimental studies in animals. Mukawa [1964a, b] studied the fiber connections of the Forel H field in cats using Marchi preparations. He found extensive centripetal or retrograde degeneration from the lesions in H fields and concluded that the Forel H fields are the crossroads of the extrapyramidal system in association with the brainstem activating system. Saper [1985] studied the organization of hypothalamic projections to cerebral cortex using retrograde and anterograde tracer methods in rats. He identified four separate populations of hypothalamic neurons, constituting a major source of diffuse cortical innervations: (1) Field of Forel (FF) neurons, which project primarily to the frontal cortex of the ipsilateral hemisphere, and which are located just ventral to the medial edge of the medial lemniscus at the level of the ventromedial basal thalamic nucleus. The more laterally placed neurons innervate the lateral frontal, insular and perirhinal cortex, whereas the more medial neurons around the mamillothalamic tract innervate the medial frontopolar, prelimbic, infralimbic and anterior cingulate cortex. (2) Tuberal lateral hypothalamic (LHAt) neurons, which innervate the cerebral cortex cluster in the perifornical region, in the zona incerta, and along the medial edge of the cerebral peduncle. Most of these neurons project to the ipsilateral cortex, only small percentages innervate the contralateral cortex. (3) Posterior lateral hypothalamic (LHAp) neurons, which form a dense

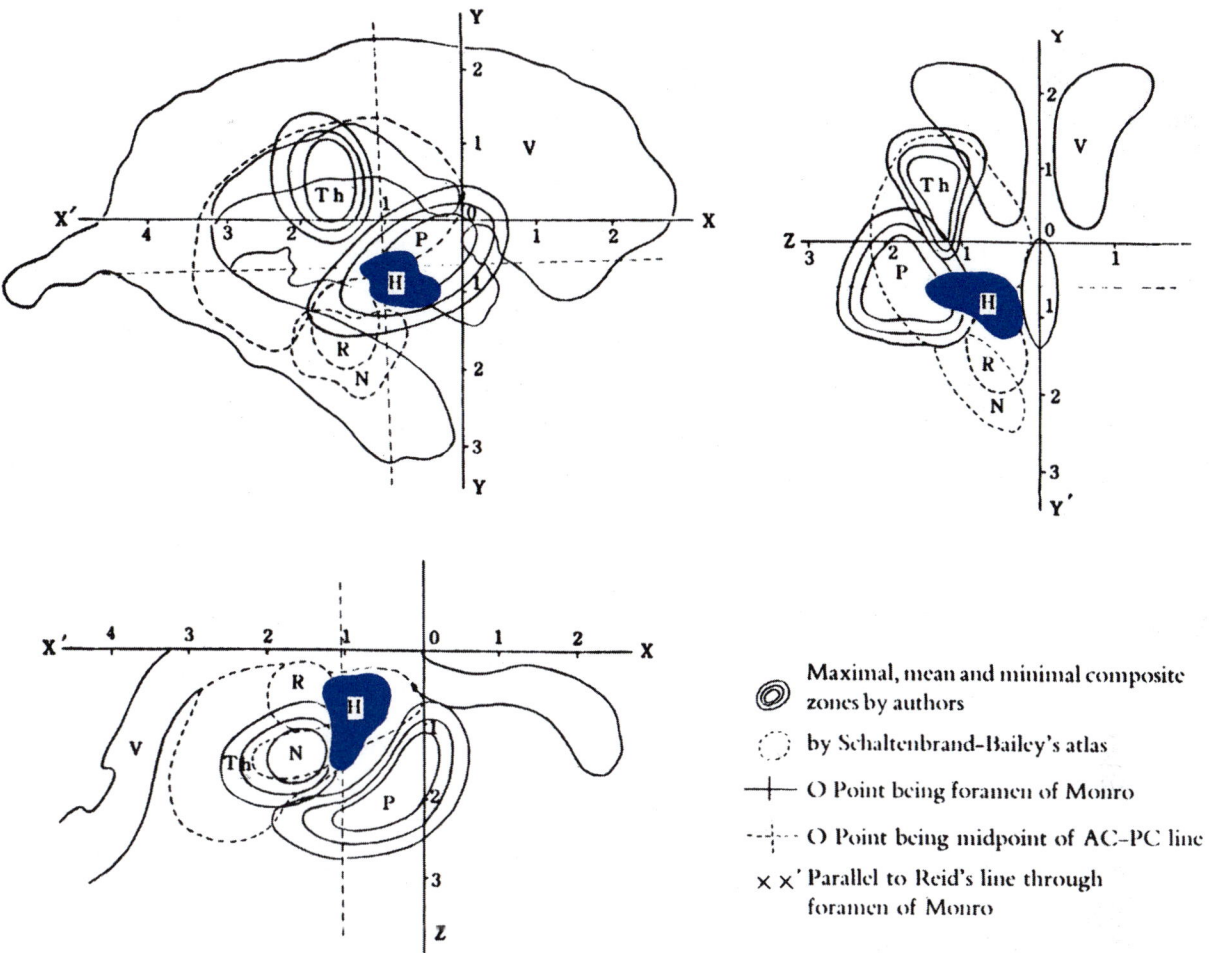

Figure 34. Stereotactic coordinates of the Forel H field, as depicted by Jinnai and Nishimoto [1963].
V, ventricles; **H**, Forel H field, **P**, globus pallidus; **Th**, lateral group of thalamic nuclei; **R**, nucleus ruber; **N**, substantia nigra.
Modified from: Jinnai D, Nishimoto A. *Stereotaxic destruction of Forel H for treatment of epilepsy.* Neurochirurgia 1963; 6: 164-176 (Fig. 5).

cluster spanning the lateral hypothalamus from the cerebral peduncle to the posterior hypothalamic area at premamillary levels, and extend into the supramamillary nucleus and the adjacent ventral tegmental area. LHAp neurons innervate the entire cerebral cortex, predominantly on the ipsilateral side. Populations of LHAp neurons projecting to different cortical target areas show considerable spatial overlap. (4) Tuberomamillary (TMN) neurons, which form a sheet along the ventrolateral surface of the premamillary hypothalamus. There is no apparent topographic organization of the TMN cortical projection system, although about twice as many TMN neurons innervate the ipsilateral, as compared to the contralateral hemisphere. Rieck *et al.* [1986] studied the organization of collicular afferents arising within the hypothalamus or the ventral thalamus using large injections of wheat germ-agglutinin-conjugated horseradish peroxidase (WGA-HRP) into the superior colliculus of the cat. The authors found retrogradely labeled neurons within the reticular nucleus of the thalamus, the zona incerta, the fields of Forel, and throughout the hypothalamus,. The dorsal hypothalamic area contains the largest number of labeled neurons. They suggested that the hypothalamic and ventral thalamic projections to the superior colliculus are separate and unrelated pathways.

Effects of Stimulation and Ablation

There is considerable evidence that the Forel H fields play an important role in the regulation of cardiovascular function. By using microinjections of DL-homocysteic acid, McCallister et al. [1988] found that electrical and chemical stimulation of the Forel H fields decrease total lung resistance in chloralose-anesthetized paralyzed dogs. The authors concluded that stimulation of cell bodies in the Forel H fields produced bronchodilation by withdrawal of cholinergic tone to airway smooth muscle. Ordway et al. [1989] confirmed that lesions made in the hypothalamus in the region of the fields of Forel abolished the increases in cardiovascular and muscle motor function evoked by stimulation, although the cardiovascular variables measured in the awake beagles at rest and during dynamic exercise were similar pre- and postlesion.

Whether and to what extent the Forel H field plays a role in voluntary vocal control is not yet clear. Afferent subcortical connections from the Forel H field into the motor cortical larynx area were found in rhesus monkeys. Simonyan and Jürgens [2005] injected the retrograde tracer WGA-HRP into the motor cortical larynx area and found retrogradely labeled cells in various brain sites including the claustrum, basal nucleus of Meynert, substantia innominata, extended amygdala, lateral and posterior hypothalamic area, Forel H field, and numerous thalamic nuclei, with the strongest labeling in the nuclei ventralis lateralis, ventralis posteromedialis, medialis dorsalis and centrum medianum, and weaker labeling in the nuclei ventralis anterior, ventralis posterolateralis, intermediodorsalis, paracentralis, parafascicularis and pulvinaris anterior. In the midbrain, labeling was found in the deep mesencephalic nucleus, ventral tegmental area, and substantia nigra. In the lower brainstem, labeled cells were found in the pontine reticular formation, median and dorsal raphe nuclei, medial parabrachial nucleus, and locus coeruleus.

Cowie and Robinson [1994] described connections between Forel H field and the subcortical gigantocellular head movement region (a medial pontomedullar area caudally to the abducens nucleus, from which a variety of head movements can be elicited by stimulation in macaques). As determined by injections of WGA-HRP, efferent fibers projected via two paths to the caudal medulla and upper cervical spinal cord, as well as to the interstitial nucleus of Cajal, Forel H field, paramedian pontine reticular formation, caudal vestibular nuclei and parvocellular reticular field. Afferent connections to the gigantocellular head movement region arose from the superior colliculus, but labeled neurons were also found in the caudal Forel H field, interstitial nucleus of Cajal, pontine medial tegmentum including the pontine paramedian reticular formation, nucleus subcoeruleus, and vestibular nuclear complex. These data indicate that the gigantocellular head movement region has the requisite efferent and afferent connections to function in the subcortical control of head, but not eye, movements.

In rats, the Forel H2 field has been studied with respect to the phenomenon reported by Leith and Barrett [1981], wherein tolerance was shown to develop to D-amphetamine-induced facilitation of self-stimulation. Anderson et al. [1978] showed that the development of such tolerance is dependent on the location of the stimulating electrode. Subsequent tolerance developed with stimulation of dorsal or medial hypothalamic structures (Forel H2 field, dorsal medial forebrain bundle, medial hypothalamic nuclei), but no tolerance was found with ventral or lateral hypothalamic stimulation (fornix, ventral medial forebrain bundle).

With the advent of improved stereotaxy, the Forel H field (and related structures, see campotomy) quickly became a target for therapeutically motivated lesions to improve symptoms of Parkinson's disease (PD), hyperkinesias and certain types of epilepsies [Spiegel et al., 1963]. Studies concerning stimulation and ablation in patients with epilepsy will be discussed in the Discussion chapter (pp. 133). Here, the issue of cervical dystonia (CD) will be shortly mentioned, in view of Hassler's initial pathophysiological model.

Historically, thalamotomy was the preferred procedure for CD, or at least for certain forms of CD. Later on, the subthalamic area was targeted more frequently with the aim of affecting pallidal outflow. In the late 1970s, functional stereotactic surgery for CD was abandoned for several reasons, including the widespread and beneficial use of botulinum toxin and the general decline in movement disorder surgery [Loher et al., 2004]. However, it is interesting to note that the rationale of subcortical stimulation and ablation for the treatment of CD was based on Hassler's pathophysiological model, which, in turn, is based on W.R. Hess' milestone neurophysiologic studies, for which he was awarded with the Nobel prize. Hassler visited Zurich to review the kinematographic data and histologic serial cuts of W.R. Hess' famous cat experiments, and concluded that the movements of the cat's head is related to circumscribed neuronal systems in the basal ganglia and the brainstem: Stimulation of the interstitial nucleus of Cajal (INC) led to head rotation towards the side of stimulation, whereas coagulation of the INC resulted in a mirror like tonic posture with the head rotated to the contralateral side. The precommissural and prestitial nuclei were thought to be associated with flexion and extension of the head: Stimulation of the precommissural nucleus led to flexion of the head, whereas its destruction resulted in tonic head extension, similar to retrocollis. Vice versa, stimulation of the prestitial nucleus led to retroflexion [Hassler and Hess, 1954; Hassler and Dieckmann, 1970]. Hassler also determined the nucleus ventrointermedius thalami as a potential target to eliminate the vestibular influence on head posture and neck muscle. Since most patients with CD presented with a combined dystonic pattern, the choice of the side to be operated on proved to be problematic. It has to be mentioned that Hassler's pathophysiological model of CD was not unanimously accepted. Sano et al. [1970a] proffered the INC region as a target for ablative stereotactic surgery. Cooper [1964] suggested targets such as the (somatosensory) ventralis posterolateralis (VPL) or ventralis posteromedialis (VPM) nuclei of the thalamus as well as the lateral portion of the centrum medianum (CM).

In 1970, Hassler and Dieckmann [1970] reported their results with interruption of pallidothalamic pathways in the thalamic fascicle H1 of Forel and lesions of the nucleus ventro-oralis internus (V.o.i.), contralateral to the side towards the chin pointed. In patients with rotational torticollis, the lesion was placed in the most posterior part of the V.o.i. and was extended caudally in order to also alter fibers from the interstitial nucleus to the V.o.i. With respect to the treatment of horizontal torticollis, the primary target was fibers in Forel field H1. Twelve of 21 patients treated according to this rationale had a good postoperative result, nine showed a moderate benefit. Ten patients suffered from ataxia and dyssynergia of the contralateral arm immediately after the operation, but ataxia recovered in all patients over the course of a few months.

The Subthalamic Nucleus

The STN is considered to be an important modulator of basal ganglia output. It is thus not surprising that the STN has emerged as an important target for functional surgery in certain movement disorders, in particular in patients with PD. In fact, chronic high frequency stimulation of the STN is currently the major surgical treatment for motor complications in advanced PD. In the last years this target also was investigated in certain types of epilepsy, as will be discussed in detail on pages 139-140.

Anatomy and Fiber Connections

The STN is a small, obliquely oriented structure of ovoid shape (like a biconvex lens) located in the ventral part of the subthalamus on the dorsal surface of the peduncular part of the internal capsule directly rostral to the substantia nigra. The STN is essentially composed of projecting glutamatergic neurons. The STN receives massive afferent projections from the lateral segment of the globus pallidus, and, somatotopically organized, from the ipsilateral motor cortex. Smaller bundle of afferent fibers arrive from the brainstem and from the centromedian nucleus of the thalamus, terminating in the rostral part of the nucleus. The STN has efferent projections to both pallidal segments, the striatum, the pars reticulata of the substantia nigra, and, to a smaller extent, also to the ipsilateral pedunculopontine nucleus. Fig. 35 depicts the basic anatomical structures and stereotactic coordinates of the STN.

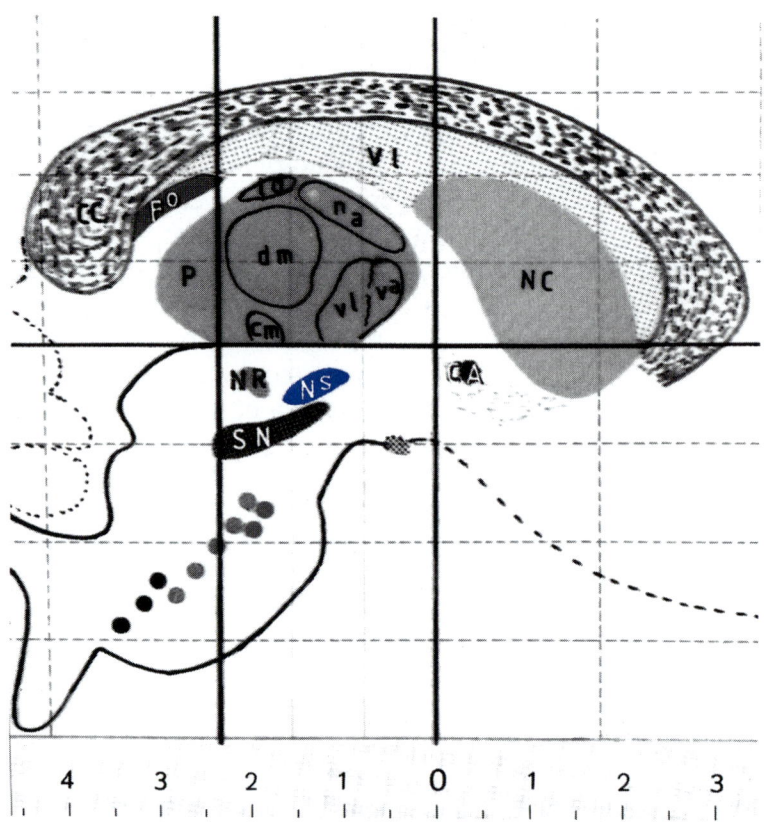

Figure 35. Stereotactic coordinates of the subthalamic nucleus, as shown in the atlas of Talairach & Tournoux, 1988.

NS, subthalamic nucleus; **SN**, substantia nigra; **NR**, red nucleus; **NC**, caudate nucleus; **FO**, fornix; **VL**, lateral ventricle; **CC**, corpus callosum; **P**, pulvinar; **dm**, dorsomedial nucleus of the thalamus; **cm**, centromedian nucleus of the thalamus; **na**, anterior nucleus of the thalamus; **ld**, laterodorsal nucleus of the thalamus; **vl**, ventrolateral nucleus of the thalamus; **va**, ventralis-anterior complex of the thalamus.

Modified from: Talairach J, Tournoux P. *Co-Planar Stereotaxic Atlas of the Human Brain* (translated by Rayport M). Stuttgart, New York: Thieme 1988 (Fig. 45).

Effects of Stimulation and Ablation

Early reports of surgery of the subthalamic region extend back to the 1960s, in a time when campotomy was performed as an alternative method to pallidotomy and thalamotomy. Campotomy was performed in an attempt to improve results with smaller lesions targeted at pallidofugal fibers, mainly in patients with advanced PD. Considering that fibers severed by campotomy passed through the Forel H field, the zona incerta, and the prerubral field (all of which situated directly dorsal to the STN), such lesions may well have involved the STN, at least to some extent. In fact, lesions of the Forel H2 field or the posterior subthalamus were reported to produce results similar to those with thalamotomy. Such lesions were reported to be safe, although provoking transient hemiballism in some of the cases. Today it is generally accepted that small lesions of the STN may induce contralateral choreiform abnormal movements and ballism, whereas lesions outreaching the boundaries of the STN by also severing the inner part of the pallidum and its fiber systems (i.e. the fields of Forel) do not induce involuntary movements disorders [Hamani et al., 2004a]. This is likely to be related to the fact that pallidal or pallidal outflow pathway lesions are highly effective in suppressing dyskinesias [Lozano, 2001]. In animals, ballism as well as choreic and athetoid movements of the contralateral hemibody have been found with lesioning or topical application of GABAergic agonists in the STN [Hammond et al., 1979].

In animal models of PD, STN is dysfunctional and neurons have been shown to fire in oscillatory patterns closely related to tremor. STN lesions or the topical administration of

GABAergic agonists into the STN regularize the firing patterns in the globus pallidus and the substantia nigra (SNr), decreasing the overall electrophysiological and metabolic activity within these structures. In non-human primates, excitotoxic lesions of the STN reduced the mean discharge rate of GPi neurons (from an average of 69.8 to 47.4 Hz) and GPe (from an average of 63.6 to 41 Hz) [see review in Hamani *et al.*, 2004a].

Aside from the size of the lesion, its precise location within the STN seems also to be important with regard to the development of abnormal movements. Experimental studies in monkeys support the hypothesis that different functional domains can be identified in the STN. A sensorimotor region innervated by M1 has been localized in the dorsolateral STN. A segregated body map with arm-related neurons located in a lateral position relative to leg-related neurons has been described, as evidenced by microelectrode recordings in patients with PD undergoing STN DBS placement [Romanelli *et al.*, 2004]. Many groups believe that intraoperative neurophysiology is essential, or at least helpful, for the determination of the optimal electrode position [Romanelli *et al.*, 2004]. However, despite the existence of a certain degree of point-to-point specificity within the STN cortical network, neurons related to specific joints (i.e. shoulder, elbow, wrist, hip, knee, ankle) may not be entirely restricted to a single region of the STN but located in various sites within the nucleus [DeLong *et al.*, 1985; Bergman *et al.*, 1994; Wichmann *et al.*, 1994a]. It has been estimated that 30 to 50% of STN neurons are movement related, and up to 20% of STN neurons are responsive to eye fixation, saccadic movements or visual stimuli. The majority of the latter units are located in the ventral part of the STN and participate in circuits that involve the frontal eye fields, the caudate nucleus, the GPe and the SNr. Activation of the STN drives SNr activity, which subsequently inhibits the superior colliculus, allowing the maintainance of eye position on an object of interest or the recovery of eye fixation once a saccade is executed [Matsumura *et al.*, 1992].

Although the method of lesioning the STN appears to be safe and effective, chronic high frequency DBS is nowadays being used as a preferred approach to ablation in patients with PD, mainly due to the potential reversibility of DBS, and due to concerns regarding intractable unilateral or bilateral hemiballism with subthalamotomy. Long term follow up studies have unequivocally shown that STN DBS markedly improves motor function, reduces the severity of dyskinesias and substantially decreases drug dosage requirements in selected patients with advanced PD for up to 5 years after implantation [Krack *et al.*, 2003; Kleiner-Fisman *et al.*, 2003]. Chronic high frequency DBS of the STN induces alterations in the levels of neurotransmitters in basal ganglia structures. Glutamate increases in the GPi and SNr and dopamine increases in the striatum, whereas the levels of GABA increase in the SNr [Windels *et al.*, 2000; Bruet *et al.*, 2001]. In primates, dyskinesias and abnormal movements have recently been described with high frequency stimulation of the STN, whereas low frequency stimulation did not induce any behavioural effects [Beurrier *et al.*, 1997; see review in Hamani *et al.*, 2004a]. With low frequency stimulation, an increase in metabolic and electrophysiological activity is generally observed not only in the STN, but also in SNr, GPi and GPe.

The Fornix

The fornix comprises an outflow white matter tract from the hippocampus and is an important element of the so-called Papez circuit, and, thus, is a part of Broca's "grand lobe limbic" (Fig. 36). Paul Broca first described and named the limbic lobe in 1878, attributing olfactory functions to these structures, which has led to naming this brain area "rhinencephalon" [Broca, 1878; Turner, 1981a; 1981b]. Papez [1937, 1958] suggested that the limbic structures in man are only partially olfactory but mainly concerned with emotional behavior (Fig. 37).

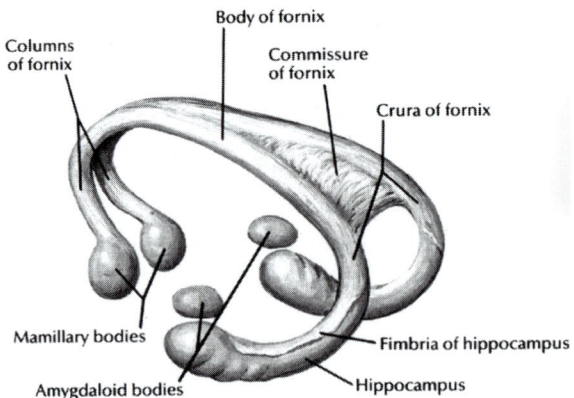

Figure 36. Scheme of the fornix.
Modified from: Netter FH. Atlas of human anatomy. Ardsley USA: CIBA-GEIGY Corp. 1989 (distributed and printed by CIBA-GEIGY Limited, Basle, 1991; Part of Plate 106).

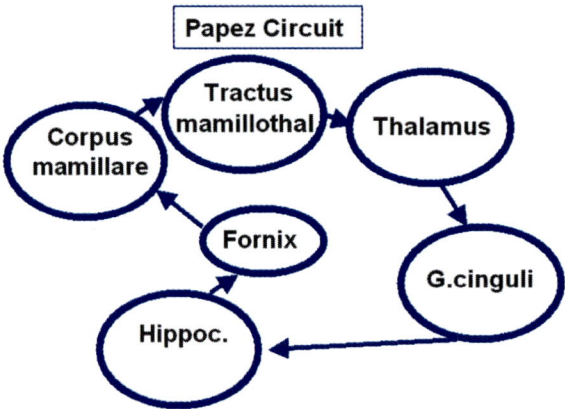

Figure 37. Core elements of the Papez circuit.

The limbic lobe was later extended by the amygdala, and MacLean [1970] added numerous other subcortical structures such as the septum, midline thalamus, habenula and hypothalamus, resulting in the concept of the so-called limbic system. Nauta [1958] further developed this concept by emphasizing the functional importance of the septum, preoptic area, hypothalamus and mesencephalon (Fig. 38). The hypothalamus serves as the link between limbic and endocrine systems, the so called "mesolimbic system", which is a mesencephalic system enabling visceral information ascending to the brainstem to influence general functioning of the limbic system [Yakovlev et al., 1960; Duvernoy, 1988].

Anatomy and Fiber Connections

The fornix is the most prominent of all myelinated fiber bundles of the hypothalamus, comprising close to one million fibers. A considerable part of the fornix fibers arises in different fields of the hippocampus and terminate in the lateral mamillary body. There is extensive crossing between the left and the right fornices. On its course through the hypothalamus, the fornix exchanges fibers with adjacent areas of gray matter, particularly with the perifornical nucleus. At the level of the precommissural septum, the fornix fibers form two distinct bundles: (1) the compact anterior column that runs posteroventrally towards the mamillary body, and (2) the more diffuse precommissural fornix that is connected with the septal gray matter. In some mammals, fibers of the precommissural fornix join the medial forebrain bundle (MFB). In rodents, the postcommissural fornix gives off the so called medial corticothalamic tract, which is directed towards periventricular hypothalamic layers. However, this tract has not

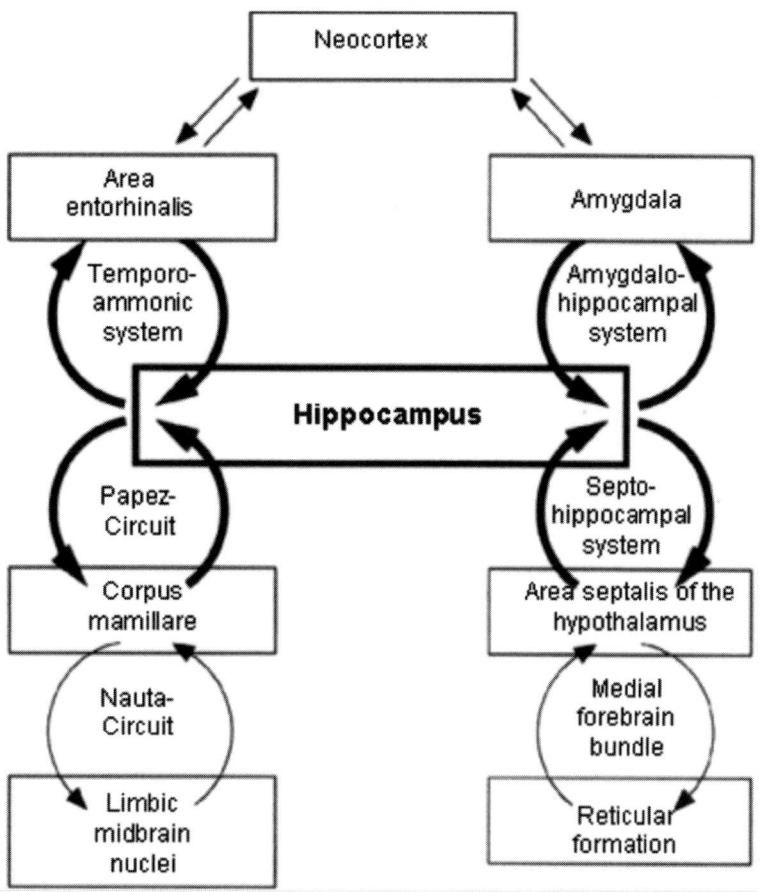

Figure 38. Simplified scheme of the most important loops of the hippocampus.
Modified from: Akert K. Limbisches System. In: Drenckhahn D, Zenker W ed. *Benninghoff Anatomie*, Band 2, 15th revised edition. Munich: Urban and Schwarzenberg 1994: 603-627 (Fig. 7), and taken from: Wieser HG. Temporal lobe epilepsies. In: Meinardi H ed. *Handbook of Clinical Neurology*, Vol. 73 (29): The Epilepsies, Part II, Amsterdam: Elsevier Science BV 2000: 53-96.

been identified with certainty in higher mammals. Some of the fornix fibers bypass the mamillary body and terminate in the periaqueductal gray matter (see p. 54-56) and the anterior tegmentum of the mesencephalon [Nauta and Haymaker, 1969; Hartwig and Wahren, 1982].

Effects of Stimulation and Ablation

Stimulation of the fornix posterior to the foramen of Monro has been shown to elicit a feeling of strangeness associated with fatigue and visual hallucinations such as an oscillating checkered pattern [Schaltenbrand and Wahren, 1982].

Fornicotomy has been evaluated with respect to the control of temporal lobe seizures already in the 1960s, based on the concept of interrupting pathways of the limbic circuit [Umbach and Riechert, 1964; Orthner and Lohmann, 1966]. Early experience indicated that lesions implicating the fornix and mamillary bodies may produce temporary memory impairment [Andy and Stephan, 1982]. Sugita et al. [1971] reported their experience with stereotactic fornicotomy in 20 patients with temporal lobe epilepsy (TLE) and associated behavioural disorders, finding that the operative results were more favourable in patients with emotional disturbances such as aggression. Burzaco [1973] reported on unilateral lesions in the fundus striae terminalis in 13 patients, based on the findings of Fernandez-Molina and Hunsperger [1959]. He found that two patients with severe behavioural disorders and TLE had a reduction in seizure frequency and were free of any behavioural disturbances for 2 years. The epilepsy data will be discussed in detail on pages 140-141.

The Mamillary Bodies

The mamillary bodies (MB) have been implicated in amnesia, learning and memory, but the importance of these nuclei and the nature of their contributions remains poorly understood.

Anatomy and Fiber Connections

The MB lie within the circuit of Papez [1937], which goes from the hippocampus to the subiculum, via fornix fibers to the MBs, via the mamillothalamic tract (MTT) to the anterior thalamic nuclei, and via the cingulate gyrus back to the presubiculum, the entorhinal cortex and the hippocampus. On cytoarchitectonic and functional grounds, the MB can be divided into lateral and medial mamillary nuclei, both of which on a rough scale are projecting to the same target regions, such as the anterior thalamic nuclei, the Gudden's tegmental nuclei or the hippocampal formation. More specifically, however, the lateral and medial mamillary nuclei have been shown to comprise two parallel systems, both anatomically and functionally [Vann and Aggleton, 2004]. The lateral mamillary nucleus contains head direction cells signaling the horizontal orientation in space of an animal. The activity of these cells is crucial for the anterior thalamic head direction signal, which, in turn, is critical for head direction signals of the hippocampal formation. The medial mamillary nucleus, on the other hand, comprises theta related cells that are thought to reflect hippocampal activity and to relay to the anterior thalamic nuclei (medial mamillary theta activity may act as a "significance signal" enabling storage of incoming theta-range information by integrating orientation information and theta).

Effects of Stimulation and Ablation

The effects of selective mamillary body lesions in animals clearly emphasize the involvement of this region in encoding spatial information and normal recall of episodic information. It has been suggested that the medial and lateral mamillary nuclei may contribute in a complementary fashion, though this assumption remains to be formally proven. Nevertheless, the effects of selective lesions within anterior thalamic nuclei (to which the MBs project) have been shown to be additive, what emphasizes the concept of two distinct but related functions. Furthermore, the severity of memory loss associated with MB damage has been shown to depend upon the extent of damage to other diencephalic regions, key amongst these being the anterior thalamic nuclei.

The amnestic syndrome, which is characterized by (1) impairment of recent memory, (2) preservation of the ability for immediate recall, and (3) preservation of remote memories, might be of special interest in this context. The amnestic syndrome has been referred to as Korsakoff syndrome, on the basis of the description of memory disturbances accompanying alcoholic peripheral neuropathy by S. S. Korsakoff in a series of papers published between 1887 and 1891. Korsakoff's classical amnestic syndrome results from a discrete inability to encode and store new memories, whereas behavior and other cognitive functions including language may remain perfectly unaffected. The syndrome has been reported in association with thiamine deficiency, but may also occur due to cerebrovascular lesions, anoxic injury or head trauma. The anatomic basis of this disorder has been a source of controversy. Pathologic studies of alcoholic patients with Korsakoff's syndrome invariably demonstrated gliotic lesions of the MB, and many authorities attributed the memory disturbance to these lesions. However, it is pertinent to note that lesions of the MBs may also occur in the absence of the amnestic syndrome. Subsequent studies demonstrated that lesions of the dorsal medial thalamic nuclei correlated with the amnestic syndrome in alcoholic patients, and the role of the MBs in the memory disorder was largely, although not entirely, dispelled [Victor, 1987]. The importance of the dorsal thalamus to recent memory acquisition was corroborated by other instances, such as the appearance of an amnestic syndrome following penetrating trauma to this region [Squire and Moore, 1979]. Yoneoka et al. [2004] reported on a patient with bilateral isolated lesions of the MTT associated with Korsakoff's syndrome, concluding that bilateral MTT lesions are sufficient to cause an amnestic syndrome. Isolated bilateral lesions of the MTT are a rare occurrence, which might explain why this association had not been previously reported. However, this finding is not particularly surprising, considering that the mamillary complex reciprocally innervates the hippocampal limbic system by way of the MTT and the fornix. The role of the hippocampal formation in the acquisition and storage of new memories is well established. Scoville and Milner [1957] reported on permanent memory impairment following bilateral medial temporal lobe resection that extended sufficiently posteriorly to damage portions of the anterior hippocampus and hippocampal gyri. D'Esposito et al. [1995] demonstrated that bilateral lesions of the fornix may also result in an amnestic syndrome. Most evidence indicates that bilateral lesions of segments of the temporal or diencephalic or both limbic systems are necessary to impair learning [Berger, 2004].

Chronic electrical stimulation of the MB and MTT in chronic refractory epilepsy has been performed by a group in Leuven, Belgium, with the hypothesis that the odds of efficacy of MB or MTT stimulation appear at least equivalent to the other targets [Raftopoulos et al., 2005; see p. 141-142]. Duprez et al. [2005] recently reported that bilateral MB and MTT electrode implantation did not induce memory dysfunction in three patients.

The Thalamic Nuclei

The human thalamus (thálamos, from Greek "bedroom", "chamber") consists of two prominent bulb shaped masses of about 5.7 cm in length, located obliquely and symmetrically on each side of the third ventricle. In a very broad sense, the human thalamus can be subdivided into three major parts: the anterior, medial and ventral complex, each containing numerous nuclei of variable size (Figs. 39-41). More specifically, more than 120 subdivisions can be delineated in the human thalamus [Hassler, 1982]. The organization of these anatomical and functional subdivisions is complex, and the terminology of thalamic nuclei is further complicated by anatomical and functional differences between the primate and human thalamus. Therefore, several nomenclatures have been introduced over the last century [Le Gros Clark, 1932; Crouch, 1934; Walker, 1938a, b; Van Buren and Borke, 1972; Hassler, 1982]. There exists a comprehensive list of American synonyms for the terminology of the Schaltenbrand-Walker atlas [1977], which, in turn, is based on a modification of Hassler's [1982] and Walker's terminology [1982]. For the purpose of this book, the nomenclature of the individual nuclei will be based on the terminology proposed by Hassler [1982]. Moreover, the focus here will be on the nuclei that are most relevant for the understanding of stereotactic thalamic interventions in patients with epilepsy, which are the nuclei of the anterior and medial complex.

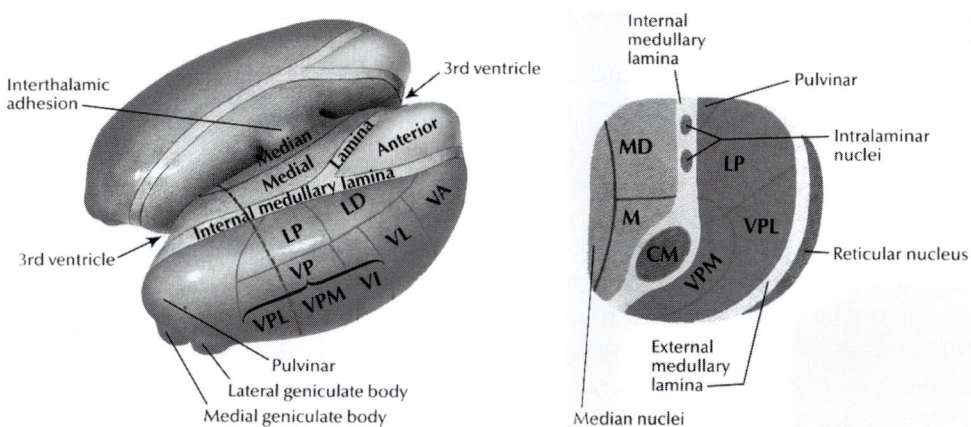

Figure 39. Schematic presentation of the thalamus with lateral, medial and anterior nuclear complex.
CM, centromedian; **LD**, lateral dorsal; **LP**, lateral posterior; **M**, medial; **MD**, medial dorsal; **VA**, ventral anterior; **VI**, ventral intermedial; **VL**, ventral lateral; **VP**, ventral posterior; **VPL**, ventral posterolateral; **VPM**, ventral posteromedial.
Modified from: Netter FH. Atlas of human anatomy. Ardsley USA: CIBA-GEIGY Corp. 1989 (distributed and printed by CIBA-GEIGY Limited, Basle, 1991; Part of Plate 105).

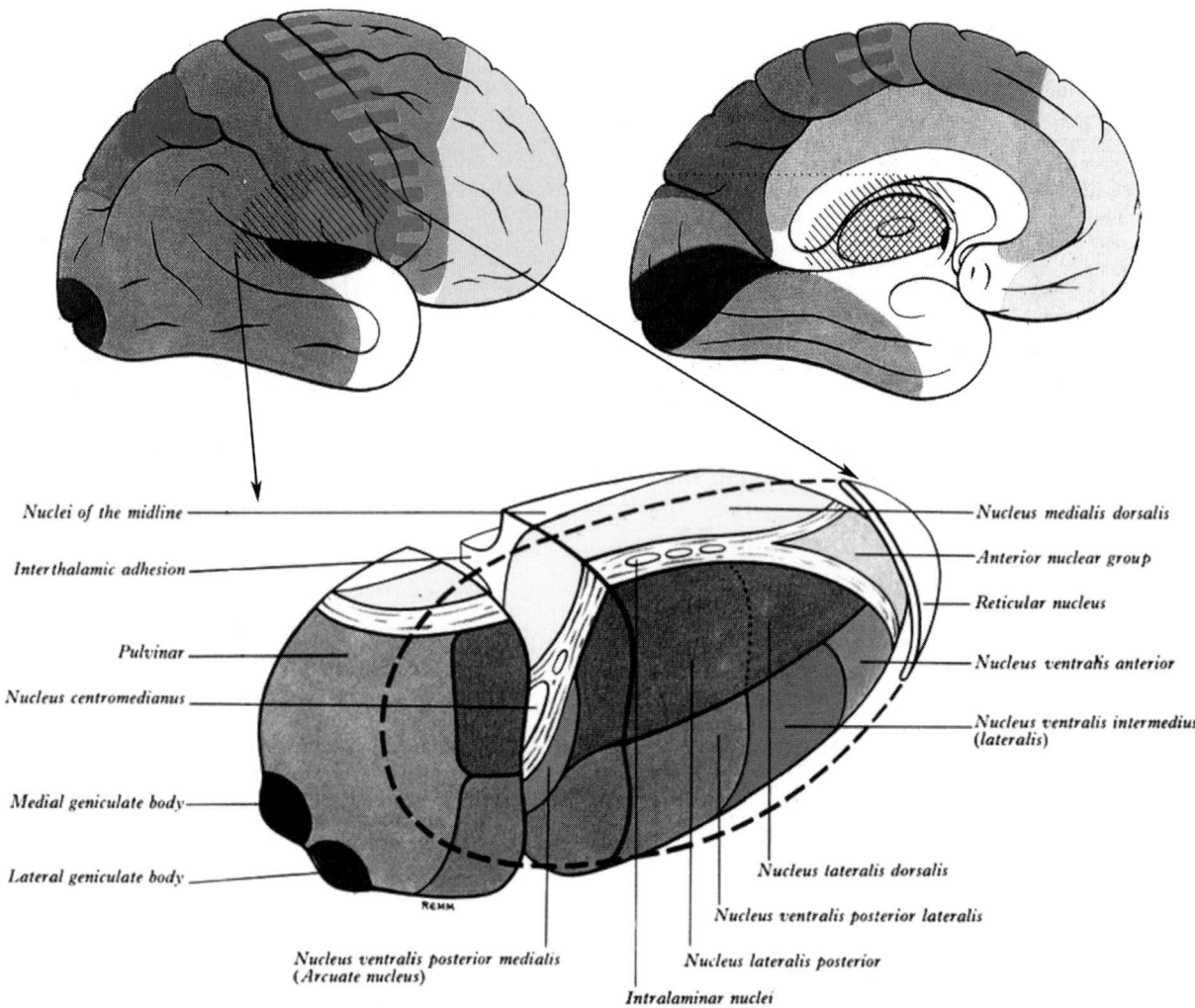

Figure 40. Scheme of the main nuclear masses of the dorsal thalamus (below) with the connected neocortical areas.
Modified from: Warwick R, Williams PL eds. *Gray's Anatomy*, 35th edition. Edinburgh: Longman 1973 (Fig. 7.101).

Technical Note regarding the nomenclature of the Schaltenbrand-Wahren atlas

Each plate bears a Roman numeral and indicates the brain; Letters F (frontal), S (sagittal) and H (horizontal) indicate the plane. Each plate has a number indicating the distance in mm of the section from its base plane and a letter to designate its orientation to the plane. a means anterior and p posterior to the midcommissural plane, l lateral to the midsagittal plane; in the horizontal sections d means dorsal and v ventral to the intercommissural plane. The base plane is always designated as 0. For example H.d+4,0 means. Horizontal plane, 4 mm above the intercommissural line. Furthermore, it should be remembered that Schaltenbrand and Wahren used the center of the commissures (maximal diameter of the anterior commissure, 3 mm; of the posterior commissure, 2 mm) to erect their intercommissural line, whereas Talairach and colleagues used the upper border of the anterior commissure and the lower border of the posterior commissure to erect the ac-pc line. In addition, Talairach and colleagues erected two perpendiculars (vca and vcp) to the ac-pc line, whereas Schaltenbrand and Wahren erected a single perpendicular at the mid point of the intercommissural line. This midcommissural plane (MCP) serves as vertical zero plane in the Schaltenbrand-Wahren system.

Plates 64-66 of the Schaltenbrand-Wahren Atlas [1977] summarize motor function and sensation with electrical stimulation (Fig. 42). The former is subdivided into "motor inhibition",

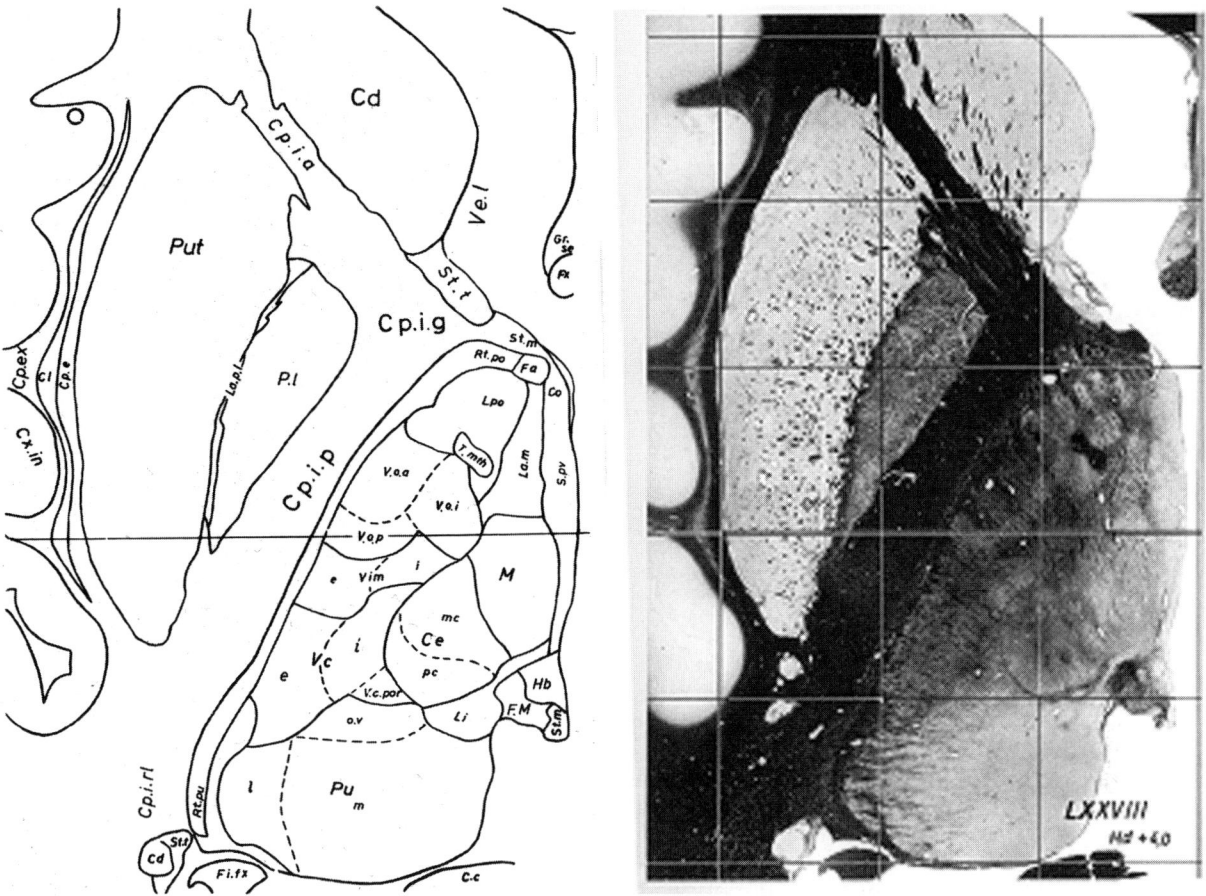

Figure 41. Schematic diagram (left) and histological preparation (right) of the thalamus.

Plate 52 LXXVIII H.d.+4,0. **Cc**, corpus callosum; **Cd**, caudatum; **Ce**, ncl. centrales thalami, centré median de Luys; **Ce mc**, ncl. centralis, magnocellularis; **Ce pc**, ncl. centralis, parvocellularis; **Cl**, claustrum; **Co**, ncl. commissuralis thalami; **Cp.ex, cp.e**, capsula externa; **Cp.i.a**, capsula interna, crus anterius; **Cp.i.g**, capsula interna, genu; **Cp.i.p**, capsula interna, crus posterius; **Cp.i.rl**, capsula interna, pars retrolenticularis; **Cx.in**, cortex insularis; **Fa**, ncl. fasciculosus thalami; **Fi.fx**, fimbria fornicis; **F.M**, fasciculus retroflexus Meynertii; **Fx**, fornix; **Gr.se**, griseum septi; **Hb**, ganglion habenulae, epithalamus, ncl. habenularis; **La.m**, lamella medialis thalami, lamella medullaris medialis, ncl. intralamellaris (medialis); **La.p.l**, lamina pallidi lateralis; **Li**, ncl. limitans thalami; **Lpo**, ncl. lateropolaris thalami; **M**, ncl. dorsomedialis; **P.l**, pallidum laterale; **Pu l**, pulvinar laterale; **Pu m**, pulvinar mediale; **Pu.o.v**, ncl. pulvinaris oroventralis; **Put**, putamen; **Rt.po**, ncl. reticularis polaris; **Rt.pu**, ncl. reticularis pulvinaris; **St.m**, stria medullaris thalami, stria habenularis, taenia thalami; **St.t**, stria terminalis, stria cornea – semicircularis; **S.pv**, substantia periventricularis, midline nuclei (Walker); **St.t**, stria terminalis; **T.mth**, tractus mamillothalamicus, fasciculus Vicq d'Azyrii; **V.c**, ncl. ventrocaudales; **V.c.e**, ncl. ventrocaudalis externus; **V.c.i**, ncl. ventrocaudalis internus; **V.c.por**, ncl. ventrocaudalis portae; **Ve.l**, ncl. ventriculus lateralis; **V.im.e**, ncl. ventrointermedius externus; **V.im.**, ncl. ventrointermedius internus; **V.o.a**, ncl. ventrooralis anterior; **V.o.i**, ncl. ventrooralis internus; **V.o.p**, ncl. ventrooralis posterior.

From Schaltenbrand G, Wahren W. Atlas for Stereotaxy of the Human Brain (architectonic organization of the thalamic nuclei by Rolf Hassler) - 2nd, revised and enlarged edition. Stuttgart: Georg Thieme Publishers 1977, including Guide to this atlas.

"motor excitation" and "torsion". Both motor function and sensation respect topographical aspects (leg, shoulder, arm, hand, head, eyes, and rump).

An abundance of data was collected with respect to vegetative and psychic effects. Schaltenbrand and Wahren [1977] summarized these vegetative effects in plates 67-69 of their atlas (not shown here), by further distinguishing vegetative phenomena I (feeling warm, sweating; feeling cold, goose skin; euphoria; depression, sadness; swallowing; respiratory arrest, respiratory stimulation; arousal; smelling sensation) and vegetative phenomena II (pupillary dilatation; illusion of movements in observed objects; tiredness; vomiting; optical hallucinations; feeling strange).

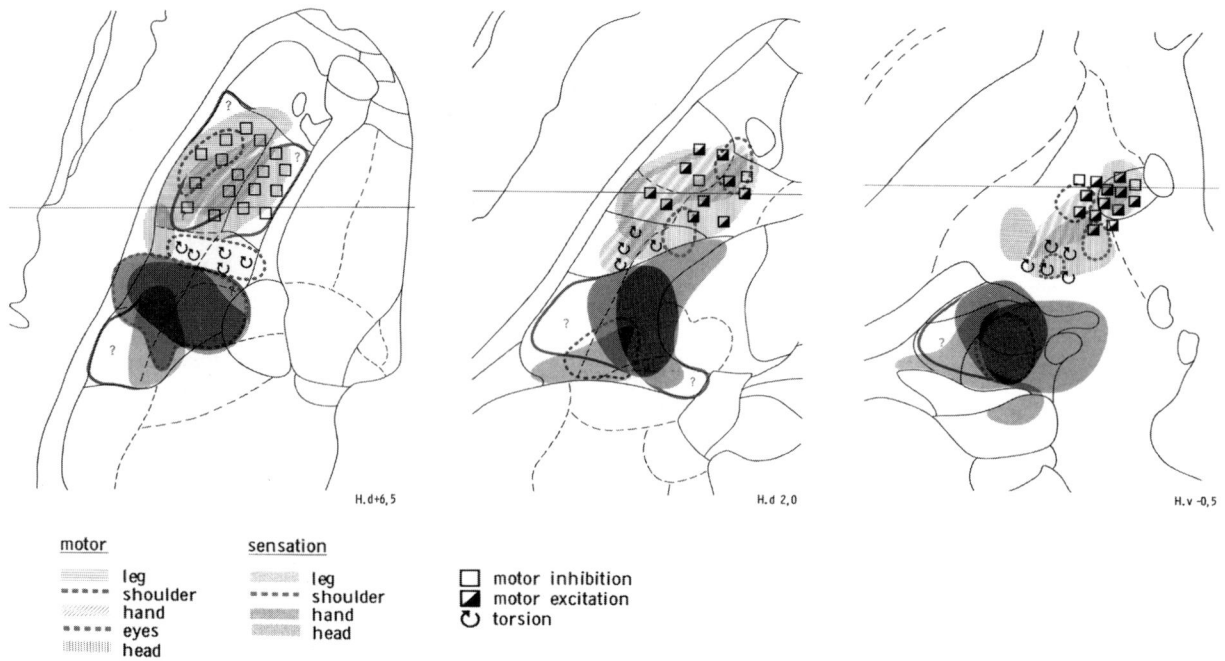

Figure 42. Summary of the electroanatomical observations with respect to motor function and sensation.

Modified from Schaltenbrand G, Wahren W. Atlas for Stereotaxy of the Human Brain (architectonic organization of the thalamic nuclei by Rolf Hassler) - 2nd, revised and enlarged edition. Stuttgart: Georg Thieme Publishers 1977; including Guide to this atlas, with permission. (Plate 66 Electroanatomical Observations: Motor function and sensation).

As outlined by the authors in their Guide to the Atlas (p. 24-25), a direct comparison of the results of the various authors (for example, Hassler and Riechert [1955], Monnier and Fischer [1951, 1955], Narabayashi [1968], Narabayashi and Ushimura [1950], Umbach [1961], Riechert and Umbach [1955], Tasker and Emmers [1967, 1969]) is clearly hampered by the use of dissimilar stimulation parameters by different authors, such as current intensity, distance of electrodes and frequency of stimulation. Schaltenbrand and Wahren [1977] performed all stimulations using a standardized technique, that is, stimulation through bipolar electrodes, separated 1/2 mm, with rectangular alternating current up to 8 V produced by the Wyss stimulator at a frequency of 16 to 30/s. In individual cases the effects are similar over an area of 3 to 4 mm, but plotting the results of many cases on the same chart results in considerably larger areas, which overlap with neighbouring regions.

The Anterior Nucleus

Anatomy and Fiber Connections

The anterior thalamic region of man consists of five individual thalamic nuclei: the large lemon-shaped *anteroventral nucleus* (also nucleus anterior principalis or anterior main nucleus) and four smaller adjacent nuclei termed *nucleus anterodorsalis* (this nucleus is clearly less developed in man than in carnivora or rodents), *nucleus anteromedialis*, *nucleus anterio-inferior* (less developed in man) and *nucleus antero-reuniens* (blending with its partner on the contralateral side within the rostral massa intermedia) [Hassler, 1982]. With respect to the stereotactic technique, the subdivision of the anterior nuclear region into its individual nuclei admittedly appears somewhat questionable, considering the small diameter of the entire anterior nuclear region of about 6 mm. Therefore, the acronym AN will henceforth be used to refer to the entire anterior nuclear region, rather than to the anterior thalamic nucleus sensu stricto. Nevertheless, it must be remembered that parts of the AN (namely the anteroventral nucleus) extend caudally above the medial nuclear group as far as the middle of the ventricular length of the thalamus (and are then replaced by the dorsal superficial nucleus).

The AN lies within the circuit of Papez [1937], as outlined on p. 40. The functionally most important ascending *afferent* connections of the anterior thalamic nuclei are those from the medial and lateral mamillary bodies (the MTT), which have received their own afferents from the subicular portion of the hippocampal formation and from the midbrain tegmentum. Additional afferent fibers ending in the nucleus anterodorsalis of the AN arise from the non-specific thalamic nuclei [Gloor, 1997].

The functionally most important *efferent* projections of the AN are those to the cingulate gyrus of the frontal lobe. These connections use the ancestral projection routes of the medial pallium (the premammalian hippocampal homologue; that is, they pass through the medial wall of the hemisphere and not through the phylogenetically younger internal capsule). Specifically, the fibers run forward in the thalamus, exit from the rostral pole of the diencephalon by crossing the anterior commissure and basal forebrain, and join the rostral end of the cingulum after piercing the genu of the corpus callosum. The thalamofugal fibers then travel through the cingulum in a caudal direction to and beyond the retrosplenial region before descending into the hippocampus, where they terminate in the stratum lacunosum-moleculare [Amaral and Cowan, 1980; Herkenham, 1978]. These thalamo-hippocampal projections of the AN are known to have a medial-to-lateral topographical organization with the most medial thalamic nuclei projecting preferentially to the hippocampal allocortex and the more lateral ones to the adjacent mesocortex [Yakovlev et al., 1960]. Fig. 43 shows a schematic representation of the thalamo-cortical projections (keeping in mind that the assignment of the thalamic nuclei to individual Brodmann areas (BA) are clearly oversimplistic and, thus, must be interpreted with circumspection). These thalamofugal connections to the hippocampal region are reciprocated by the descending corticothalamic, polysynaptic connections that originate in the entorhinal cortex and presubiculum, but also in more distant regions such as the temporopolar, cingulate, retrosplenial, and parahippocampal cortices.

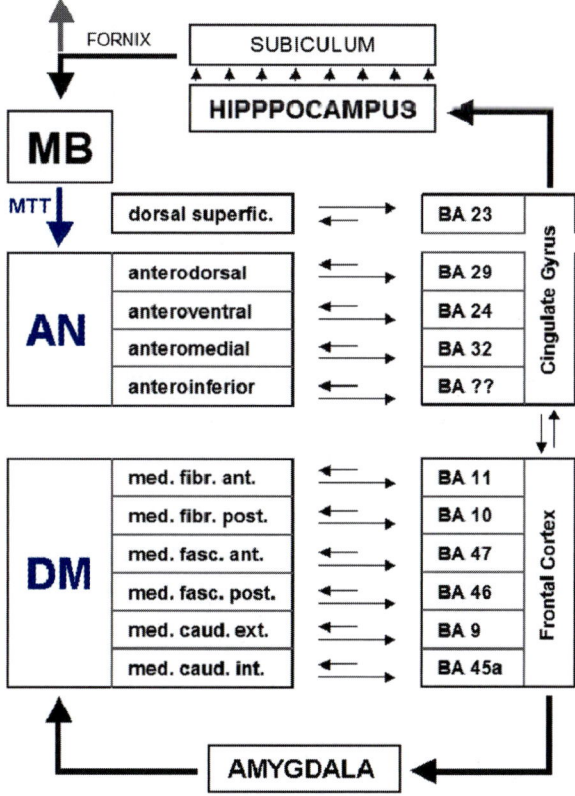

Figure 43. Schematic (and clearly oversimplistic) assignment of the reciprocal thalamocortical connections to individual Brodmann areas (BAs) of the cortex.

MB, mamillary bodies; **MTT**, mamillothalamic tract; **AN**, anterior nuclear region of the thalamus; **DM**, medial nuclear region of the thalamus.

[Gudden, 1881; Nauta, 1956; Valenstein and Nauta, 1959; Powell, 1973; Sikes et al., 1977; Poletti and Creswell, 1977; Kaitz and Robertson, 1981; Aggleton et al., 1986; Yeterian and Pandya, 1988; van Groen and Wyss, 1990a; van Groen and Wyss, 1990b; Witter and Groenewegen, 1990; Witter et al., 1990].

Effects of Stimulation and Ablation

It has been shown that single pulse stimulation of the AN (and other thalamic nuclei) leads to the generation of cerebral responses (ERs)[1] and that low frequency stimulation may synchronize the pattern of EEG activity, mediated either by direct stimulation of specific and unspecific thalamic nuclei or by direct or antidromic excitation of pathways connecting these structures with the cortex [Jasper and Droogleever-Fortuyn, 1947; Hunter and Jasper, 1949; Penfield and Jasper, 1954; Steriade, 1997; Ingram et al., 2001]. As early as 1942, Dempsey and Morison developed the dichotomous concept of a specific and unspecific thalamic projection system [Dempsey and Morison, 1942; Morison and Dempsey, 1942, 1943]. However, the validity of this strict dichotomous anatomical and physiological separation of the thalamus into specific and unspecific thalamic projection systems causing either augmenting or recruiting responses has been repeatedly questioned and the occurrence of mixed responses has been suggested [Jasper, 1961; Schlag and Villablanca, 1967; Sasaki et al., 1970; Zumsteg et al., 2006a, 2006b]. There is evidence that ERs to suprathreshold electrical stimulation are complex in form and may spread far beyond their specific projection areas [Ganglberger, 1982]. Zumsteg et al. [2006a, 2006b] demonstrated that suprathreshold single pulse stimulation of the AN led to robust and highly reproducible time locked ERs consisting of a sequence of components with latencies between 20 and 320 ms post stimulus, both when analyzed with scalp and depth electrode EEG recordings. Morphologically, these ERs showed a marked inter- and intraindividual heterogeneity, indicating a certain degree of thalamocortical point to point specificity. Statistical nonparametric mapping (SNPM) of low resolution electromagnetic tomography (LORETA) values [Pascual-Marqui et al., 1994; Pascual-Marqui, 1999; Nichols and Holmes, 2002] indeed revealed a very heterogeneous pattern of cortical activation (reflecting the presumed cortical sources of the ERs), depending primarily on the site of stimulation [Zumsteg et al., 2005, 2006a]. In general, AN stimulation led to responses of limbic (especially cingulate and insular) and neocortical lateral temporal areas, and, to a much lesser extent, the parahippocampal gyrus. This pattern of cortical activation corresponds well with the thalamocortical connections (hodology) of the anterior thalamus. Due to the divergence of thalamocortical pathways (or convergence of corticothalamic pathways, respectively), small differences in electrode localization within thalamic structures might correspond to large differences with respect to cortical activation.

Previous studies have shown that low frequency (> 5 Hz) electrical stimulation of the thalamus may cause rhythmic EEG synchronization. The generation of such synchronization has been suggested to predict clinical efficacy of stimulation in patients with epilepsy [Velasco et al., 2001; Hodaie et al., 2002], but thus far, there is no definite evidence for this prognostic role of rhythmic EEG synchronization. Zumsteg et al. [2006c] have challenged this assumption and suggested that rhythmic EEG synchronization with low frequency stimulation primarily reflects spatiotemporal summation (interference) of single pulse ERs, based on their finding that the magnitude of low frequency rhythmic EEG synchronization was positively related to the amplitudes of single pulse ERs, and simple temporal superposition of single pulse ERs by mathematical calculation resulted in "modeled" responses with strikingly similar morphology and scalp voltage distribution.

Taking into consideration that single pulse stimulation of the AN led to ERs/cortical activation with a certain degree of point to point specificity within the thalamocortical circuitry, it is reasonable to question whether high frequency stimulation of the same structures may reveal effects that are "mirroring" the findings with low frequency stimulation (by showing an opposite, modulatory or inhibitory, effect with a similar point to point specificity within the

---

1. Although brain responses to electrical stimulation have also been referred to as evoked potentials (EPs), we clearly prefer the term evoked response (ER), considering that brain responses evoked by afferent volleys elicited by direct or antidromic electrical stimulation of subcortical (or cortical) structures should be strictly distinguished from brain responses to stimulation of a peripheral sense organ or a sensory nerve, as already suggested by Ganglberger [1982].

thalamocortical circuitry). Zumsteg et al. [2006d] studied the effects of high frequency stimulation in a patient undergoing presurgical evaluation who had simultaneous deep brain stimulation (DBS) and depth electrodes positioned bilaterally in the AN and the mesial temporal structures. The authors found a predominant "inhibition" of ipsilateral mesial temporal structures (namely a significant decrease in cross power spectral density) and concluded that this finding is a) in keeping with a certain degree of point to point specificity within the thalamocortical circuitry, b) corresponds well with the findings obtained with single pulse stimulation, c) is in line with the results from previous neuroanatomical studies, and d) is in keeping with the hypothesis that the decrease in seizure severity and frequency with AN stimulation might be related to the connectivity and functional relations of the AN to limbic structures.

There is good evidence from animal studies that lesioning of AN afferents, the application of muscimol to inhibit neuronal firing, or electrical high frequency stimulation of the AN may increase the seizure threshold or reduce frequency of generalized seizures in the pentylenetetrazol seizure model [Mirski and Ferrendelli, 1984a, 1986a, 1987; Mirski and Fisher, 1994; Mirski et al., 1986, 1997]. Hamani et al. [2004b] showed that bilateral lesioning or high frequency stimulation of the AN are protective against pilocarpine induced seizures and status epilepticus in animals. In humans, AN stimulation for the treatment of epilepsy was pioneered by Cooper et al., who reported a > 60% seizure reduction in five of six patients [Cooper et al., 1984; Cooper and Upton, 1985; Upton et al., 1985, 1987]. Subsequent unblinded pilot trials confirmed that chronic AN stimulation may result in a significant decrease in seizure frequency in the long term (the results of these unblinded pilot trials will be discussed in more detail in the Discussion section) [Sussman et al., 1988; Hodaie et al., 2002; Kerrigan et al., 2004; Andrade et al., 2006]. To date there are no controlled studies on the therapeutic efficacy of chronic AN stimulation in patients with epilepsy, but a multicenter clinical is currently underway [SANTE trial, Graves et al., 2004].

The Dorsomedial Nucleus

Anatomy and Fiber Connections

The medial nuclear region is a large structural element of the median thalamus showing a length of 18 to 20 mm in humans and comprising two main nuclei, that is, the large *dorsomedial nucleus* (also nucleus medialis dorsalis) and the smaller *medioventral nucleus* (also nucleus medialis caudalis). According to Hassler [1982], the human dorsomedial nucleus can be further subdivided into a medial part containing larger cells within a fiber network (the pars magnocellularis, comprising the nucleus medialis fibrosus), and a larger lateral part with smaller nerve cells between thicker nerve bundles (the pars parvocellularis, comprising the nucleus medialis fasciculosus). These two nuclei may themselves be further subdivided into an anterior and posterior part. The medioventral nucleus, on the other hand, may be subdivided into an inner (nucleus medialis caudalis internus) and outer portion (nucleus medialis caudalis externus). Please note that the acronym DM will henceforth be used to refer to the entire medial nuclear region, rather than to the dorsomedial nucleus sensu stricto. Immunohistochemically, the DM is a "mixed" region, showing a distinctive heterogeneous "patchy" pattern of immunoreactivity for the three calciumbinding proteins [Münkle et al., 2000]. However, unlike the AN, the DM is generally quite dense for parvalbumin, but only moderate for calbindin and weak for calretinin immunoreactivity.

The DM is the source of extensive reciprocal thalamic connections to the prefrontal cortical region and, to a lesser extent, also to the amygdala and the anterobasal temporal cortex. Widespread connections from the amygdala to the prefrontal cortex, in particular to the mesocortical and proisocortical areas in the medial posterior orbital and perigenual and subcallosal mesial frontal cortex, complete the so-called circuit of Yakovlev (see Fig. 44) [Yakovlev, 1948; Yakovlev et al., 1960, 1966]. Anterograde and retrograde cell degeneration studies have shown that the most relevant thalamocortical projections of the DM go to the prefrontal cortical areas 9,

10, 11, 45, 46 and 47, showing a rostral to caudal and medial to lateral topographical organization, where rostral and medial in the thalamus corresponds to rostral and medial in the cortex (Fig. 43) [Freeman and Watts, 1947; Hassler, 1948; Angevine *et al.*, 1964]. Area 8 might also receive fibers from the lateral paralaminar portion [Walker, 1982]. The thalamofugal projections of the DM comprise both thicker specific (myelinated) and thinner unspecific (unmyelinated) fibers. The thinly myelinated or unmyelinated corticothalamic fibers, originating from deeper layers of the prefrontal cortical areas, close the "reverberating" circuit between the DM and the prefrontal cortex [Chang, 1950]. In addition to these prefrontal projections, there also exist reciprocal projections of the medial (magnocellular) parts of the DM to mesial temporal structures such as the amygdalar complex and the entorhinal and perirhinal cortex, as well as to the temporal pole, in part directly, in part through the septum [Akert, 1964; Angevine *et al.*, 1964; Freeman and Watts, 1947; Creutzfeldt and Wieser, 1987]. The lateral part of the DM, however, receives few if any fibers from the temporal lobe [Russchen *et al.*, 1987]. Minor reciprocal connections also exist to and from the subiculum, the ventral insula and the superior and inferior temporal gyri. Afferent fibers to the DM also arise from the inferior thalamic peduncle, partly from the pallidum and partly from the basal nucleus [Walker, 1982].

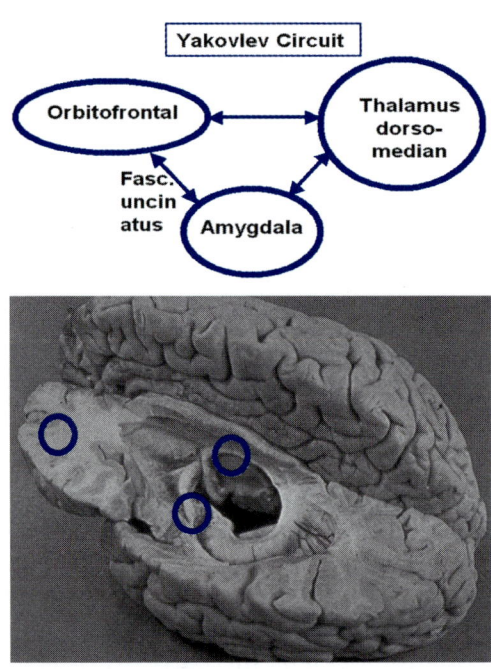

Figure 44. Main components of the Yakovlev circuit.

Effects of Stimulation and Ablation

Lesions of the DM have been performed with the aim of relieving psychoneurotic disorders and pain. Such lesions have been shown to produce transient slowing of the EEG, transient decrease of intelligence and memory scores, vegetative disturbances such as hypotension, increased appetite, and incontinence of urine. The majority of the vegetative changes were only transient, but in some cases obesity persisted for years. By means of its anatomical connections, the DM has the capabilities of integrating the convergent visceral impulses from the hypothalamus with emotional discharges - fear, rage, pleasure, both somatic and sexual - from the amygdala [Yakovlev, 1948; Yakovlev *et al.*, 1960; 1966; Walker, 1982]. Stimulation of the DM has been shown to elicit a variety of clinical responses including feelings of weakness, dizziness, floating, uncertainty, spinning, and anxiety.

Zumsteg *et al.* [2006a] have shown that suprathreshold single pulse stimulation of the DM led to SNPM LORETA source signals within orbital (BA 11, 47, and 25), mesial frontal (BA

6 and 8), lateral frontal cortical areas (BA 10, 45 and 46), and, to a lower extent, also within ipsilateral mesial temporal structures such as the amygdala, the hippocampus and the entorhinal cortex (BA 28 and 34). Depth EEG recordings during monopolar cathodic or bipolar single pulse stimulation of the DM revealed large ERs in ipsilateral orbitofrontal areas and smaller ERs in ipsilateral mesial temporal structures [Zumsteg et al., 2006b]. This pattern corresponds well to the most relevant thalamocortical connections of the DM (as previously established by retrograde cell degeneration studies by Freeman and Watts [1947], Hassler [1948] and Angevine et al. [1964]), but, as with AN stimulation, it is not clear whether the cortical activation was mediated by direct orthodromic activation of thalamofugal fibers (fiber tracts comprising both thicker specific, myelinated and thinner unspecific, unmyelinated fibers) or by antidromic activation of corticothalamic fibers (fiber tracts originating from deeper layers of the prefrontal cortical areas, and closing the "reverberating" circuit between the DM and the prefrontal cortex [Chang, 1950]). Notwithstanding this limitation, it must be emphasized that the pattern of cortical activation following high intensity stimulation of the DM could be clearly differentiated from the pattern elicited by AN stimulation. In this respect, it is important to note that the deepest contacts of the DBS electrodes in patients with anterior thalamic stimulation for the treatment of epilepsy are generally situated in the medial parts of the DM, due to the small diameter of the entire anterior nuclear region (~ 6 mm) in comparison to the substantial size of the DBS electrode (10.5 mm, model 3387, Medtronic, USA).

The Centromedian Nucleus

Anatomy and Fiber Connections

The CM is the largest cell complex of all truncothalamic nuclei. The human CM consists of ventral and caudal parts that are composed of small cells (parvocellular), and dorsal and rostral parts comprising larger cells (magnocellular). Together with other nuclei of the intralaminar nuclear complex, the CM is considered to be prototypic for the unspecific thalamic projection system. It most likely exerts an integratory function by influencing impulses arising from specific projection systems (or spontaneous cortical rhythms) via polysynaptic pathways [Dempsey and Morison, 1942; Sano et al., 1970b].

Efferent bundles of both parts of the CM emerge laterally to the nucleus. The parvocellular parts of the CM project to the ipsilateral putamen, the magnocellular to the ipsilateral striatum [Vogt and Vogt, 1941; Hassler, 1949a, b]. Kamikawa et al. [1967] also described efferent fibers projecting to the contralateral striatum and to the CM of the opposite side. According to Simma [1951], the basolateral parvocellular part of the CM projects to the putamen, whereas the dorsal magnocellular portion heads to the nucleus caudatus. In any case, it is important to realize that the CM most likely does not reveal direct connections with the cortex. This is corroborated by the fact that the cells of the CM have been shown to remain intact after decortication [Walker, 1937] or deafferentation of the cortex of one hemisphere [Vogt and Vogt, 1941].

Afferent fibers to the CM arise from the basal ganglia, showing a topographical organization similar to that of the thalamofugal projections [Schulman and Auer, 1957] and from all the adjacent thalamic nuclei [Hassler, 1982]. Afferent fibers may also arise from cerebellar nuclei such as the emboliform nucleus via the brachium conjunctivum [Uemura, 1917; Hassler, 1950]. Other afferent fibers that originate in the spine, brainstem and midbrain have been described, but it is questionable whether these fibers actually terminate in the CM, or simply pass through the CM on their way to adjacent thalamic nuclei, such as the nuclei of the centrolateral complex, for example.

Effects of Stimulation and Ablation

Electrophysiological experiments by Albe-Fessard and Gillett [1958] have shown that the CM is related to pain experience (fibers of Forel's tegmental fascicles approach the CM caudally and ventrally and, in part, pass through its ventral region. These fiber bundles come from the midbrain and constitute the dorsal secondary trigeminal pathway of Wallenberg [1900], which is the only ipsilateral trigeminal pathway). Furthermore, the CM might serve a generalized alerting function for the diencephalic motor integrations associated with the elaboration of hand and vocal cord activity.

Lesioning of the intralaminar nuclei (thalamolaminotomy) has been applied for the relief of behavioral disturbances, such as aggressiveness, destructiveness, anxiety or obsessive compulsive states. For the relief of intractable pain, lesions of the intralaminar region have proved to be more satisfactory than lesions within primary sensory thalamic nuclei. Side effects after unilateral or bilateral lesioning of the intralaminar region may include mild to moderate confusion and memory impairment (in particular, if the lesions are made bilaterally at one sitting), but these signs and symptoms tend to clear up within two weeks. Subtle changes in verbal learning are common, and are particularly pronounced after left sided lesions [Walker, 1982]. Electrical stimulation of the posterolateral portion of the CM may induce a variety of head sensations.

Zumsteg *et al.* [2006a] found that high intensity CM stimulation revealed a very diffuse, though still mainly ipsilateral and highly significant cortical activation, as revealed by SNPM LORETA. This diffuse pattern is in good accordance with the presumed widespread and polysynaptic pathways responsible for modulation of cortical activity by the CM. With single pulse stimulation of the ventro-caudal parvocellular part of the CM, ERs have been elicited over the second somatosensory cortex [Sano *et al.*, 1970b]. Zumsteg *et al.* [2006a] also found cortical activation of ipsilateral somatosensory areas (BA 1-4, and 40) with stimulation through the deepest contacts of the CM electrodes (which was in keeping with the contralateral sensory symptoms experienced by the patient during stimulation through these contacts). The activation of distinct cortical somatosensory areas with deep CM stimulation might be best explained by excitation of fibers of the medial lemniscal system that are passing through or by the CM on their way from the brainstem to the neighboring ventral nucleus, or by direct stimulation of the adjacent specific ventral nucleus [Mountcastle and Henneman, 1952].

The Lateral Nuclear Region

Anatomy and Fiber Connections

The lateral nuclear region occupies the region between the lamellae medialis and lateralis from the anterior pole to the plane of the commissura posterior [Hassler, 1982]. Several different functional systems must be distinguished. The *ventral thalamic nuclei* receive extrathalamic fibers and comprise primary receptive (sensory) or cortical relay nuclei. The *dorsal thalamic nuclei*, in contrast, do not receive such extrathalamic fibers and denote association or integration nuclei. The nucleus lateropolaris, which is the rostral pole of the lateral nuclear mass, is important with respect to the pathways of the reticular activating system to cortical fields. Hassler also distinguished the zentrolateral nuclei (that are the nucleus zentrolateralis caudalis, intermedius, and oralis).

For the functions of the distinct ventral thalamic nuclei of man, Hassler [1982] designed six homunculi representing six functionally different localizations, each of which revealing a somatotopic arrangement (Figs. 45 and 46). Almost all of the different afferent systems have terminals in five to six thalamic structures. In summary, the ventrobasal complex constitutes the thalamic component of a somatic sensory circuit feeding into the sensory S1 cortex. Throughout the system, the topical and modality organization is maintained, and at different neuronal levels, the signals undergo an elaboration by facilitatory and inhibitory inputs that provide a mechanism for coding. These inputs may originate on the same or opposite side of the spinal cord, brainstem, cerebellum, thalamus or cortex.

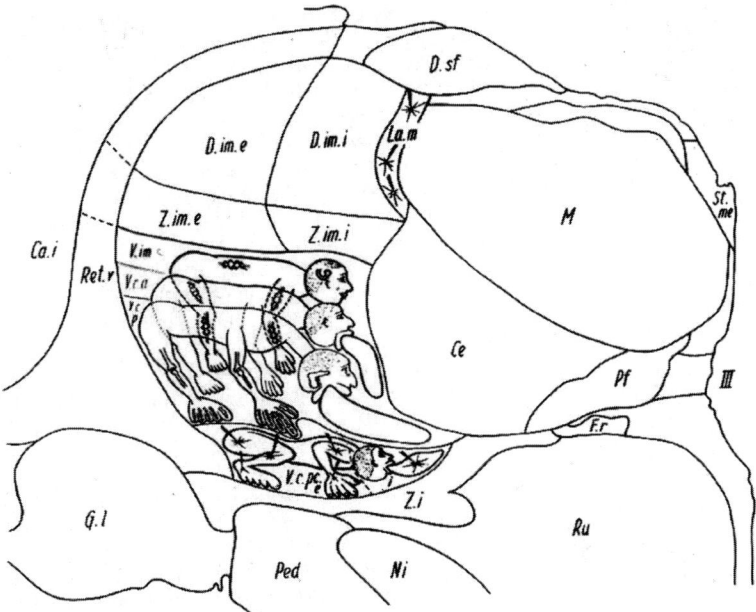

Figure 45. Schematic drawing of the representation of different somatosensory modalities in the human thalamus and their somatotopic arrangement based on findings from stereotactic operations involving fiber connections of the somatosensory systems and circumscribed stimulations.

The most ventral nuclei are the ventrocaudalis parvocellularis externus and internus **(V.c.pc.e and V.c.pc.i)**. These nuclei have a representation of cortical pain perception. The ventrocaudal posterior nucleus **(V.c.p.)** is related to joint sensibility of the fingers, elbows and knees. In the nucleus ventrocaudalis anterior **(V.c.a.)** the homunculus represents tactile sensibility with the receptors in the small hairs of the skin. Most rostrally, the representation of the muscle spindles is situated in the nucleus ventrointermedius externus **(V.im.e)**. The representation of the vestibular excitations is in the nucleus ventrointermedius internus **(V.im.i)**.

Modified from: Hassler R. Architectonic organization of the thalamic nuclei. In: Schaltenbrand G, Walker AE eds. *Stereotaxy of the Human Brain*. Stuttgart, New York: Thieme 1982: 140-180 (Fig. 9-5).

The oral segment of the lateral nuclear region receives two large afferent fiber bundles, the thalamopetal fibers of the brachium conjunctivum and the fasciculus thalamicus (the Forel bundle H1) originating from the inner part of the pallidum, ending - one in front of the other - in the oral ventral nuclei. The anterior part (V.o.a.) is supplied by pallidal fibers, the posterior part (V.o.p.) by fibers of the brachium conjunctivum. The nucleus ventro-oralis internus (V.o.i.) contains a large contingent from the nucleus interstitialis. All these ventral oral nuclei (V.o.p., V.o.a., V.o.i.) send out specific projections to the motor and premotor cortex, as indicated in the scheme. In front of these oral ventral nuclei is the lateropolar nucleus (L.po.), the nucleus ventralis anterior (VA), and the anterio- and posterio-oral ventral nuclei.

Effects of Stimulation and Ablation

The lateral nuclear region was used as a target for lesions in order to relieve tremor and rigidity in patients with PD. Both thalamotomy and posteroventral pallidotomy (PVP) have been shown to be effective means to alleviate motor symptoms in PD. Rigidity and dopa-induced dyskinesia are improved and abolished by either of the two procedures, but tremor is more markedly improved by thalamotomy than by PVP. Lesions in the nucleus ventralis lateralis or the ventrointermedius abolished preexisting tremor and rigidity, without resulting in paresis. Electrical stimulation of these nuclei has been shown to produce muscle sensations without concomitant movement or autonomic effect, and spontaneous tremor, if present, was aggravated in 40% of cases and suppressed in 60%. Albe-Fessard [1973] recorded rhythmic burst discharges that were temporally related to the tremor. "Kinesthetic neurons" responding to passive movements of the joints have been found rostrally to tactile neurons of the nucleus

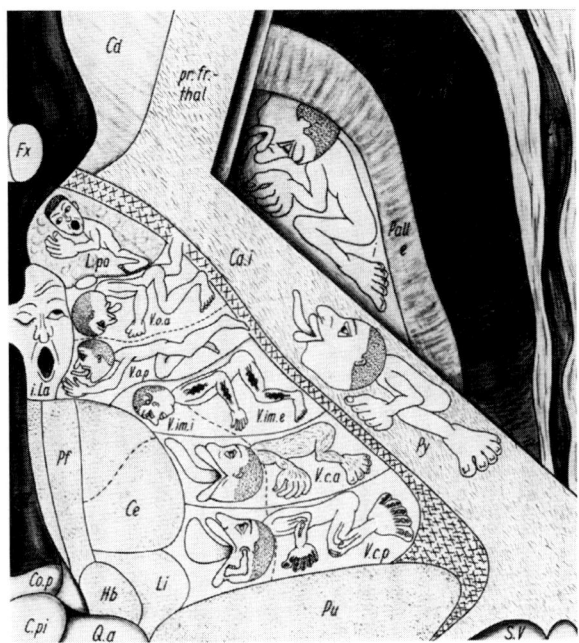

Figure 46. Diagram of the right human thalamus with the six functionally different ventral relay nuclei in a representative horizontal section (see also Fig. 45).

In addition to Fig. 45, this figure shows the "sprinter homunculus" of the fast muscle action induced by cerebellar afferents to the nucleus ventro-oralis posterior **(V.o.p.)**. The homunculus of slow and lasting muscle action by pallidum locomotor afferents is represented in the nucleus ventro-oralis anterior **(V.o.a.)**. The homunculus of turning to the contralateral side, raising of the contralateral arm, and vocalization is shown in the pole of the nucleus lateropolaris **(L.po)**. Furthermore, the sleepy and awake face expressions of the homunculi symbolize the sleep-waking regulation by the intralaminar nuclei **(i.La)**. The homunculus of the inner segment of the thalamus is in connection with the homunculus of the lasting muscle action in V.o.a. Finally, the homunculus in the internal capsule **(Ca.i)** indicates voluntary motor action of pyramidal fibers.

Modified from: Hassler R. Architectonic organization of the thalamic nuclei. In: Schaltenbrand G, Walker AE eds. *Stereotaxy of the Human Brain.* Stuttgart, New York: Thieme 1982: 140-180 (Fig. 9-6).

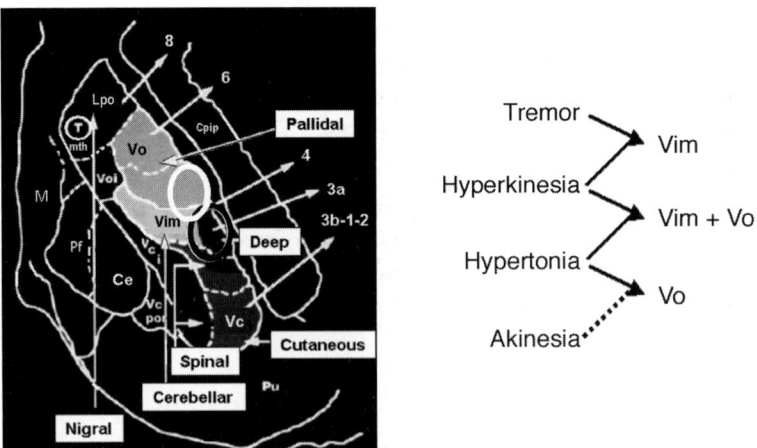

Figure 47. Semischematic illustration of the functional organization of the ventral motor nuclei of the human thalamus and the respective input-output relations in a horizontal section (left), and thalamic targets for different kinds of movement disorders, as proposed by Ohye [2000 – right].

The punctuated line (right) indicates that improvement of akinesia after Vo thalamotomy cannot be guaranteed. The anterior white circle denotes the optimal target area for the relief of rigidity (or hypertonic disorders) and the blue posterior circle that for tremor (or hyperkinetic movement).

Modified from: Ohye C. Use of selective thalamotomy for various kinds of movement disorder, based on basic studies. *Stereotact Funct Neurosurg* 2000; 75: 54-65.

ventralis posterior (this area was located between 5 and 10 mm anterior to the plane of the posterior commissure, between 7-8 mm above and 1-2 mm below the intercommissural line, and between 10-16 mm lateral to the midline). Electrical stimulation of these neurons usually evoked an "electrical sensation". Stereotaxic lesions have also been performed for the relief of dyskinesia. A transient disuse or apraxia of the formerly shaking extremity has been described. Speech disturbances such as impairment of repetitive speech with prolonged reaction time, aphasia, anomic errors, usually misnaming or perseverations have been noted after thalamotomy for PD, especially after left thalamic lesions.

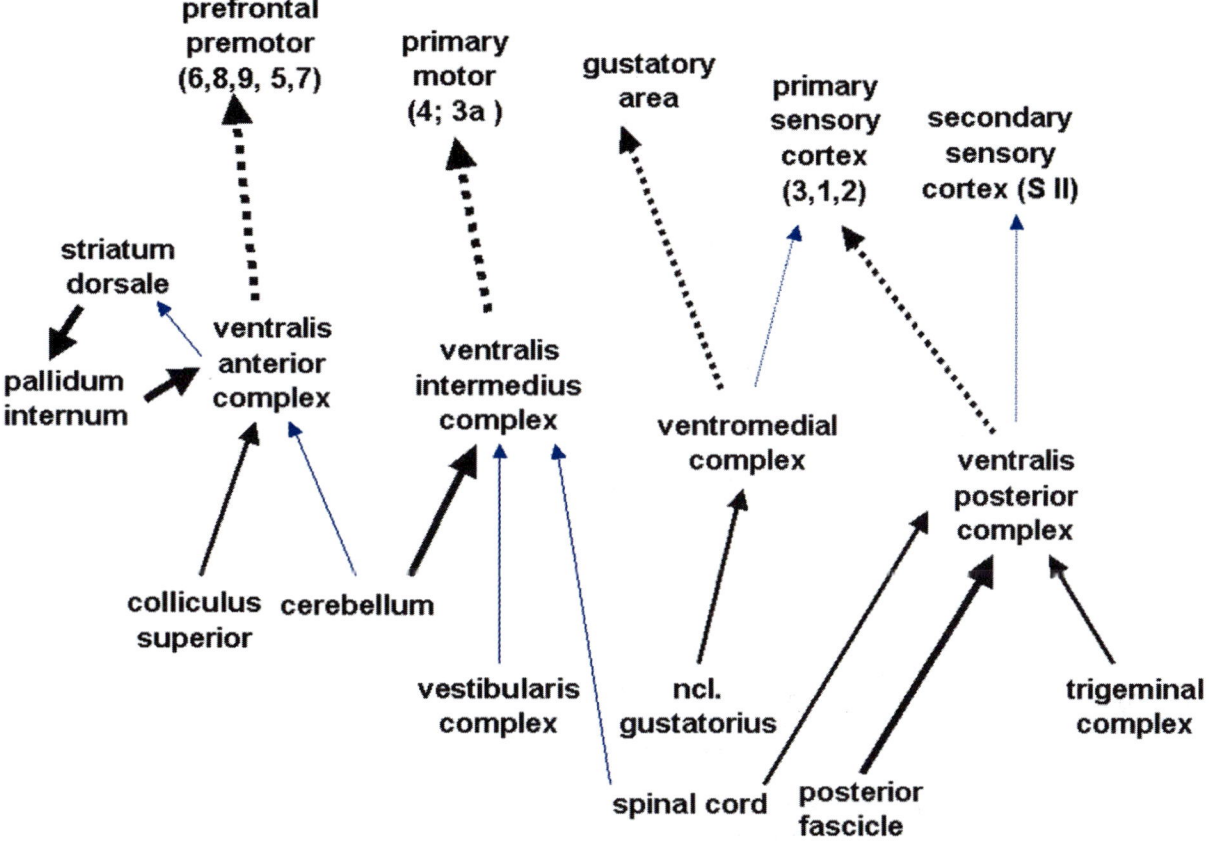

Figure 48. Ventral nuclear complexes of the thalamus with main afferents and efferents. Neglected are reciprocal corticothalamic connections.
Modified from: Künzle H. Aufbau und Verbindungen des Zwischenhirns. In: Drenckhahn D, Zenker W eds. Benninghoff Anatomie. Volume 2, 15th. revised edition. München, Wien, Baltimore: Urban & Schwarzenberg 1994: 544-571 (Fig. 16.16-18).

The Pulvinar

Anatomy and Fiber Connections

The pulvinar extends from the bottom of the trigonum of the lateral ventricle rostrally almost to the middle of the central nuclei and fronto-dorsally to the intermediate dorsal nuclei (Fig. 41). On its dorsal, medial and ventral surface, it is covered by a zonal lamina of fibers [Hassler, 1982]. In humans, the pulvinar can be roughly divided into five larger complexes of nuclei, namely the nucleus pulvinaris superficialis, supranucleus pulvinaris lateralis, supranucleus pulvinaris medialis, supranucleus pulvinaris ventralis (composed of the nuclei pulvinaris intergeniculatus and suprabrachialis), and supranucleus pulvinaris oralis [Vogt, 1909; Chow et al., 1950].

The pulvinar is considered to be a subcortical coordinating apparatus for high level gnostic and praxic functions. The largest influx to the pulvinar is the stalk of the lateral geniculate body. Efferent fibers of the pulvinar go to both subcortical and cortical, mainly iscortical, structures. The nucleus pulvinaris superficialis might be considered a lower integration nucleus of the auditory system. The supranucleus pulvinaris medialis has widespread connections with cingulate, posterior parietal, and prefrontal cortical areas. The medioposterior extension of the dorsomedial nucleus in the nucleus pulvinaris medialis projects into to the zone between the premotor and prefrontal cortex, that is, BA 8. It can be assumed that visual and auditory afferents from the medial pulvinar complex have direct access to the prefrontal and premotor cortex through these connections. The supranucleus pulvinaris lateralis has widespread connections with visual cortical association areas. The supranucleus pulvinaris intergeniculatus probably projects to BA 18 (these optic fiber connections are more direct than those to the lateral and medial pulvinar nuclei). The supranucleus pulvinaris oralis, finally, has connections with somatosensory cortical association areas [Hassler, 1982].

Effects of Stimulation and Ablation

The electrogram of the pulvinar is characterized by a regular 8-10/s rhythm and spontaneous spindling of 12-16/s, similar to the alpha rhythm of the occipital cortex and the nucleus lateralis posterior. Electrical stimulation of the pulvinar may enhance (or induce) the cortical occipital alpha rhythm and visual evoked potentials [Crighel and Kreindler, 1974]. Pulvinar lesions have been shown to relieve intractable chronic pain without changing the perception of acute pain [Waltz et al., 1966; Yoshii et al., 1970]. Furthermore, pulvinar lesioning and stimulation has been shown to induce disconjugate eye movements, predominantly of the contralateral eye [Ungerleider and Christensen, 1977]. Few investigators have reported phosphenes and hallucinations with pulvinar stimulation [Sano et al., 1970b]. Ojeman [1974] found that pulvinar stimulation, particularly in the posterosuperior part, modified object naming.

The Periaqueductal Gray Matter

Anatomy and Fiber Connections

The periaqueductal gray matter (PAG, PGM, substantia grisea centralis; zentrales Höhlen-Grau) comprises the central gray matter surrounding the cerebral aqueduct in the mesencephalon. The PAG may be divided into a medial (surrounding the canal and situated posterior to the dorsal raphe nucleus), dorsal and lateral division. The latter may be further subdivided into a dorsal and ventral part. The ventral lateral and, to a lesser extent, also the lateral dorsal division of the PAG comprise glutamatergic neurons. Inhibitory GABA neurons are most prominent in the dorsal and ventral parts of the lateral division, but can be found throughout the PAG. Inhibitory glycine neurons are mostly found in the dorsal part of the lateral division. Substance P has been found to cause enkephalin release from the PAG. Other neuropeptides include vasoactive intestinal peptide (VIP), cholecystokinin, and somatostatin.

The heaviest cortical input to the PAG arises from the mediofrontal cortex. Moderate to weak projections come from the insula, lateral prefrontal, and premotor cortex as well as the superior and middle temporal cortex. Subcortical moderate to weak projections reach the PAG from the central and medial amygdala, nucleus of the stria terminalis, septum, nucleus accumbens, lateral preoptic region, lateral and posterior hypothalamus, globus pallidus, pretectal area, deep layers of the superior colliculus, the pericentral inferior colliculus, mesencephalic trigeminal nucleus, locus coeruleus, substantia nigra pars compacta, dorsal and ventral raphe, vestibular nuclei, spinal trigeminal nucleus, solitary tract nucleus, and nucleus gracilis.

In the last decades, the PAG has received much attention with respect to pain treatment. Fig. 49 depicts a scheme of pain pathways, as proposed by Sugita and Kobayashi [1982]. It appears that there is a much stronger projection from pain related fibers to the PAG than to the thalamus (despite the fact that the so-called spinothalamic pathway is much better known than the spinoperiaqueductal gray pathway). The radiations from the PAG involved in pain inhibition generally do not reach the pain receptors of the spinal cord in a direct fashion. At the level of the facial nuclei, two large nuclei associated with inhibition of motor (muscle) contraction are considered to be the main relay structures for the input of the PAG on pain signals in the cord. These two nuclei, known as the nuclei raphe magnus (NRM) and the nuclei raphe pallidus (NRP), send inhibitory fibers that descend through the entire length of the cord. These fibers appear to function through serotonin and are not arranged topographically. Most of the PAG sends fibers to the NRM, which is located more toward the center of the brainstem, and to an area of the medulla known as the medullary reticular formation. The lateral PAG sends descending fibers to the NRP, which displays some level of somatotopy or organization in fiber connection. Anti-pain fibers join not only the NRM and reticular formation, but also project to the tegmentum of the lateral pons and the paralemniscal cell group. The very lowest part of the PAG projects to the lowest part of the medulla oblongata to the nucleus retroambiguus, which connects to motor neurons in the pharynx, palate, larynx, ribs and abdomen. Afferent fibers to the dorsolateral PAG, important for the perception of pain, arise in the cingulate gyrus and prefrontal cortical areas. Moreover, the PAG also has reciprocal projections to the reticular nucleus, the midline and intralaminar thalamic nuclei, and the hypothalamus.

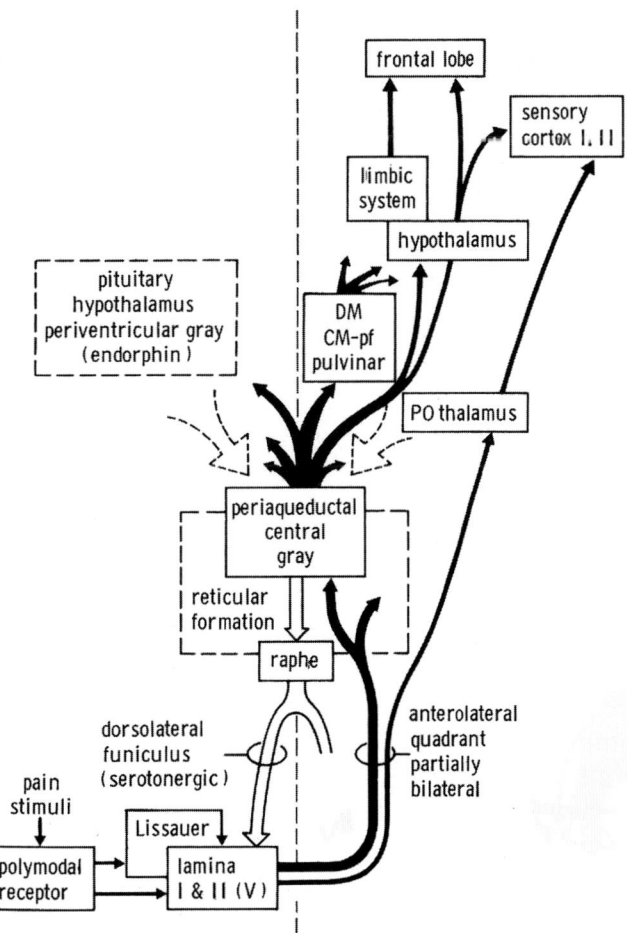

Figure 49. Pain pathway (solid arrows) and pain inhibition systems (open arrows).
From: Sugita K, Kobayashi S. General considerations of pain. In: Schaltenbrand G, Walker AE eds. *Stereotaxy of the Human Brain*. Stuttgart, New York: Thieme 1982: 462-468 (Fig. 26-1).

Effects of Stimulation and Ablation

Electrical stimulation of the PAG has been shown to produce potent analgesic effects in animals [Reynolds, 1969; Mayer et al., 1971; Liebeskind et al., 1973; Goodman and Holcombe, 1975] and humans [Richardson and Akil, 1977a, b; Hosobuchi, 1977]; a finding that has led to the stereotactic treatment of pain by electrical stimulation of the PAG. There is evidence that opiate diminution of pain may be, at least in part, dependent on activation of the PAG. In this respect, it is pertinent to note that stimulation of the PAG may only stop pain, that is opiate responsive.

Furthermore, PAG stimulation has also been shown to play an important role in the "emotional motor" system, which regulates behaviors that are heavily influenced by emotions and important for the survival of the individual or the species [De Oca et al., 1998; Mouton, 1999; Amorapanth et al., 1999; Depaulis and Bandler, 1991]. Some examples of these behaviors elicited by electrical stimulation are aggressive behavior, sexual behavior, freezing, micturation, cardiovascular control, breathing, tone in the gut and bladder, reaction to temperature, vocalization, as well as feelings of strong fear. Aggressive behavior and vocalization are probably mediated by the involvement of NRM/NRP/reticular/tegmentum/paralemniscal areas. Aggressive head movements have been found to be mediated by PAG projections to the ventral part of the cervical cord, namely the funiculus. Vocalization is influenced by stimulation of projecting fibers to the retroambiguus. The input of the PAG vocalization eliciting regions is dominated by limbic, motivation controlling afferents (see above), but also comes from sensory, motor, arousal controlling, and cognitive brain areas [Dujardin and Jurgens, 2005].

Patients undergoing PAG stimulation for the treatment of "central pain" may show hyperresponsiveness in blood pressure increase with stress and, very commonly, an overreaction to room temperature (making extremes of hot or cold very uncomfortable and causing them a sense of overheating or chilling with minor changes in temperature). Moreover, these patients frequently report feelings of not breathing fully, fear, fright, anxiety, foreboding, and, quite commonly, a feeling of "overfulness" in the gut and severe bladder cramps (intestinal activity has been shown to be diminished with morphine injection into the PAG). Some patients also report disorders in the pharynx and larynx, mainly changes in swallowing (PAG connections to the motor neurons of the pharynx travel via the nucleus retroambiguus). The fact that these symptoms do not occur universally in all patients suggests a certain point specificity within the PAG.

The Reticular Formation

Anatomy and Fiber Connections

The reticular formation comprises a region extending from the pons and medulla oblongata through the mesencephalon. It is characterized by a diversity of neurons of various sizes and shapes that are arranged in different aggregations and enmeshed in a complicated fiber network. Although this netlike collection of cells may not be easily divisible into separate nuclei on morphological grounds, it may be dissected into separate hodological and biochemical groups. Well-known examples are, for example, the small group of noradrenergic cells in the locus coeruleus or the small group of serotonergic cells in the raphe nuclei. These cells with their widespread ascending projections to cerebral cortical areas play an important role in activation and the sleep waking cycle. The reticular formation with its ascending projections (the ascending reticular activation system, ARAS) is continuous with the diffuse cell groups of the zona incerta, the reticular thalamic nucleus, and possibly the intralaminar thalamic nuclei. The descending pathways of the reticular formation are continuous with the intermediate zone (Rexed's layer V-VIII) located between the dorsal and ventral horns throughout the entire length of the spinal cord.

The simplest division of the reticular formation is into three zones, that is, (1) a small midline region made up primarily of the raphe nuclei, (2) a large medial tegmental field, and (3) a large lateral tegmental field. The raphe nuclei and the medial tegmental field are considered effector regions due to the long descending and ascending fibers that primarily originate here. The lateral tegmental field is often considered a sensory or receptive field because it receives many secondary sensory projections. It has also many projections to the ipsilateral cranial motor nuclei [Holstege *et al.*, 1977] and, thus, must be considered a motor region as well [Van der Kooy, 1987].

The role of the reticular formation in epilepsy has been revisited by Fromm *et al.* [1977]. The interested reader is referred to this book.

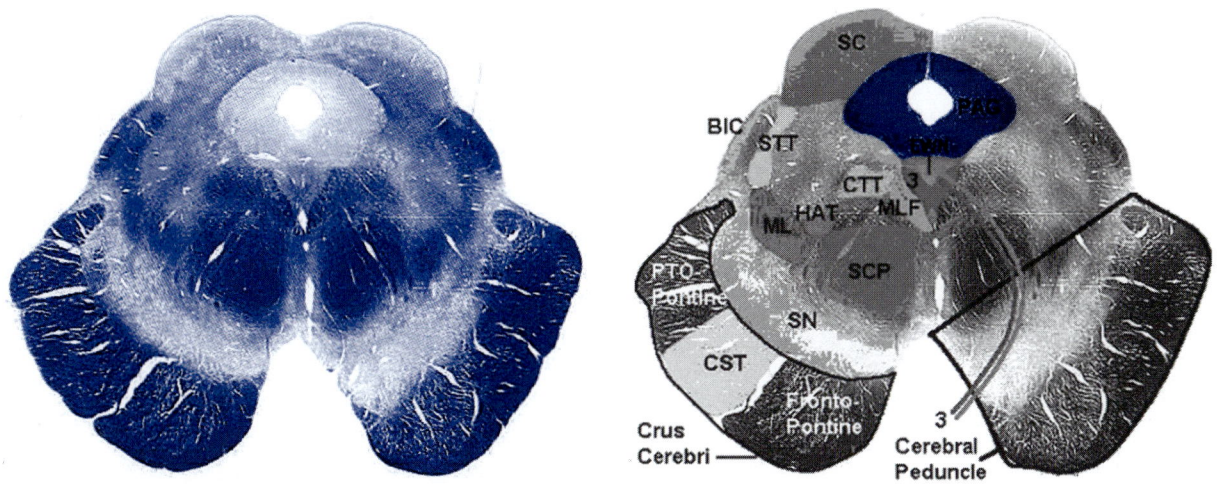

Figure 50. Transverse section of midbrain.

SC, superior colliculus; **BIC**, Brachium of the Inferior colliculus; **SN**, substantia nigra; **SCP**, superior cerebellar peduncles; **CTT**, central tegmental tract; **HAT**, hypothalamo-autonomic tract; **ML**, medial lemniscus; **STT**, spinothalamic tract; **PAG**, periaqueductal gray; **3**, oculomotor nucleus; **EWN**, Edinger-Westphal nucleus of 3; **MLF**, medial longitudinal fasciculus.

Taken from: http://braininfo.rprc.washington.edu/Scripts/indexothersite.aspx?ID=501&type=h&term=central_gray_substance_of_midbrain&thterm=PAG&city=Chicago&country=USA&institue=Loyola%20University&namesite=Medical%20Neuroscience&URL=http://www.meddean.luc.edu/lumen/meded/Neuro/frames/nIBSsL/nl18fr.htm.

Case studies

Case 1

Patient History

This 37 year-old man with a history of drug abuse had intractable left temporal lobe epilepsy (TLE) with frequent psychomotor seizures (~ 15 per month) since childhood. His seizures were characterized by cephalic and occasional auditory auras. Pregnancy and birth were uneventful and subsequent neonatal and childhood development was normal. He had no family history of epilepsy. Seizure onset was at age 4 with status epilepticus, which was reportedly associated with right dominant clonic activity. CT-scan at age 37 showed an unclear, small, calcified lesion in the left posterior parahippocampal gyrus.

SEEG Exploration

Ten auras and seven complex partial seizures were recorded during chronic SEEG with eight depth electrodes (Fig. 51). The spontaneous seizures originated in the posterior parts of the left superior temporal gyrus (T1) and were spreading to the left posterior cingulate gyrus, the left amygdaloid nucleus, the left anterior cingulate gyrus, and finally to the contralateral temporal lobe.

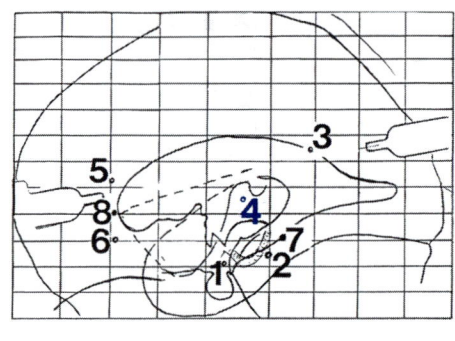

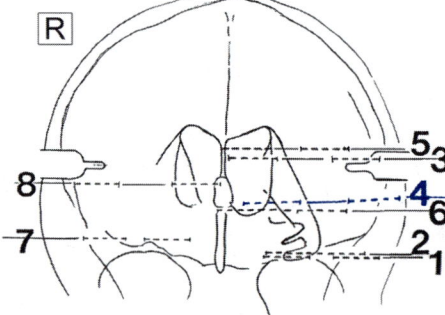

Figure 51. Location of depth electrodes in the proportional Talairach system.
The deepest contacts of electrode 4 (contacts 1-2) were in the left subthalamic area, presumably in or next to the Forel H field.

Surgery

A palliative left selective AHE was performed at age 38. Histological examination of the resected specimen was not performed.

Outcome

The initial postsurgical outcome was moderate (Engel class III). Later, the situation worsened to outcome class IV despite treatment with various AEDs. At age 41, the patient was re-evaluated at the Montreal Neurological Institute, Canada. At this time, the seizures showed bilateral temporal onset and, thus, no surgery was recommended. At age 43, the patient was again reevaluated with noninvasive long-term video-/EEG-monitoring at our institution, the University Hospital Zurich. We recorded 21 complex partial seizures with presumable right hemispheric onset and surgery was still not recommended. The patient remained dependent on social insurance.

Spontaneous Seizure Activity

Figures 52 and 53 depict the EEG recordings of a spontaneous habitual psychomotor seizure. The seizure began with a high voltage spike wave complex (inlay A) in the left hippocampus [2/2-3] with fast projection to the posterior cingulate gyrus [3/2-3], and, with a latency of

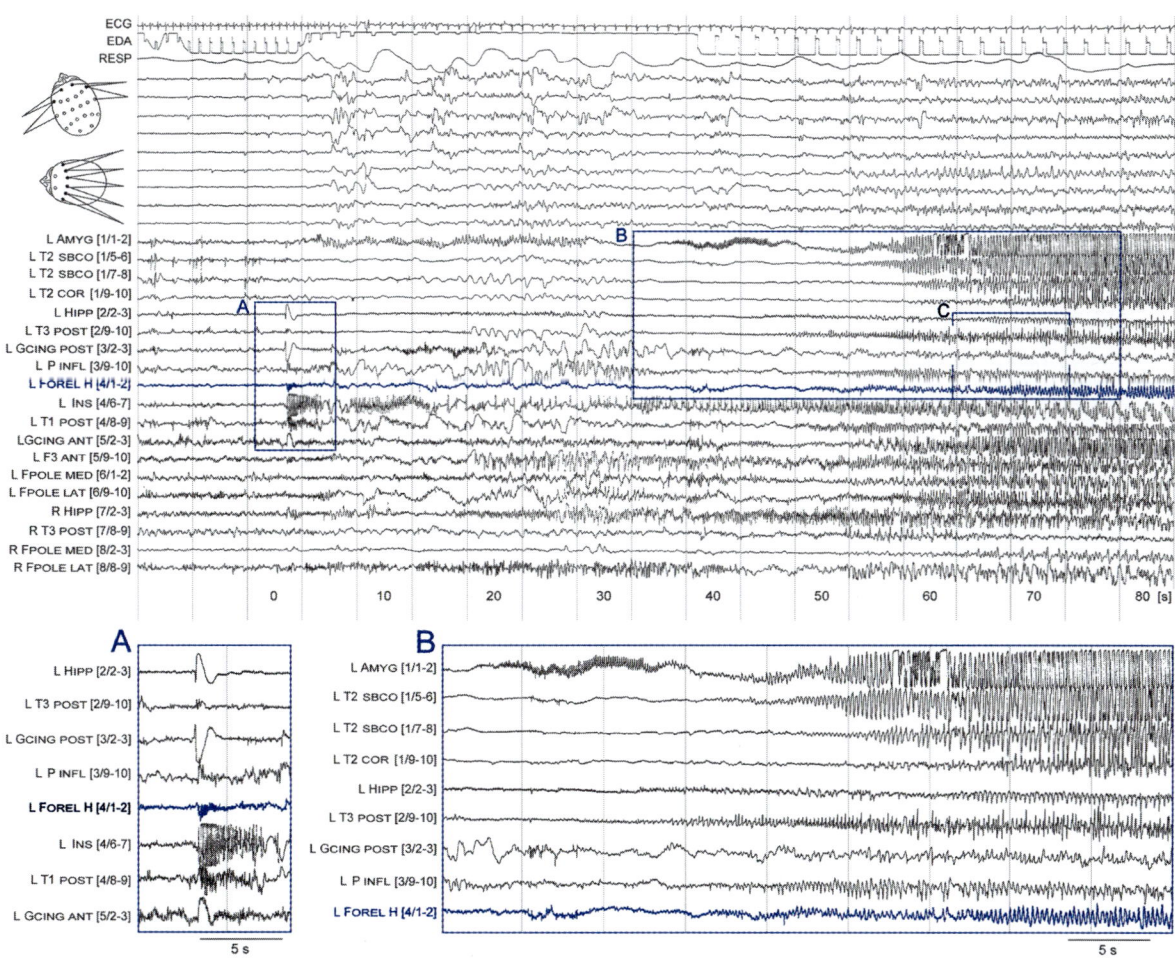

Figure 52. Combined scalp (upper traces) and intracerebral (lower traces) EEG recording of a spontaneous habitual psychomotor seizure.

Inlay A depicts the initial complex of the seizure in greater detail. Inlay B shows the early 10 Hz activity ([1/1-2], upper left corner) of the amygdala and the early propagation of the seizure to the ipsilateral hippocampus and the temporal neocortex. Inlay C and the continuation of the seizure are shown in Fig. 53. Note the marked bradycardia of about 36/s within 60 seconds from seizure onset. The electrode sites recorded from are indicated left to the traces by anatomical designations (based on the Talairach atlas) and numbers (electrode/contacts, cf. Fig. 51).
ECG, electrocardiogram; **EDA**, electrodermal activity, **RESP**, respiration; **AMYG**, amygdala; **T2**, middle temporal gyrus; **HIPP**, hippocampus; **T3**, inferior temporal gyrus; **GCING**, cingulate gyrus; **PINFL**, parietal inferior lobule; **FOREL H**, subthalamic area; **INS**, Insula; **T1**, superior temporal gyrus; **F3**, inferior frontal gyrus; **FPOLE**, frontal pole; **SBCO**, subcortical; **COR**, cortical; **POST**, posterior; **ANT**, anterior; **MED**, medial; **LAT**, lateral; **R**, right; **L**, left.

about 170 ms, propagation to the anterior cingulate gyrus [5/2-3]. This discharge was immediately followed by a high frequency discharge in the sylvian region, maximally recorded from the circuminsular cortex [4/6-7] and the posterior parts of the superior temporal gyrus [4/8-9]. Of note is the marked and immediate slowing of the heart rate within five seconds after seizure onset (see traces on top of the figures). Seizure activity was then spreading to the left amygdala [1/1-2], where a 10 Hz activity dominated for about 10 seconds (left upper corner of inlay B). In the following, the seizure evolved into a rhythmic 4 Hz theta activity, which was spreading to the ipsilateral hippocampus [2/2-3], the temporal neocortex [1/5-6, 1/7-8, 1/9-10, 2/9-10, and 3/9-10] and to the contralateral hippocampus [7/2-3]. Simultaneously with the spreading to neocortical temporal structures, the left subthalamic area [4/1-2] became also involved, showing rhythmic 4 Hz theta activity that was in almost perfect synchrony with the rhythmic activity recorded from left temporal neocortical structures (inlay C). As much as can be said by sole visual inspection, the subthalamic activity was also in synchrony with the ipsilateral hippocampus, though to a lesser extent. Furthermore, the subthalamic rhythmic activity rather led than followed the hippocampal activity.

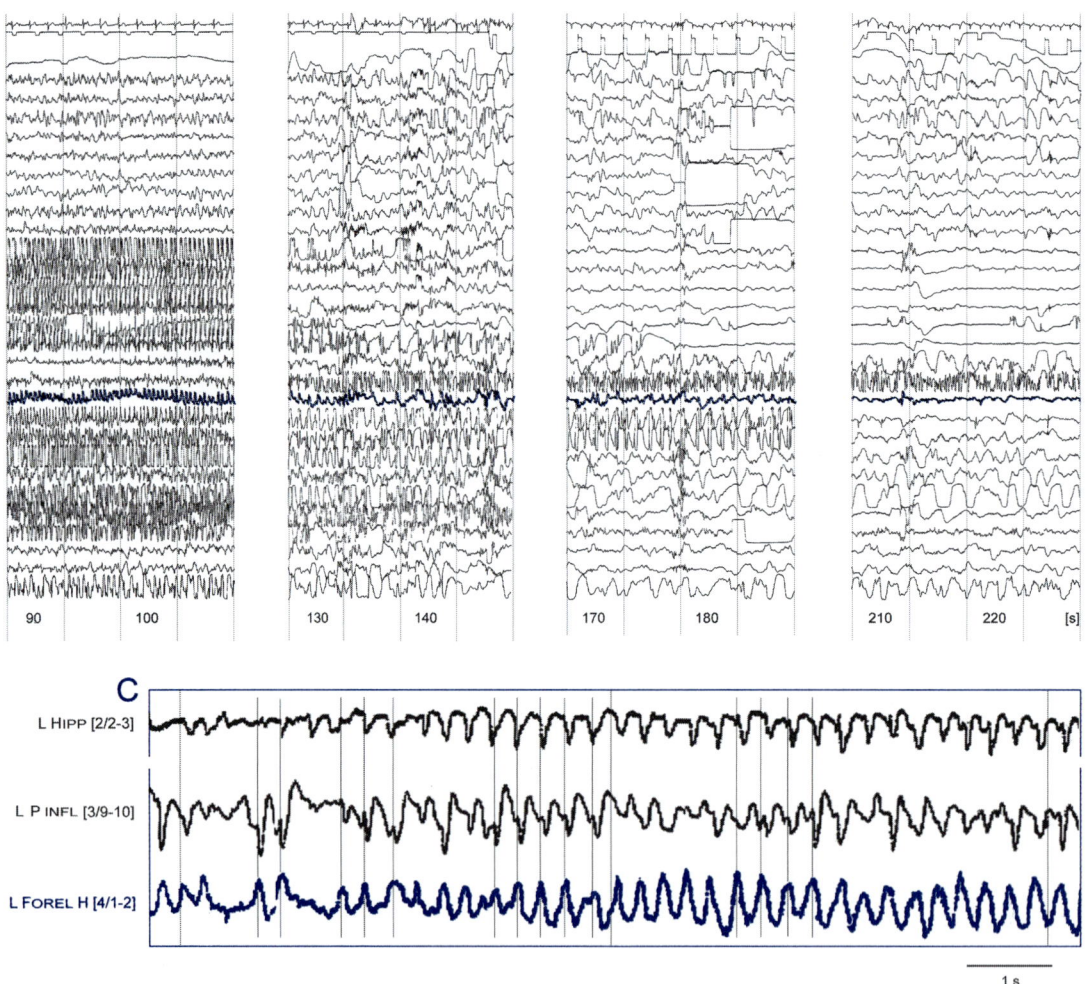

Figure 53. Continuation of the seizure shown in Fig. 52.

Each segment of 20 seconds duration is interrupted by 20 seconds that are not shown. Note the normalization of the heart rate to 72/s at the end of the seizure. Inlay C shows the ictal 3.5 Hz activity of the subthalamic area [4/1-2, lower trace], the parietal inferior lobule [3/9-10, middle trace] and the left hippocampus [2/2-3, upper trace] during seconds 60 to 70 of the seizure in greater detail. Note the synchrony between the subthalamic rhythm (lower trace) and the tiny neocortical spikes (middle trace), as pointed out by the thin gray lines, whereas the synchrony between the subthalamic rhythm and the positive hippocampal deflections (upper trace) appears less impressive. Electrode sites were identical to those given in Fig. 52.

Electrically Induced Seizure Activity

The electrical stimulation of the left amygdala [1/1-2] induced a seizure with cluster like high voltage spike bursts in the left amygdala of a duration of about 70 seconds (Figs. 54 and 55). These amygdalar spike bursts were spreading to the ipsilateral hippocampal formation [2/2-3] and posterior cingulate gyrus [3/2-3], but not to the ipsilateral sylvian region [4/6-7, 4/8-9 and 3/9-10] or subthalamic area [4/1-2]. The periamygdaloid cortex [1/5-6] and subcortical or cortical temporal structures lateral to the amygdala [1/7-8 and 1/9-10] showed irregular high voltage delta-/subdelta activity that was outlasting the amygdalar seizure activity. No bradycardia was observed during this seizure (the left circuminsular cortex was not involved). Of note is the left mydriasis that was occurring at about 30 seconds after the onset of the seizure.

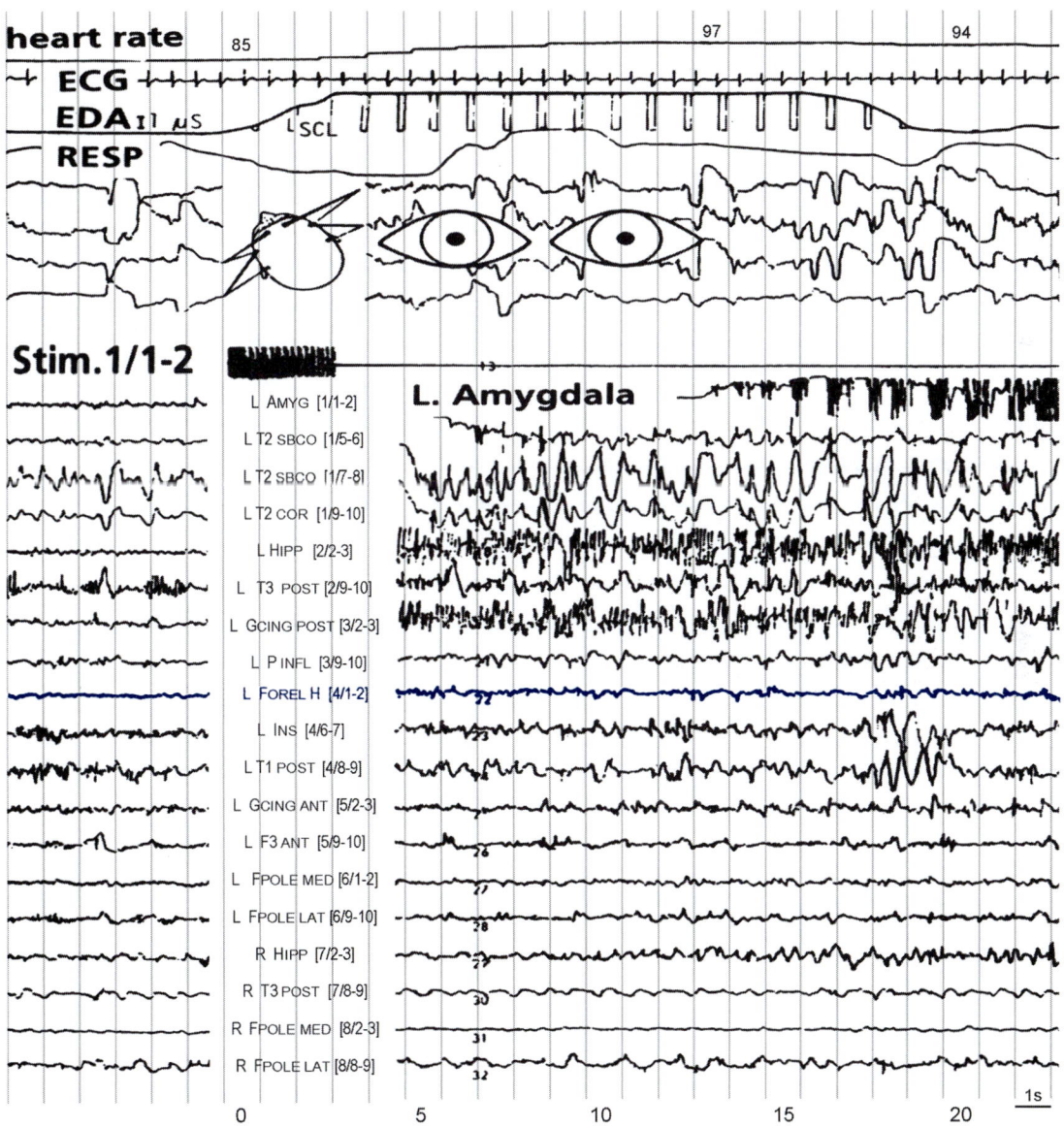

Figure 54. Electrically induced seizure following train stimulation (50 Hz, 4 V, 0.7 ms pulse width) of the left amygdala [1/1-2].

The continuation of the seizure is shown in Fig. 55. The electrode sites recorded from are indicated left to the traces by anatomical designations (based on the Talairach atlas) and numbers (electrode/contacts, cf. Fig. 1).
ECG, electrocardiogram; **EDA**, electrodermal activity; **RESP**, respiration; **AMYG**, amygdala; **T2**, middle temporal gyrus; **HIPP**, hippocampus; **T3**, inferior temporal gyrus; **GCING**, cingulate gyrus; **PINFL**, parietal inferior lobule; **FOREL H**, subthalamic area; **INS**, Insula; **T1**, superior temporal gyrus; **F3**, inferior frontal gyrus; **FPOLE**, frontal pole; **SBCO**, subcortical; **COR**, cortical; **POST**, posterior; **ANT**, anterior; **MED**, medial; **LAT**, lateral; **R**, right; **L**, left.

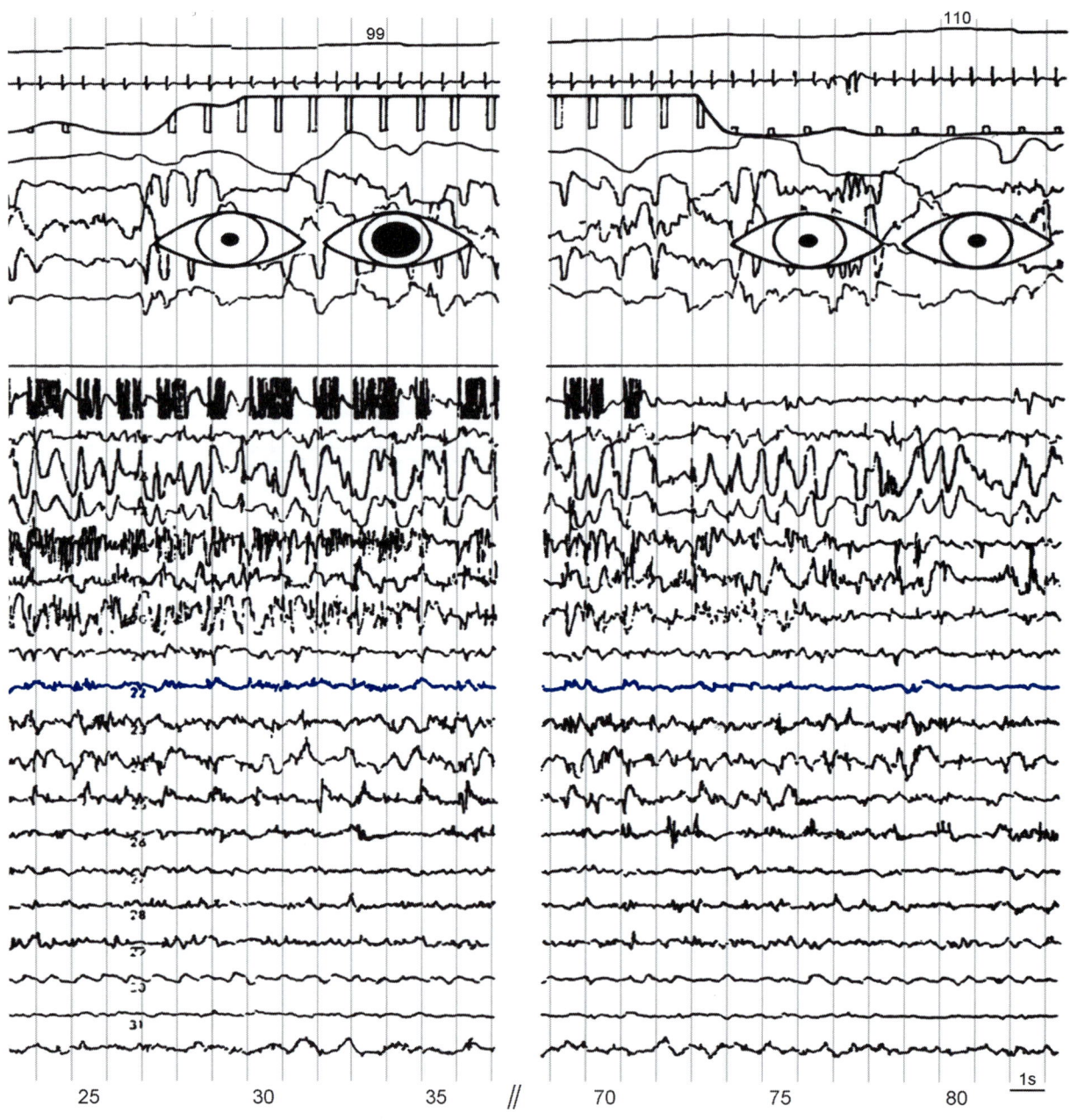

Figure 55. Continuation of the seizure shown in Fig. 54.

The segments of about 12 seconds duration are interrupted by 33 seconds that are not depicted. Note the left mydriasis, occurring about 30 seconds after onset of the seizure. Electrode sites were identical to Fig. 54.

Modified from Stodieck SRG, Wieser HG. Autonomic phenomena in temporal lobe epilepsy. *J Autonom Nerv Syst* 1986; 611 (Suppl.): 611-621 (Fig. 6).

Single Pulse Stimulation

A complex cerebral response could be recorded from the left subthalamic area [4/1-2] with repetitive single pulse stimulation of the left amygdala [1/1-2] (Fig. 56). The response consisted of two negative-positive low amplitude short latency deflections, followed by two larger positive potentials with latencies of 35 ms (A) and 85 ms (B).

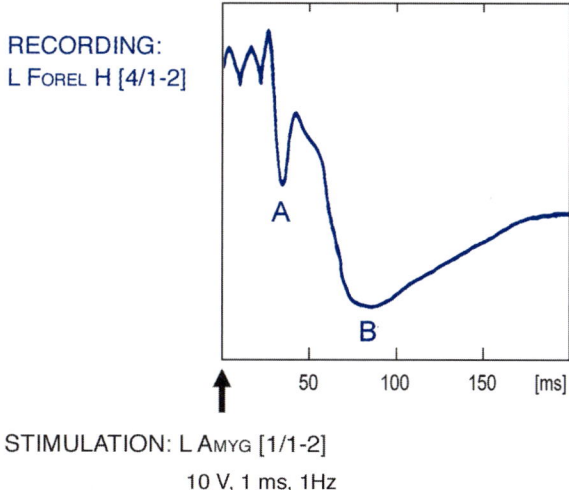

Figure 56. Averaged cerebral response recorded from the left subthalamic area [4/1-2] following repetitive single pulse stimulation of the left amygdala [1/1-2].
A and B denote positive deflections with latencies of 35 ms and 85 ms.
Modified from: Wieser HG. Selective amygdalohippocampectomy: Indications, investigative technique and results. In: Symon L, Brihaye J, Guidetti B, Loew F, Miller JD, Nornes H, Pàsztor E, Pertuiset B, Yasargil MG eds. *Advances and Technical Standards in Neurosurgery* 1986a; 13: 39-133 (Fig. 21), and from: Wieser HG. The phenomenology of limbic seizures. In: Wieser HG, Speckmann E-J, Engel J Jr eds. *The Epileptic Focus*. Current Problems in Epilepsy 3. London, Paris: John Libbey 1987 (Figs. 4 and 7).

The source generator of this complex response remains unclear. However, when taking into consideration the mode of seizure propagation in this patient (Figs. 52 and 53), this cerebral response most likely reflects volume-conducted activity originating in left temporal neocortical structures (with the positive deflections A and B reflecting the positive ends of the dipoles). Yet, the ictal activity recorded from the subthalamic area did not show inverse polarity to the tiny spikes that were imbedded in the rhythmic 3.5 Hz activity recorded from the temporal neocortex. The cerebral responses might as well have reflected "hard-wired" propagation within the limbic circuit (e.g. through fornix fibers), a possibility that cannot be ruled out with certainty. However, as much as can be said by sole visual inspection of a paper recorded EEG (Figs. 52 and 53, inlay C), the synchrony between the ictal activities recorded from the subthalamic area and from the hippocampus was not perfect (if at all, the subthalamic activity led rather than followed the hippocampal rhythmic ictal activity). Recordings from lateral temporal neocortical sites following amygdalar single pulse stimulation, which could have had clarified this issue by disclosure of an electrical near-field (i.e. phase reversal), have not been performed.

Summary

This case illustrates left subthalamic recordings during (1) a spontaneous seizure originating in the left temporal neocortex with fast propagation to the ipsilateral amygdala, the circuminsular cortex and the hippocampus, (2) an electrically induced seizure with unilateral pupillary dilation following train stimulation of the left amygdala remaining virtually restricted to ipsilateral mesial temporal structures, and (3) repetitive single pulse stimulation of the left amygdala.

While the subthalamic area clearly was involved during the spontaneous seizure, no such participation could be observed during the seizure that was electrically induced and accompanied by ictal anisocoria (the latter denoting a very rare clinical ictal sign) [Pant *et al.*, 1966]. This finding can be best attributed to the extensive involvement of temporal neocortical structures during spontaneous seizures. Whether the ictal and single pulse evoked activity recorded from this patient's subthalamic area reflected autochthonous subthalamic activity (e.g. originating from fornix fibers), or whether it simply echoed volume conducted activity originating from remote sites such as the temporal neocortex, remains unclear.

Case 2

Patient History

This 22 year-old woman with intractable MTLE had frequent psychomotor and occasional secondarily generalized seizures since age 10. Her delivery was complicated by perinatal asphyxia, but subsequent childhood development was normal. She had no family history of epilepsy. Her psychomotor seizures were characterized by fear, motor arrest, and complex oral and manual automatisms. At age 20, she made a suicidal attempt. Neurological examination demonstrated a right homonymous hemianopsia, but was otherwise normal. Her CT scan showed a left occipital porencephalic cyst (Fig. 57). Her interictal EEG showed bitemporal EEG abnormalities.

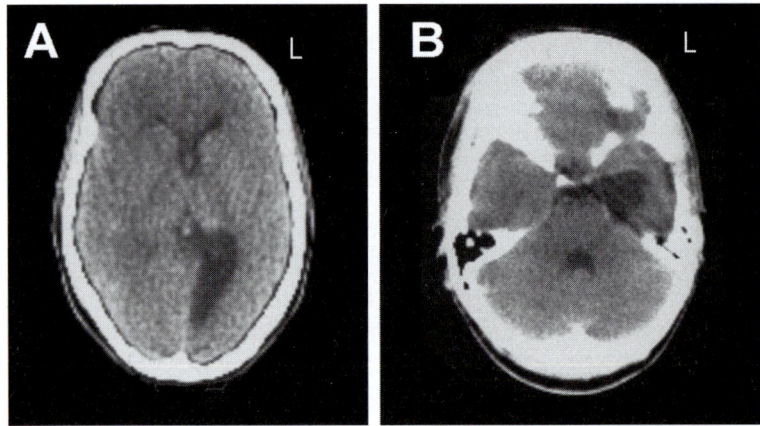

Figure 57. **A,** preoperative CT scan at age 22 showing a left occipital porencephalic cyst. **B,** postoperative CT scan after left selective AHE at age 23, showing the site of resection.

SEEG Exploration

Chronic SEEG was carried out with eight depth electrodes, with electrode 6 located in or next to the right Forel H field (Fig. 58). Two seizures were recorded during exploration, one occurring spontaneously and one electrically induced. The spontaneous psychomotor seizure clinically presented with her habitual signs and symptoms (the initial symptom was fear) and electrographically showed a simultaneous onset in the left amygdala and the left hippocampus, spreading to the posterior and anterior ipsilateral cingulate gyrus, the left lateral temporal neocortex, the right posterior and anterior cingulate gyrus, and finally affected all recording sites. The electrically induced seizure showed a right neocortical temporal onset.

Surgery

A left selective AHE was performed at age 23. The histology showed reactive gliosis.

Outcome

The initial outcome was Engel class II, and treatment with AEDs could be stopped at age 26. However, auras recurred at age 28 (Engel class IB), and due to the occurrence of an "amnestic episode" at age 39 antiepileptic treatment with carbamazepine was finally resumed (another "amnestic episode" occurred at age 40).

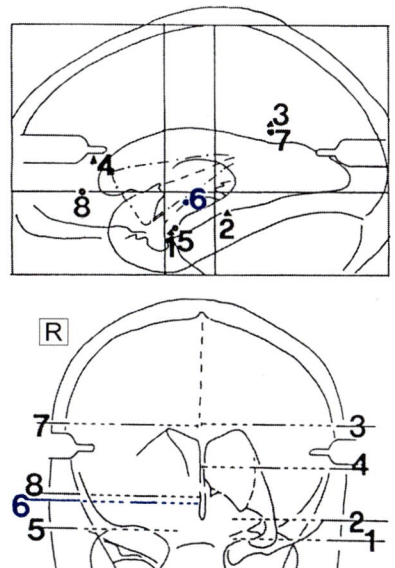

Figure 58. Location of depth electrodes in the proportional Talairach system.

The deepest contacts of electrode 6 (contacts 1-2) were in the right subthalamic area, presumably in or next to the Forel H field.

Spontaneous Interictal Activity

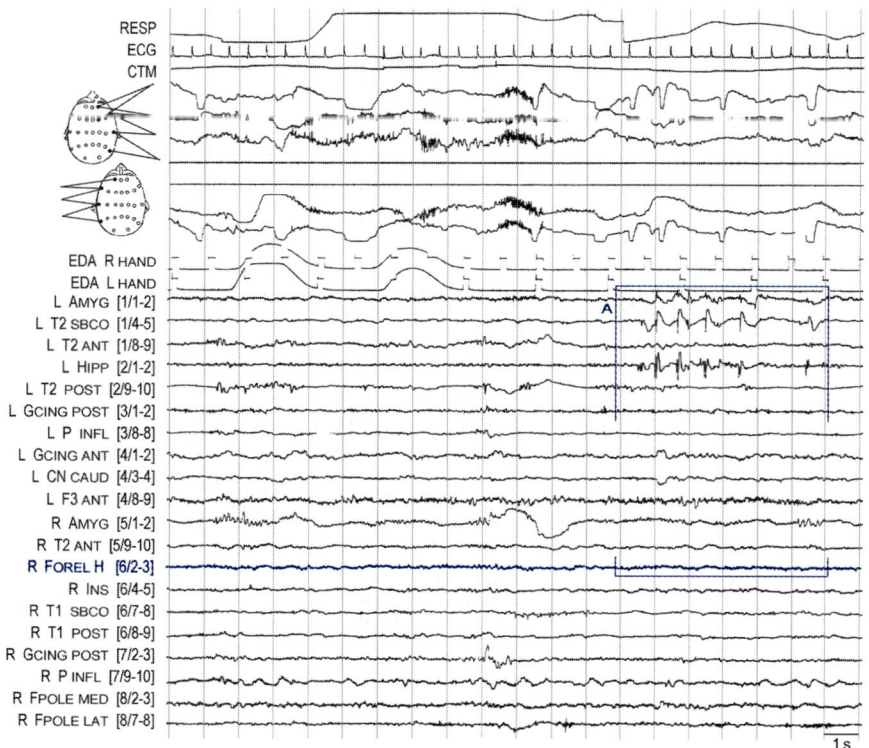

Figure 59. Spontaneous interictal left mesiobasal temporal spike train involving the amygdala and the hippocampus.

Detail A is shown in greater detail in Fig. 60. The electrode sites recorded from are indicated left to the traces by anatomical designations (based on the Talairach atlas) and numbers (electrode/contacts, cf. Fig. 58).
RESP, respiration; **ECG**, electrocardiogram; **CTM**, cardiotachymeter (heart rate frequency); **EDA**, electrodermal activity; **AMYG**, amygdala; **T2**, middle temporal gyrus; **HIPP**, hippocampus; **T3**, inferior temporal gyrus; **GCING**, cingulate gyrus; **P INFL**, parietal inferior lobule; **CN**, caudate nucleus; **F3**, inferior frontal gyrus; **FOREL H**, subthalamic area; **INS**, insular cortex; **T1**, superior temporal gyrus; **FPOLE**, frontal pole; **SBCO**, subcortical; **ANT**, anterior; **POST**, posterior; **MED**, medial; **LAT**, lateral; **R**, right; **L**, left.

Case studies

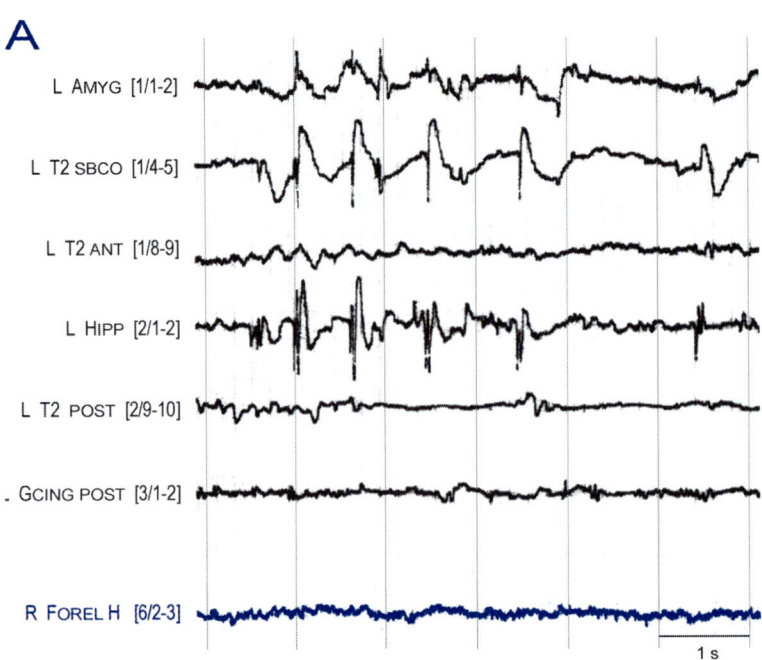

Figure 60. Detail A of Fig. 59, showing the spontaneous interictal left mesiobasal temporal spike train in greater detail.

The electrode sites recorded from are indicated left to the traces by anatomical designations (based on the Talairach atlas) and numbers (electrode/contacts, cf. Fig. 58).
AMYG, amygdala; **T2**, middle temporal gyrus; **HIPP**, hippocampus; **GCING**, cingulate gyrus; **FOREL H**, subthalamic area; **ANT**, anterior; **POST**, posterior; **R**, right; **L**, left.

Spontaneous Seizure Activity

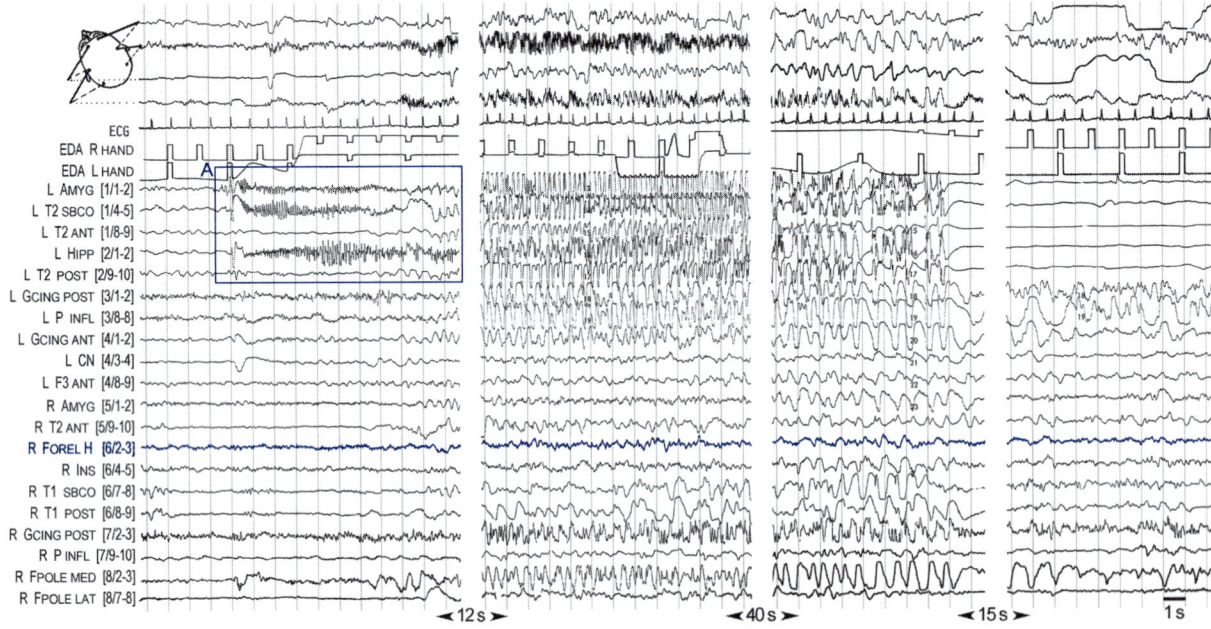

Figure 61. Spontaneous psychomotor seizure with onset in left mesiobasal temporal structures (inlay A is shown in greater detail in Fig. 62) and with propagation to the contralateral hemisphere, finally also affecting the Forel H field on the contralateral side.

Electrode sites were identical to those in Fig. 59.

Modified from: Wieser HG, Psychomotor seizures of hippocampal-amygdalar origin. In: Pedley TA, Meldrum BS eds. *Recent Advances in Epilepsy*, Number 3. Edinburgh London: Churchill Livingstone 1986b: 57-79 (Fig. 4.7).

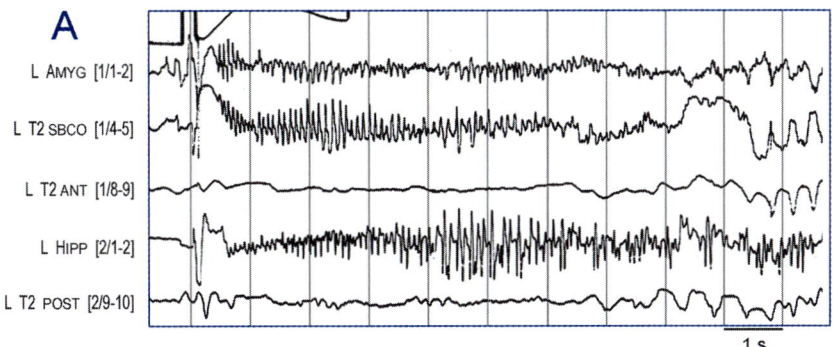

Figure 62. Detail of seizure onset of the spontaneous psychomotor seizure shown in Fig. 61.
AMYG, amygdala; **T2**, middle temporal gyrus; **HIPP**, hippocampus; **ANT**, anterior; **POST**, posterior; **SBCO**, subcortical; **R**, right; **L**, left.
Modified from: Wieser HG. Psychomotor seizures of hippocampal-amygdalar origin. In: Pedley TA, Meldrum BS eds. *Recent Advances in Epilepsy*, Number 3. Edinburgh London: Churchill Livingstone 1986b: 57-79 (Fig. 4.7).

Electrically Induced Afterdischarges

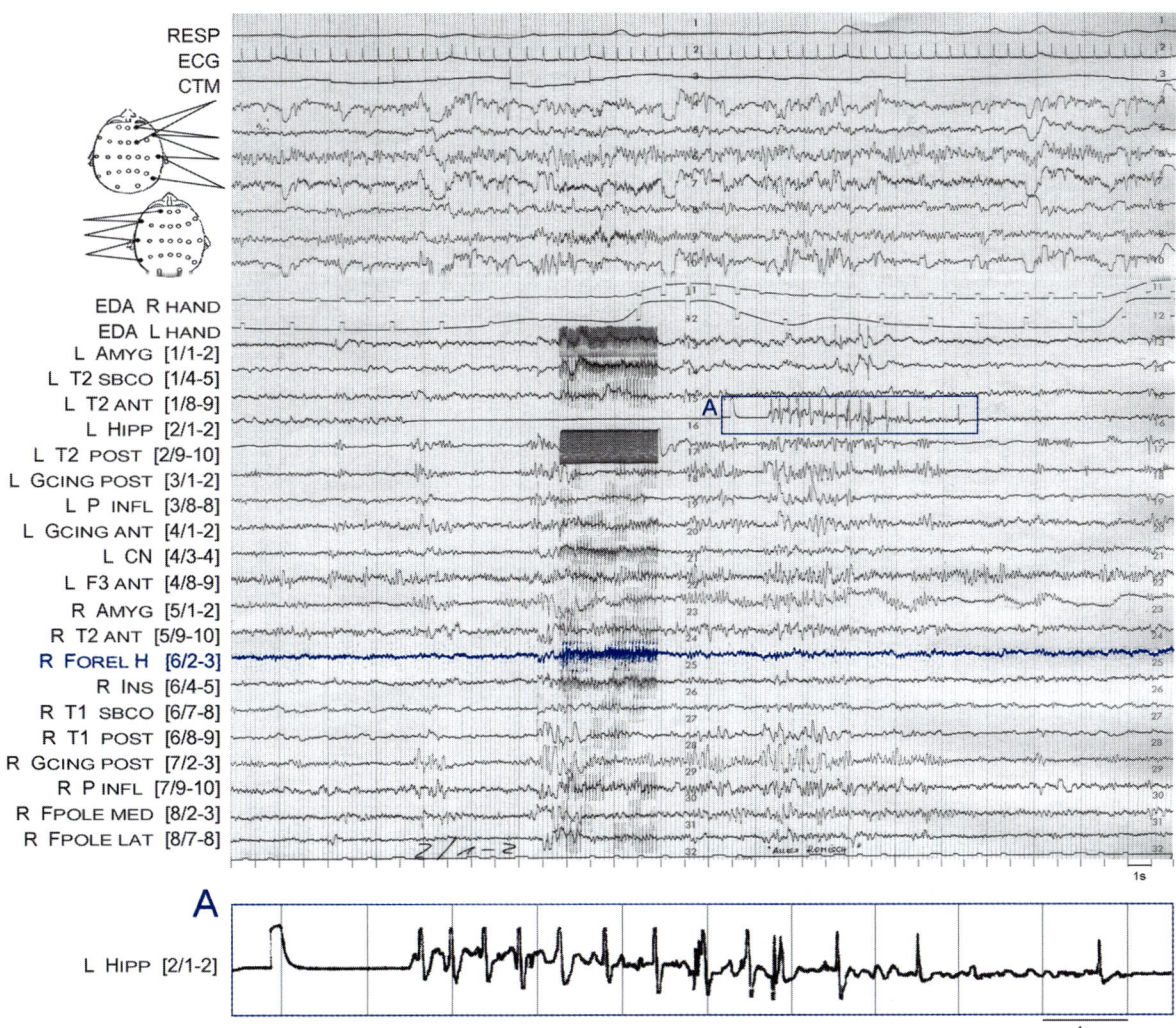

Figure 63. Electrically induced afterdischarge in the left hippocampus [2/1-2] following 50 Hz train stimulation (4 V, 1 ms) of the same site.
The afterdischarge is shown in greater detail in inlay A. Coinciding with the afterdischarge, the patient spontaneously remarked that "everything is funny". See Fig. 59 for electrode legend.

Case studies

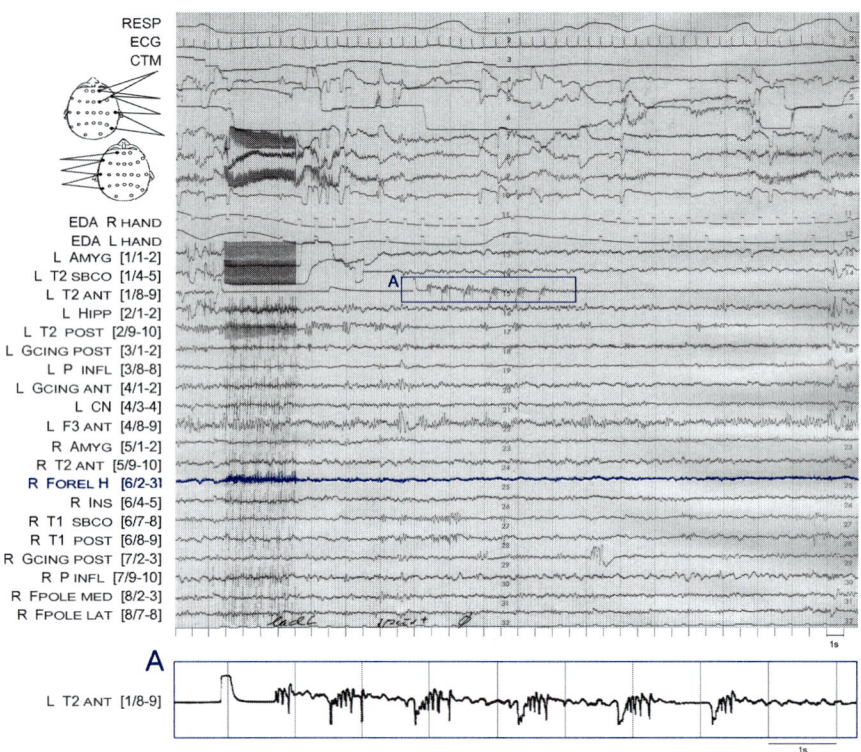

Figure 64. Electrically induced afterdischarge in the posterior parts of the left middle temporal gyrus [1/8-9] following 50 Hz train stimulation (4 V, 1 ms) of the same site.
The afterdischarge is shown in greater detail in inlay A. There were no signs and symptoms but laughing. See Fig. 59 for electrode legend.

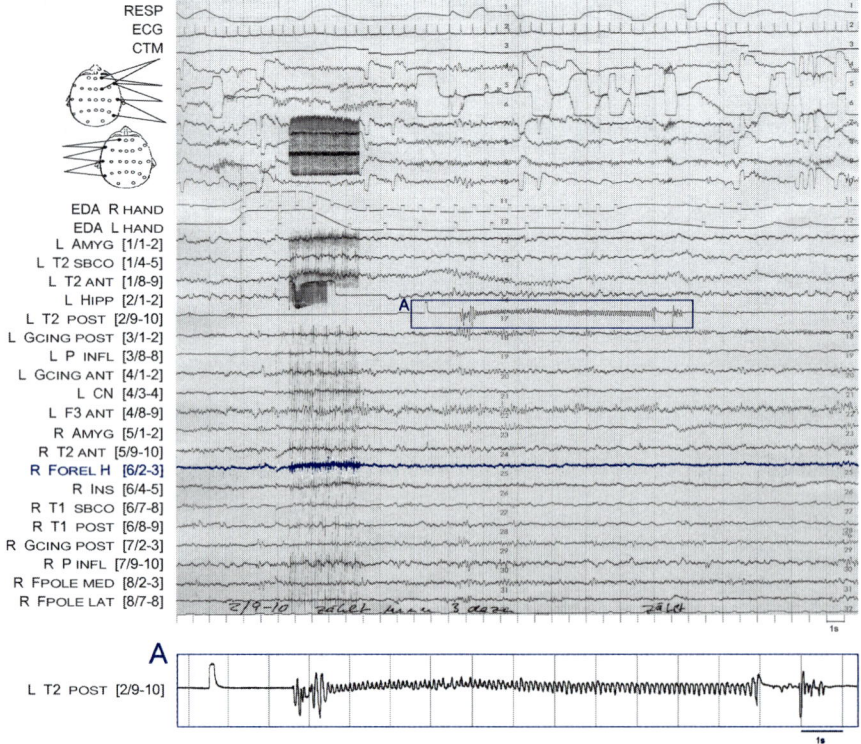

Figure 65. Electrically induced afterdischarge in the posterior parts of the left middle temporal gyrus [2/9-10] following 50 Hz train stimulation (4 V, 1 ms) of the same site.
The afterdischarge is shown in greater detail in inlay A. There were no signs and symptoms, and the patient was counting without hesitation or errors. See Fig. 59 for electrode legend.

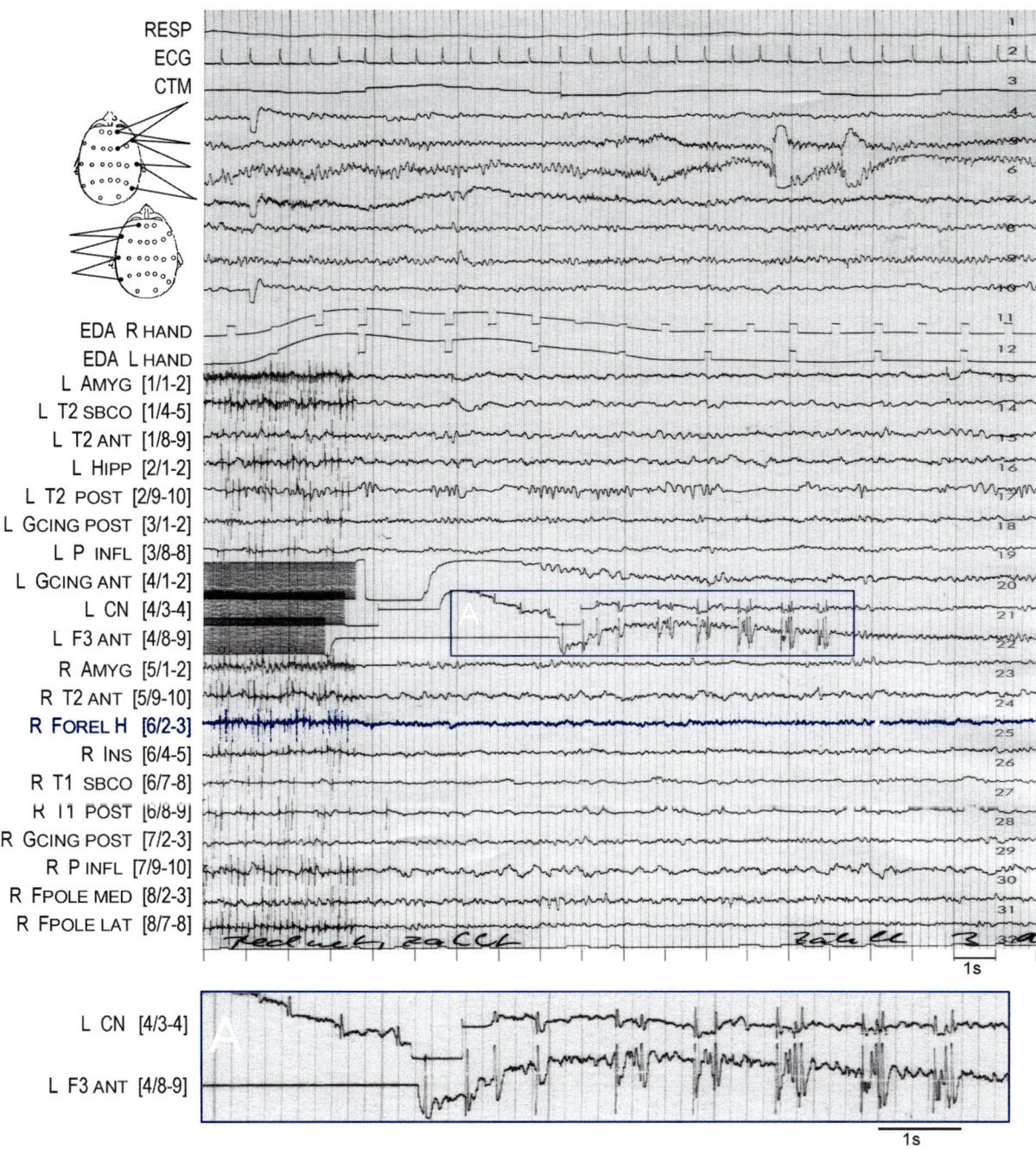

Figure 66. Electrically induced afterdischarge in the left inferior frontal gyrus [4/8-9] following 50 Hz train stimulation (4 V, 1 ms) of the same site.

The afterdischarge is shown in greater detail in inlay A. There were no signs and symptoms, and the patient was counting and calculating without problems. See Fig. 59 for electrode legend.

Summary

This patient with a left occipital porencephalic cyst in consequence of perinatal asphyxia had "classical" MTLE psychomotor seizures (characterized by fear, motor arrest, and complex oral and manual automatisms) and right homonymous hemianopsia. This case convincingly demonstrates that selective surgical removal of the seizure generating zone (that is, the left amygdala and hippocampus) by selective AHE is highly effective, despite the occurrence of widespread anatomopathological findings and bilateral interictal epileptogenesis. It also illustrates the different morphology of afterdischarge patterns, which is obviously depending on

Electrically Induced Seizure Activity

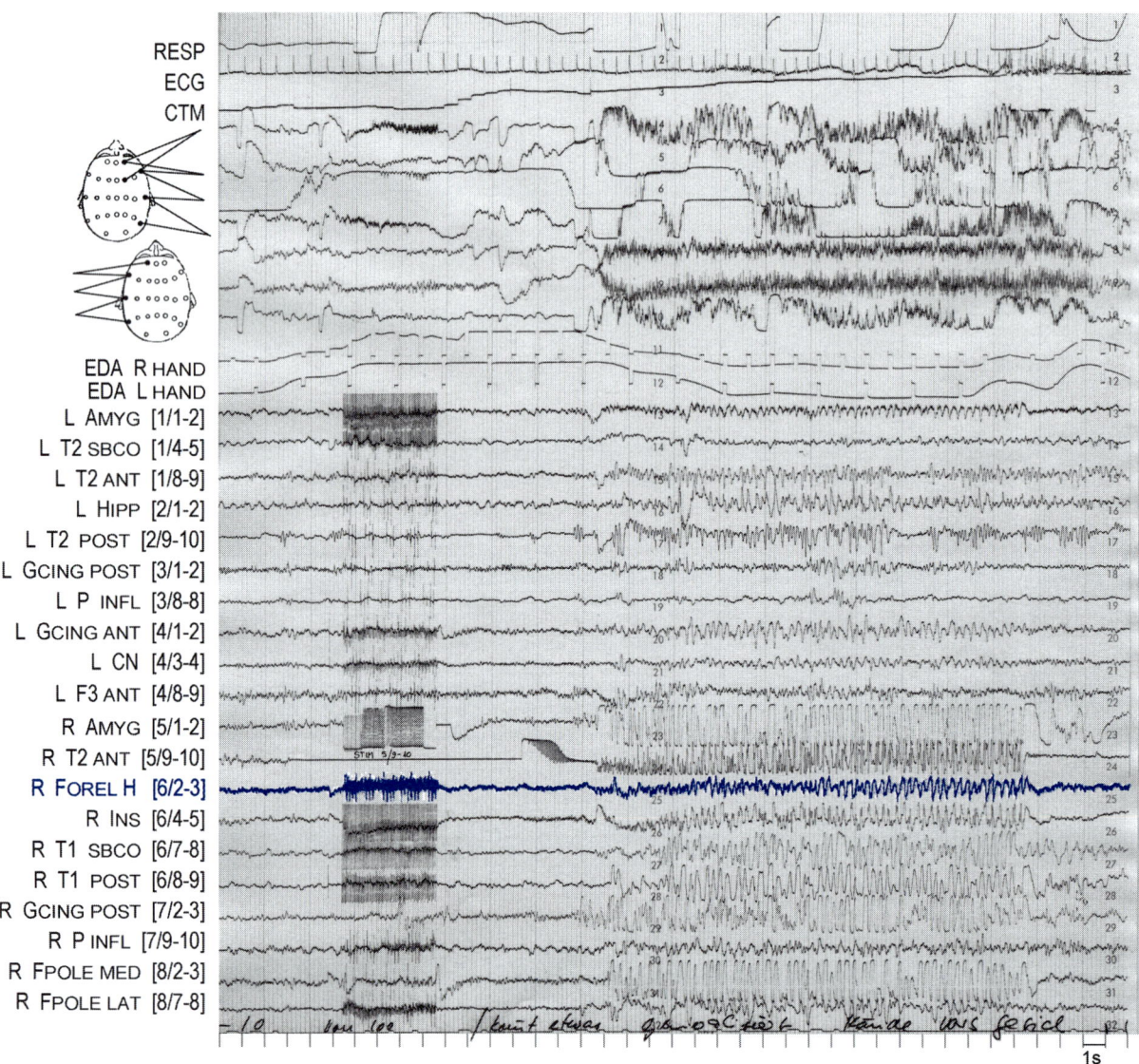

Figure 67. Electrically induced right neocortical seizure. 50 Hz train stimulation (4.5 V, 1 ms) of the anterior parts of the right middle temporal gyrus [5/9-10] provoked a seizure with propagation to the left temporal cortex and to the right Forel H field [6/2-3].

Clinically, the patient was warning that "something is coming", was bringing her hands before the face, was crying "don't touch me", and was suffering extreme fear. Note the tachycardia and the changes of electrodermal activity (EDA). See Fig. 59 for electrode legend.

the brain structures that are stimulated. The electrode located in the Forel H field was only involved if widespread ipsilateral neocortical discharges were present (these seizures were clinically accompanied by strong fear and vegetative signs). Single pulse stimulation of the anterior right temporal neocortex evoked cerebral responses in the ipsilateral insular cortex and, to a lesser degree, in the ipsilateral posterior cingulate and frontopolar cortex, as well as in Forel H field.

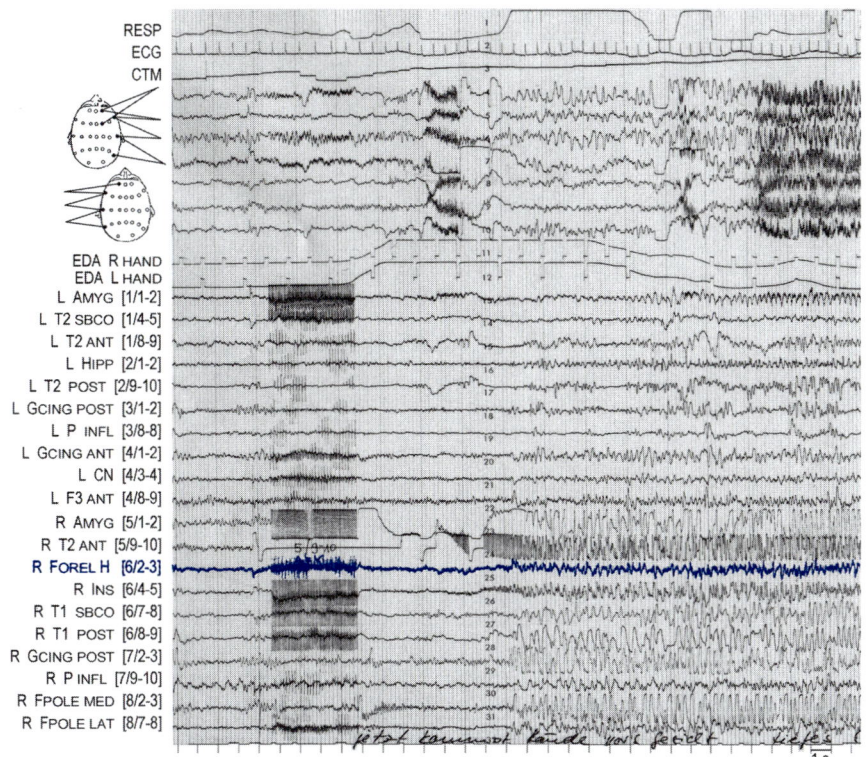

Figure 68. Electrically induced right neocortical seizure by 50 Hz train stimulation (4.5 V, 1 ms) of the anterior parts of the right middle temporal gyrus [5/9-10] provoked a seizure with propagation to the left temporal cortex and to the right Forel H field [6/2-3], similar but longer than the seizure shown in Fig. 67.

Clinical signs and symptoms were as described in Fig. 67, with marked flushing in addition. The seizure is continued in Fig. 69. See Fig. 59 for electrode legend.

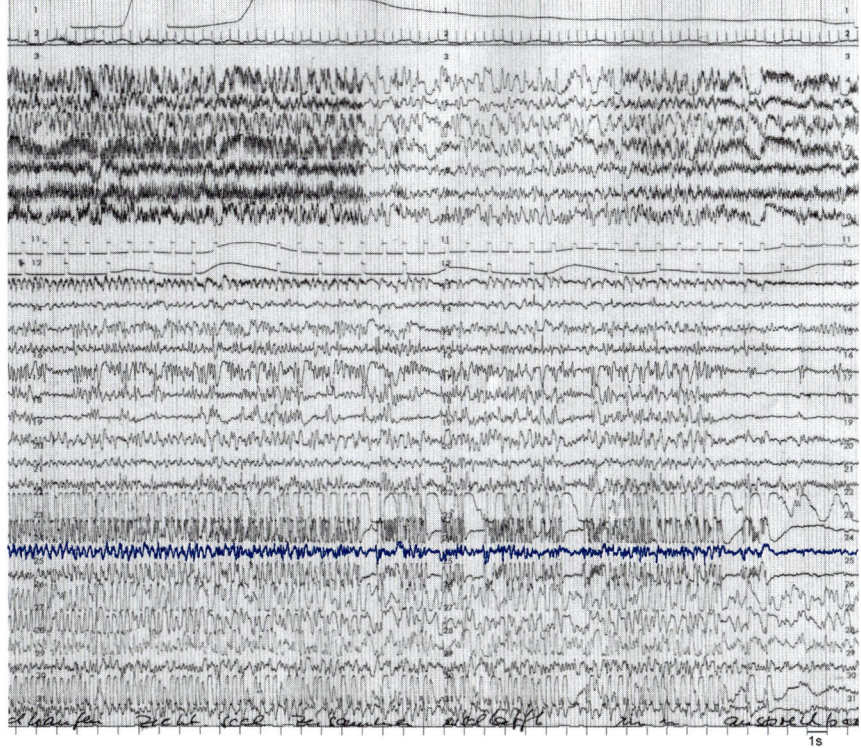

Figure 69. Continuation of the induced seizure shown in Fig. 68.

Case studies

Single Pulse Stimulation

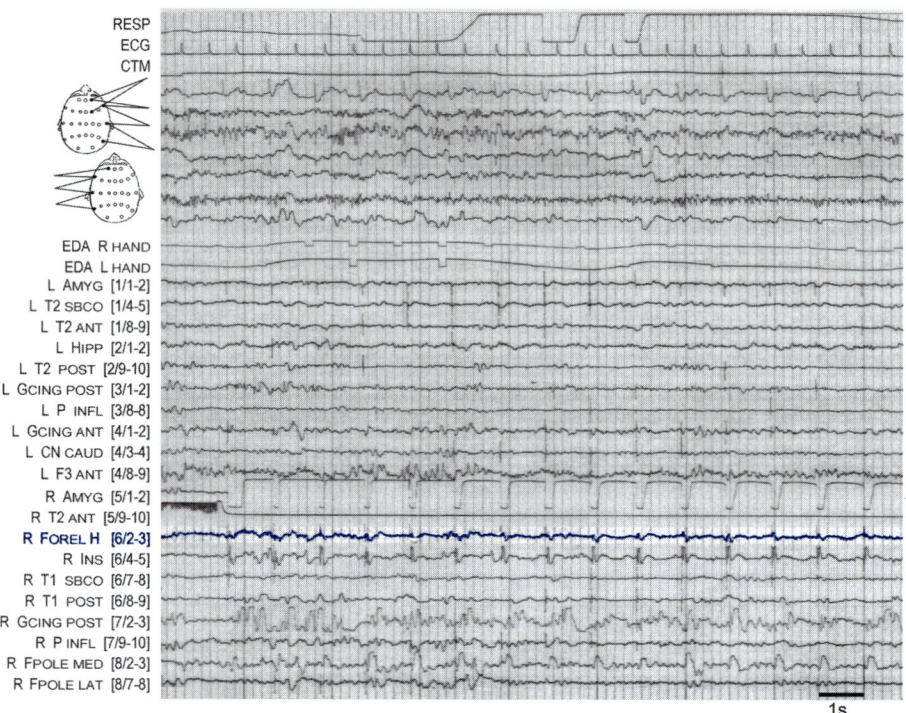

Figure 70. Single pulse stimulation (1 Hz, 4-10 V, 0.7 ms) of the anterior parts of the right middle temporal gyrus [5/9-10] evoked paroxysmal responses, mainly within the insular cortex [6/4-5] and, to a lesser extent, also in the right Forel H field [6/2-3] and the right posterior cingulate gyrus [7/2-3]. Clinically, the patient reported the feeling of a right eyelid flutter.

Case 3

Patient History

This 38 year-old man had a history of intractable epilepsy with frequent (5-10 per week) psychomotor seizures and occasional generalized seizures since age 9. Pregnancy and birth were uneventful and subsequent neonatal and childhood development was normal. He had no family history of epilepsy. Clinically, his psychomotor seizures presented with sudden fear, nausea, ascending head sensation, motor arrest (unresponsive staring), perioral myoclonia and complex oroalimentary and gestual automatisms.

SEEG Exploration

Chronic SEEG was carried out with eight depth electrodes at age 19, with electrode 3 located in or next to Forel H field (Fig. 71). Habitual auras with nausea and fear either originated in the right hippocampus (Fig. 74) or were associated with repetitive spiking in the right amygdala and Forel H field (Fig. 75). Spontaneous habitual psychomotor seizures characterized by fear and nausea as initial symptoms originated in the right hippocampus, and were subsequently spreading to the right amygdala and the right Forel H field, before finally involving the right temporal lobe, the anterior ipsilateral cingulate cortex and the left temporal lobe (Figs. 76 and 77). Electrical 50 Hz train stimulation (3 V, 0.7 ms) of the right Forel H field [3/1-2] was accompanied by a sensory sensation (crawling/itching) and slight motor weakness in the left hand and arm. Repetitive 1 Hz single pulse stimulation (5 V, 1 ms) of the right Forel H field produced pulse locked cloni of the left arm.

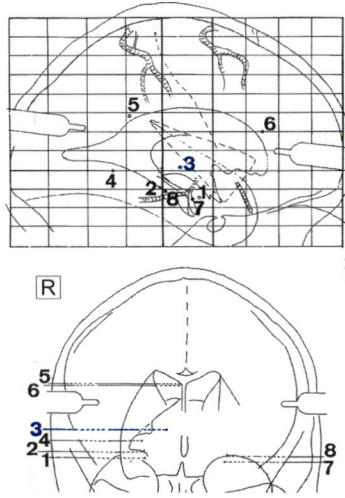

Figure 71. Location of the depth electrodes in the proportional Talairach system.
The deepest contacts of electrode 3 (contacts 1-2) were in the right subthalamic area, presumably in or next to the Forel H field.

Surgery

A right selective AHE was performed at age 20. Histological investigation of the resected specimen revealed gliosis.

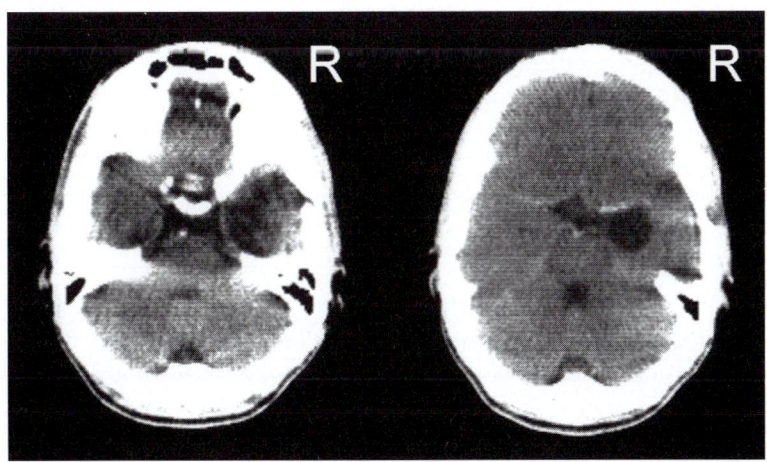

Figure 72. CT scan following right selective AHE showing the site of resection.

Outcome

This patient showed an excellent postsurgical outcome (Engel class IA). AED treatment was stopped at age 24 (that is, four years after operation). The patient is now fully employed as a consulting engineer.

Spontaneous Interictal Activity

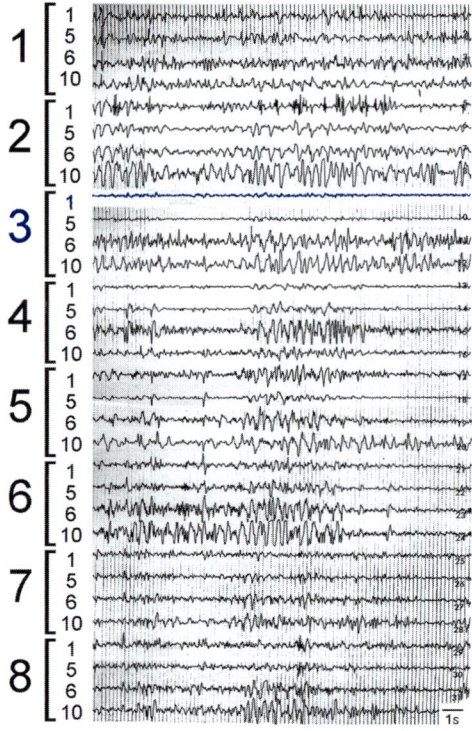

Figure 73. Interictal monopolar EEG recording (common average reference).
Note the rather "flat" EEG traces in the right subthalamic area [contact 3/1]. See Fig. 71 for electrode legend.

Spontaneous Seizure Activity

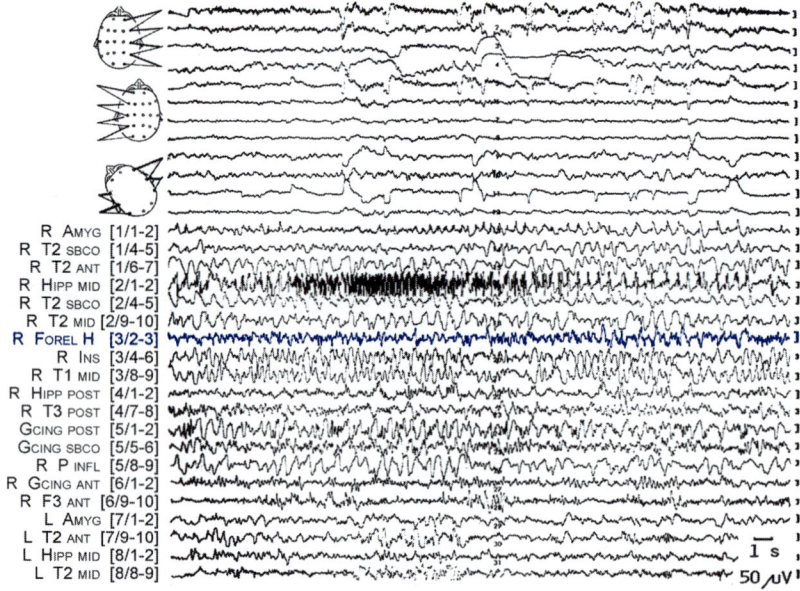

Figure 74. Spontaneous aura with nausea and fear associated with an epileptic discharge in the right hippocampus [2/1-2].

The electrode sites recorded from are indicated left to the traces by anatomical designations (based on the Talairach atlas) and numbers (electrode/contacts, cf. Fig. 71).
AMYG, amygdala; **T2**, middle temporal gyrus; **HIPP**, hippocampus; **FOREL H**, subthalamic area; **INS**, Insula; **T1**, superior temporal gyrus; **T3**, inferior temporal gyrus; **GCING**, cingulate gyrus; **PINFL**, parietal inferior lobule; **F3**, inferior frontal gyrus; **SBCO**, subcortical; **ANT**, anterior; **MID**, medial; **POST**, posterior; **LAT**, lateral; **R**, right; **L**, left.

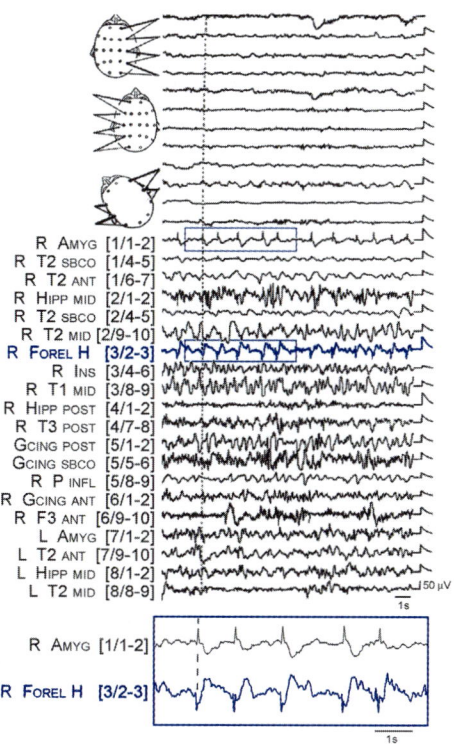

Figure 75. Spontaneous aura with fear associated with repetitive spikes in the right amygdala and Forel H field.

Modified from: Wieser HG. Selective amygdalohippocampectomy: Indications, investigative technique and results. - In: Symon L, Brihaye J, Guidetti B, Loew F, Miller JD, Nornes H, Pasztor E, Pertuiset B, Yasargil MG eds. *Advances and Technical Standards in Neurosurgery* 1986a; 13: 39-133 (Fig. 21).

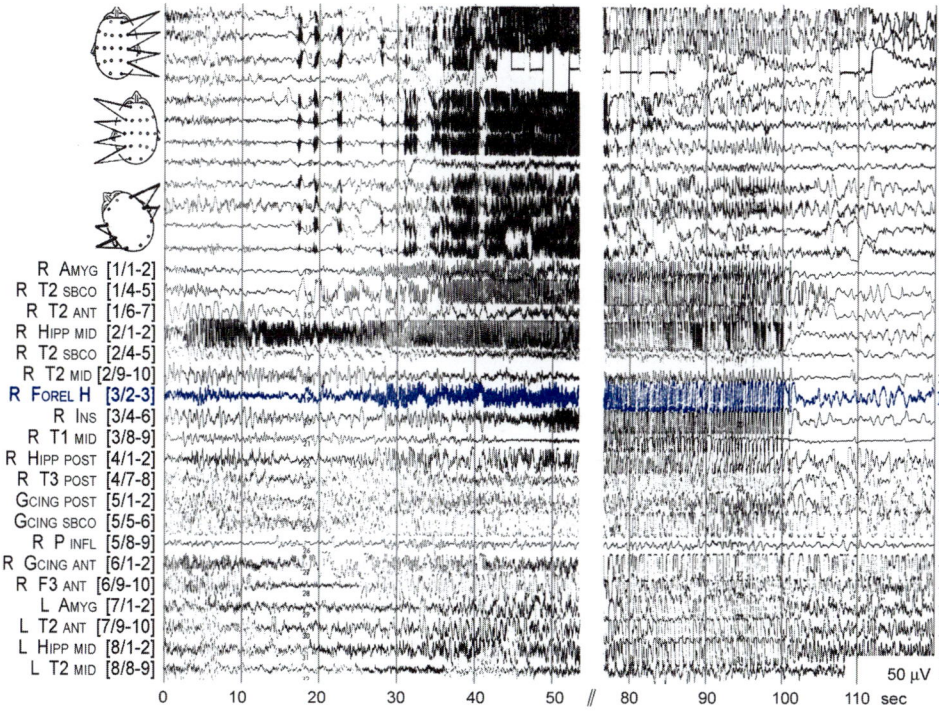

Figure 76. Spontaneous habitual psychomotor seizure with fear and nausea as initial symptoms associated with seizure discharge in the right hippocampus, spreading to the right amygdala and the right Forel H, finally involving the right temporal lobe and spreading to the anterior ipsilateral cingulate cortex and left temporal lobe.

The EEG segments are interrupted by about 25 seconds. Electrode sites were identical to those given in Fig. 74.

Case studies

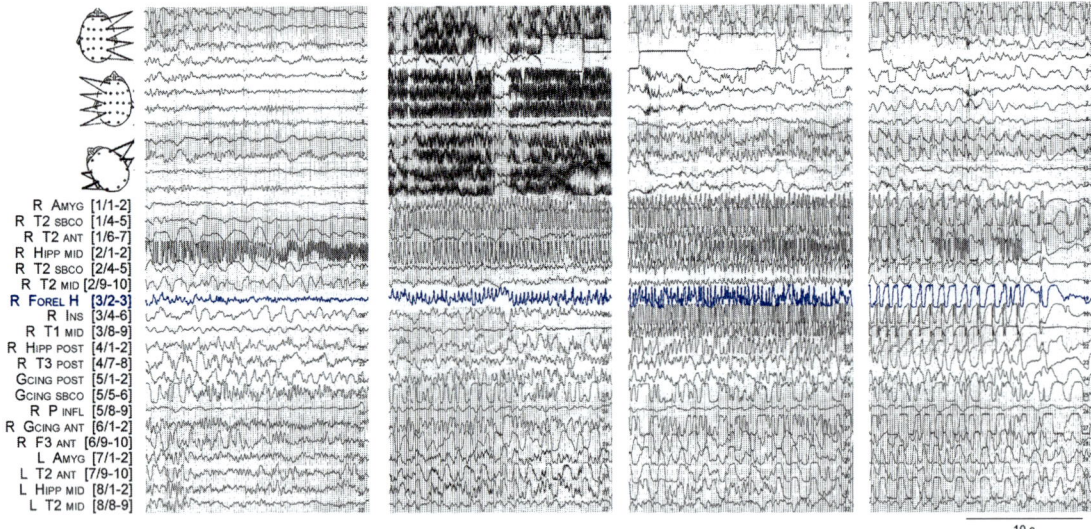

Figure 77. Spontaneous habitual psychomotor seizure with fear and nausea as initial symptoms originating from the right hippocampus, spreading to the right amygdala, the right Forel H, the right temporal lobe, the anterior ipsilateral cingulate cortex and finally to the left temporal lobe.
Electrode sites were identical to those given in Fig. 74.

Somatosensory Evoked Potentials (SEP)

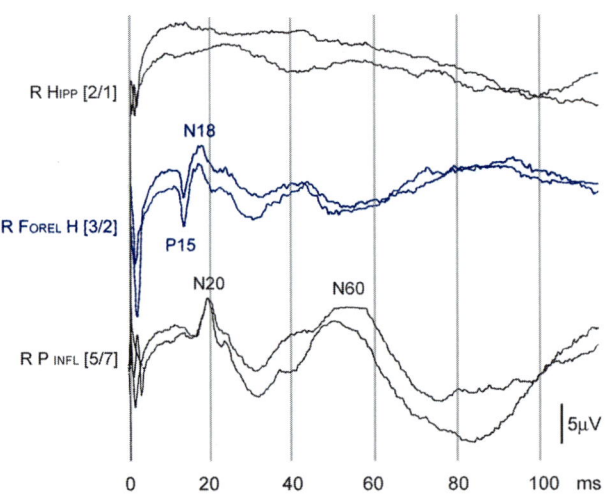

Figure 78. Somatosensory evoked potentials (SEP) following stimulation of the left median nerve.
Note the VPL-generated P15 component recorded in the right Forel H.
Hipp, hippocampus; **Forel H**, subthalamic area; **P infl**, parietal inferior lobule; **R**, right.

Summary

This patient suffering from MTLE with hippocampal sclerosis and excellent postsurgical outcome (Engel class I) after right selective AHE is interesting because (1) his spontaneous seizures originating in the right hippocampus with progressive spread to ipsilateral and finally contralateral depth electrode recording sites displayed marked ictal discharges in the right Forel H field (in this context it should be noted that this patient also had secondarily generalized seizures), because (2) electrical 50 Hz train stimulation of the right Forel H field was accompanied by sensory sensations such as crawling and itching, as well as a mild motor weakness in the left hand and arm, and because (3) repetitive 1 Hz single pulse stimulation of the right Forel H field led to pulse locked cloni of left arm. Moreover (4), a spontaneous aura with fear was accompanied by repetitive spiking in the right amygdala and, time locked, in the right Forel H field. This finding might emphasize the preferred propagation pathway of amygdalar efferents (efferent fibers from the amygdala are the stria terminalis and, to a lesser degree, the ventro-fugal bundle to overlapping areas in the medial and rostral hypothalamus (Ncl. ventromedialis and dorsomedialis hypothalami, regio preoptica) and to the regio septalis (Ncl. lateralis septi, "bed nucleus" of the stria terminalis, diagonal band - see Wieser [2000], Fig. 2). Finally (5), left median SEP revealed the recording of the VPL generated SEP component P15 in the right Forel H field, but not from other depth electrode recording sites.

Case 4

Patient History

This 16 year-old woman had intractable epilepsy of presumable right frontal onset since age 4. Delivery was complicated, but subsequent neonatal and childhood development was normal. She had no family history of epilepsy. Her seizures were characterized by left clonic motor activity. After initiation of AED treatment, she was seizure free for two years. However, seizures recurred at age six, evolving with gradually increasing frequency and intractability (up to 4 seizures per day). At this time, her seizures were characterized by tonic extension of the left arm, reclination and deviation of the head to the right, hyperextension of the trunk, and sudden atonic falls (backwards or forwards, frequently associated with injuries). There was no aura with this type of seizures, although she also reported occasional isolated auras that were characterized by the feeling of paralysis in the left arm, acoustical hallucinations (she heard people talking), while being fully aware. Progressive decline in school performance, the development of a marked behavioral syndrome and a high seizure frequency finally led to hospitalization in a specialized institution for patients with epilepsy at age 15. At this time, neurological examination demonstrated a slight left sensorimotor hemisyndrome.

SEEG Exploration

Chronic SEEG was carried out at age 16 with six depth electrodes, electrode 4 located in or next to Forel H field (Fig. 79). The SEEG exploration was restricted to the right temporal lobe, because both parents and involved physicians would have only agreed on temporal, but not on extratemporal lobe epilepsy surgery. Four spontaneous seizures were recorded, the most representative example of which is shown in Fig. 81. Ictal activity in depth electrode sites was virtually restricted to the subthalamic area [4/1-2], with, to a much lesser extent, involvement of right neocortical temporal areas [2/6-7]. Electrical 1 Hz single pulse stimulation of the Forel H field [4/1-2] provoked time-locked cloni of the left leg and arm (Figs. 82 and 83).

Surgery

Taking into consideration the SEEG findings, a second SEEG evaluation with additional exploration of the frontal lobes was suggested but not agreed upon.

Outcome

No surgery was performed in this patient. She continued to have relatively frequent seizures, but seizures associated with severe falls clearly diminished with AED treatment using a combination of valproic acid (2,100 mg daily), phenobarbital (100 mg daily), vigabatrin (2 g daily), benzodiazepine (15 mg daily) and acetazolamide (250 mg 3 times per week). Further follow up was not available, because the patient had left the country.

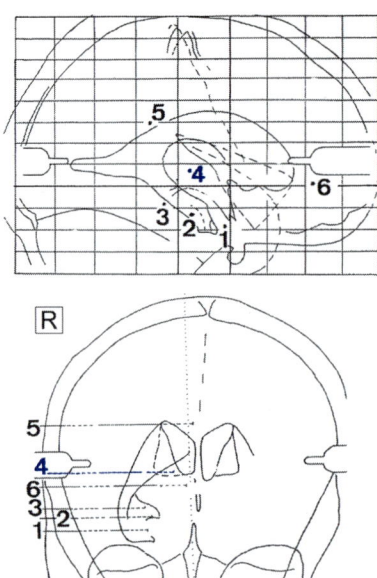

Figure 79. Location of depth electrodes in the proportional Talairach system.

The deepest contacts of electrode 4 (contacts 1-2) were in the left subthalamic area, presumably in or next to the Forel H field.

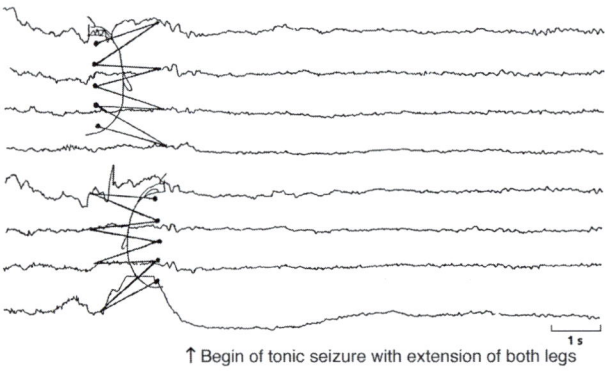

↑ Begin of tonic seizure with extension of both legs

Figure 80. Scalp EEG recording showing the EEG onset of a typical tonic seizure of this patient, characterized by a generalized decrement for 15 s (or even longer duration in other seizures) that was usually followed by a number of rhythmic slow waves over both frontal regions with a right fronto-temporal predominance.

There were no clear-cut spikes or sharp-slow waves, neither during the seizures nor between the seizures.

Summary

Despite insufficient frontal exploration (dictated by clinical arguments), the recordings of this patient with intractable seizures of presumably right frontal lobe onset is interesting because the surface EEG recordings showed a long lasting ictal decrement at the beginning of the seizure, whereas the depth electrode recording in the Forel H field showed a electrographic decrement that was followed by a rhythmic, progressively slowing high frequency spike discharge. One Hz single pulse stimulation of the ipsilateral hippocampus evoked cerebral responses in the Forel H field, and 1 Hz single pulse stimulation of the Forel H field provoked pulse locked cloni of the left leg and arm. Hence, the strong participation of the Forel H field in this presumably right frontal lobe epilepsy, and the evocation of left sided cloni by repetitive 1 Hz single pulse stimulation of the Forel H field, is in line with the spontaneous seizure semiology, which was characterized by tonic extension of the left arm, reclination and deviation of the head to the right, hyperextension of the trunk and sudden atonic falls.

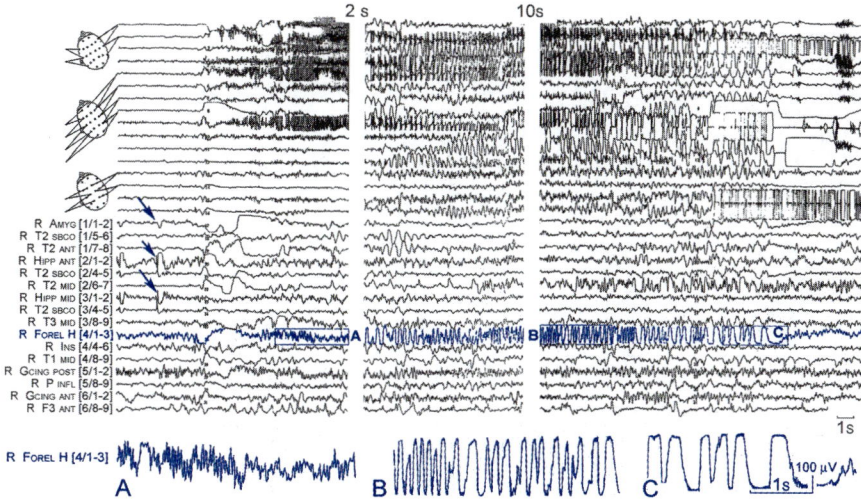

Figure 81. Spontaneous tonic seizure recorded with scalp electrodes (Hess system) and depth electrodes.

The beginning of the seizure was characterized by the occurrence of spike-wave complexes in right mesial temporal structures, that is, in the anterior [2/1-2] and mid to posterior hippocampus [3/-12], and, to a lesser extent, also in the amygdala [1/1-2] (blue arrows). Coinciding with the tonic posturing (as reflected by artifacts and muscle activity in the scalp EEG recording), the electrode contact within or next to the right Forel H field [4/1-3] showed a decrement of about 1 s duration followed by a rhythmic high frequency discharge of about 20 Hz (A), which was then slowing down to a frequency of about 4 Hz (B) and 2 Hz (C). To a lesser extent, the lateral temporal cortex [2/6-7] was also involved. – The electrode sites recorded from are indicated left to the traces by anatomical designations (based on the Talairach atlas) and numbers (electrode/contacts, cf. Fig. 79).

Amyg, amygdala; **T2**, middle temporal gyrus; **Hipp**, hippocampus; **T3**, inferior temporal gyrus; **Forel H**, subthalamic area; **Ins**, Insula; **Gcing**, cingulate gyrus; **T1**, superior temporal gyrus; **Pinfl**, parietal inferior lobule; **F3**, inferior frontal gyrus; **SBCO**, subcortical; **ANT**, anterior; **MID**, medial; **POST**, posterior; **R**, right.

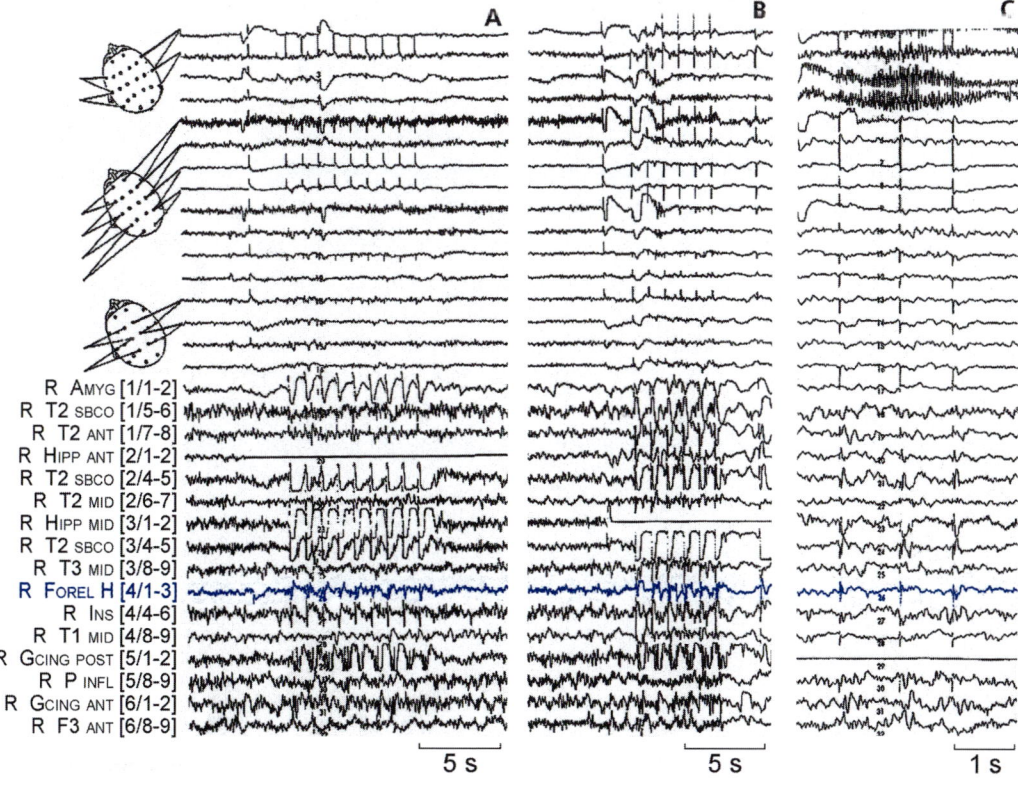

Figure 82. Single pulse stimulation (1 Hz, 4-10 V, 0.7 ms) of the right anterior hippocampus [2/1-2] **A**, the right mid to posterior hippocampus [3/1-2] **B**, and the right posterior cingulate gyrus [5/1-2] **C** with their EEG responses.

Electrode sites were identical to those given in Fig. 81.

Case studies

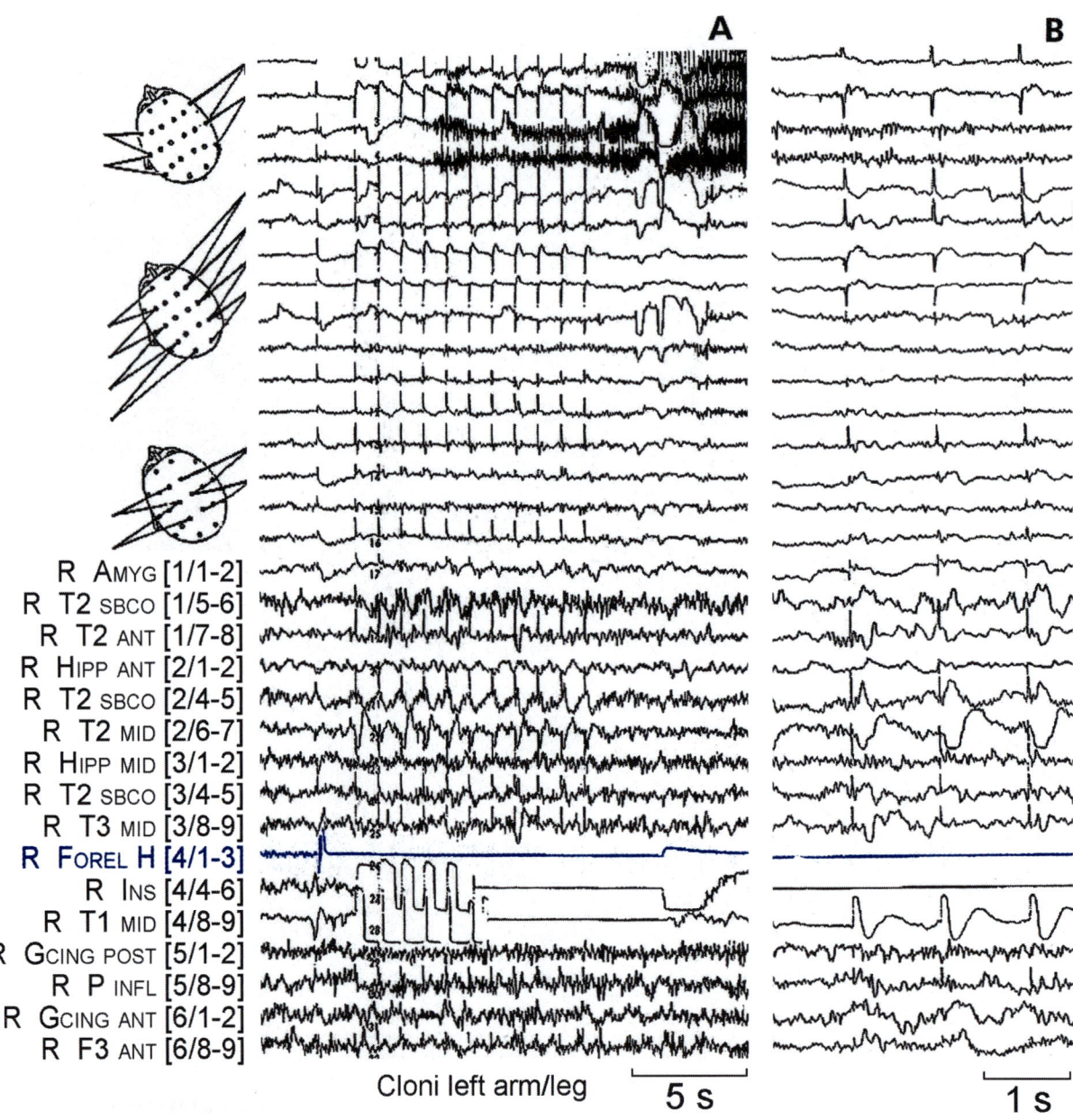

Figure 83. Single pulse stimulation (1 Hz, 4-10 V, 0.7 ms) of the right Forel H [4/1-3] depicted in two different time resolutions (**A, B**).

Clinically, the stimulation of the right Forel H field [4/1-3] provoked cloni of the left leg and arm. Electrode sites were identical to those given in Fig. 81.

Case 5

Patient History

This 15 year-old man had intractable TLE since age 5. Pregnancy was complicated by pre-eclampsia, but birth was uneventful and subsequent neonatal development was normal. His first febrile seizure occurred at age 5 months. At age 8 months, he had to be hospitalized due to a status epilepticus lasting for about 7 hours. At age 3, he had numerous febrile and non-febrile "spells". At age 5, he had a cluster of generalized seizures. At age 15, his seizures consisted of psychomotor signs and symptoms, with "absence like" or "migraine like" symptoms at the very beginning of the seizures, and with frequent secondary generalization. His father had a history of febrile seizures, and his mother suffered from migraine.

SEEG Exploration

Chronic SEEG with 10 depth electrodes was carried out at age 15, with electrode 6 located in the right thalamus and electrode 9 in or next to the left Forel H field (Fig. 84). Unfortunately, no spontaneous habitual seizure occurred during this recording, but several spontaneous seizure discharges of short duration could be recorded in left temporo-occipital cortical areas [10/8-9]. Repetitive 1 Hz stimulation at this site led to a long lasting seizure of a total duration of 23.6 minutes. This seizure showed a habitual semiology, characterized by a left sided cephalic aura, difficulties with naming and recognition of verbal items, altered thinking, strange feeling, marked vegetative signs (tachycardia and respiratory irregularities), hyperventilation, fear, aphasia and water drinking. Towards the end of the seizure, coinciding with water drinking, there were high frequency low amplitude discharges in the ipsilateral subthalamic area [9/1-2] (Fig. 85). Fifty Hz train stimulation of the left hippocampus [8/1-2] elicited a "strange feeling" around the nose. Repetitive 1 Hz stimulation of the left subthalamic area [9/1-2] during a spontaneous subclinical discharge in the left neocortical temporo-occipital region [10/8-9] resulted in "grouping" or "synchronization" of the discharge and elicited time locked EEG responses in the left superior temporal gyrus [9/9-10], while the patient reported a "pulsating" sensation in his right thumb and index finger (Fig. 86). Fifty Hz train stimulation (3.5 V, 1 ms) at this site [9/1-2] provoked an "electrical tingling sensation" in the right hand. No cognitive evoked potentials could be recorded in thalamic and subthalamic sites using a tachistoscopic paradigm presenting geometric figures and faces.

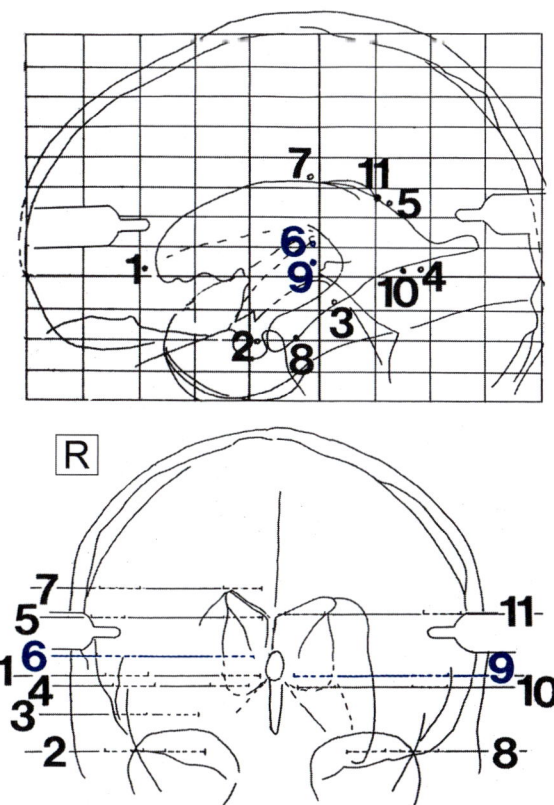

Figure 84. Location of depth electrodes in the proportional Talairach system.

The deepest contacts of electrode 6 (contacts 1-2) were in the right thalamus, presumably in or next to the dorsomedial nucleus. The deepest contacts of electrode 9 (contacts 1-2) were in the left subthalamic area, presumably in or next to the Forel H field.

Surgery

A palliative left selective AHE was performed at age 16. Histological examination of the resected specimen revealed dysplasia (atypical cortical lamination).

Outcome

The initial postsurgical outcome was moderate (Engel class III), and the situation subsequently worsened to Engel class IV despite treatment with AEDs in various combinations. At age 30, a re-evaluation was performed at another surgical center, but supplementary surgery was not recommended. At age 34, a Vagus Nerve Stimulating (VNS) device was implanted at another center, but a beneficial effect was lacking. The patient worked as an office clerk (technical drawing). He died in a generalized tonic clonic status epilepticus during night at age 35, 14 months after implantation of the VNS device.

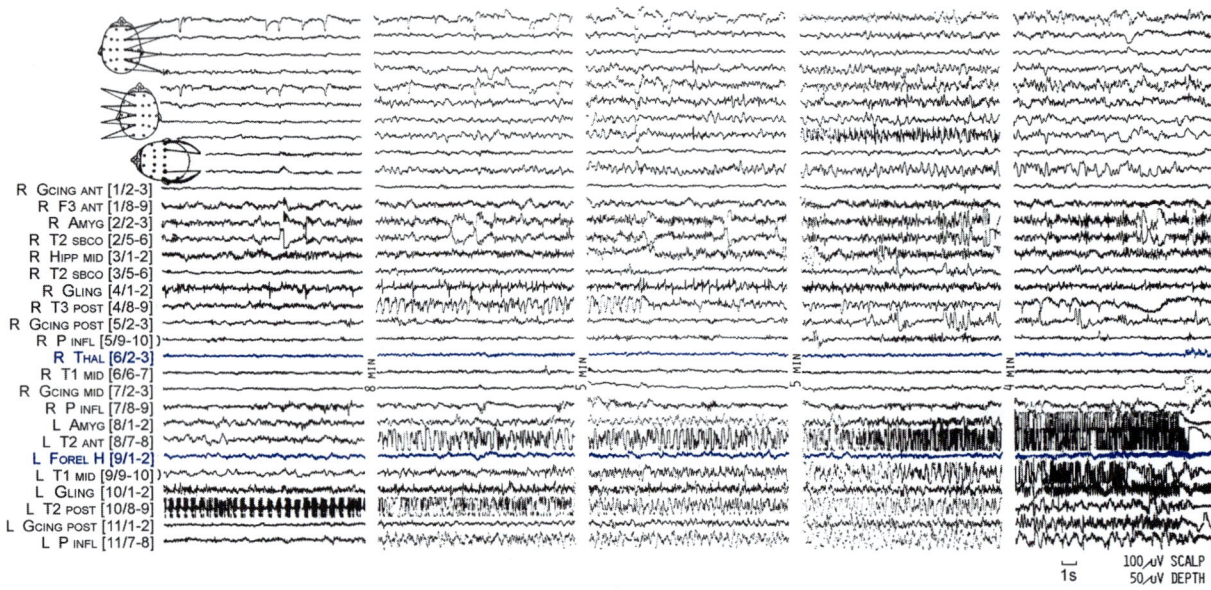

Figure 85. Single pulse stimulation (1 Hz, 3.5 V, 1 ms) of the left neocortical temporo-occipital region [10/8-9] induced a left neocortical temporo-occipital seizure with late high frequency low amplitude discharges in the subthalamic area [9/1-2].

This electrically induced seizure had a duration of 23.6 min and was associated with the typical habitual seizure symptoms of this patient, including left sided cephalic sensation, difficulties with naming and recognition of verbal items, altered thinking, strange feeling and excessive vegetative signs (tachycardia, irregular respiration, hyperventilation). With progressive spread to the left amygdala fear was the predominant symptom. In the late course of the seizure, ictal behavior predominantly was aphasia and water drinking. The electrode sites recorded from are indicated left to the traces by anatomical designations (based on the Talairach atlas) and numbers (electrode/contacts, cf. Fig. 84).

GCING, cingulate gyrus; **F3**, inferior frontal gyrus; **AMYG**, amygdala; **T2**, middle temporal gyrus; **HIPP**, hippocampus; **GLING**, lingual gyrus; **T3**, inferior temporal gyrus; **PINFL**, parietal inferior lobule; **THAL**, thalamus; **T1**, superior temporal gyrus; **FOREL H**, subthalamic area; **ANT**, anterior; **SBCO**, subcortical; **MID**, middle; **POST**, posterior; **R**, right; **L**, left.

Modified from: Wieser HG, Hailemariam S, Regard M, Landis T. Unilateral limbic epileptic status activity: Stereo-EEG, behavioural, and cognitive data. *Epilepsia* 1985b; 26: 19-29.

Summary

This patient with intractable epilepsy with "absence like" and "migraine like" seizures of presumably left neocortical posterior temporal lobe onset and with dysplasia (atypical lamination) in the palliatively resected mesial temporal lobe structures did neither profit from left palliative AHE nor from VNS. He died in generalized convulsive status epilepticus at age 35 during night. This case is interesting because of an electrically induced very long lasting

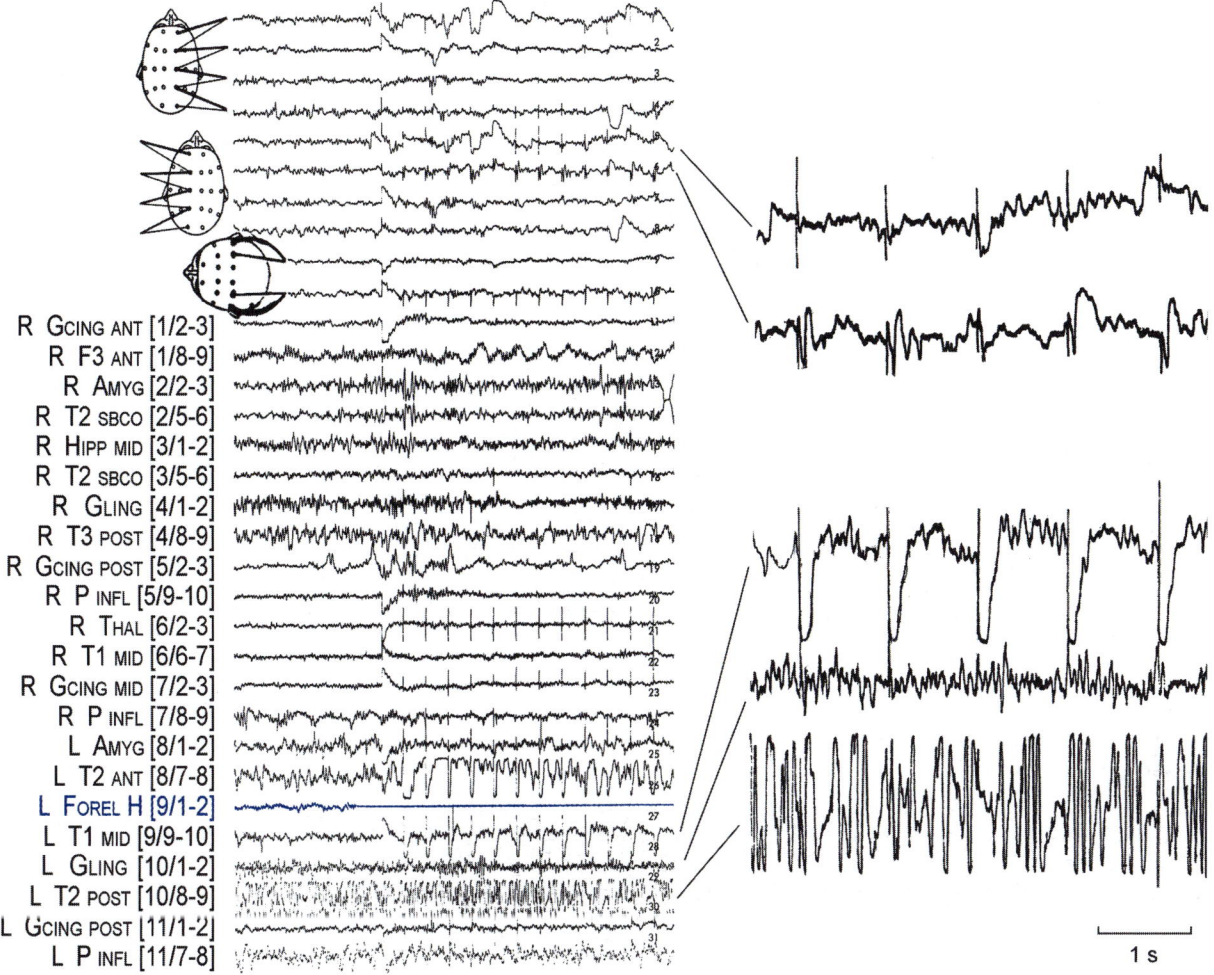

Figure 86. Repetitive 1 Hz single pulse stimulation of the left subthalamic area [9/1-2] during a spontaneous discharge in left neocortical temporo-occipital cortical areas [10/8-9] resulted in "grouping" or "synchronization" of the discharge to some extent, but otherwise failed to show a significant effect on the discharge (lower trace to the right, [10/8-9]).

Note the time-locked EEG responses in the left superior temporal gyrus [9/9-10]. Electrode sites were identical to those given in Fig. 85.

seizure associated with water drinking that was originating in left neocortical temporal structures before successively spreading to anterior neocortical temporal areas, to the ipsilateral amygdala and, to a lesser extent, to the Forel H field. However, repetitive 1 Hz electrical stimulation of the Forel H field during spontaneous discharges restricted to the left neocortical posterior temporal lobe did not significantly influence the neocortical epileptic discharge, although there was a tendency of "grouping/synchronization" of the spike discharges time locked to the stimulus. Marked cognitive cerebral evoked potentials were found in both lingual gyri but not in the right thalamic and left Forel H field recordings. With tachistoscopic presentation of rotated geometric figures, the component N300 of the cognitive evoked potential was more apparent in the left lingual gyrus if the rotated figure was presented in the right visual field. In contrast to cognitive evoked potentials with the presentation of rotated geometric figures, the tachistoscopic presentation of faces presented in the left visual field produced a pronounced P200 component in the right lingual gyrus and a prominent N300 component with predominance in the left lingual gyrus.

Case studies

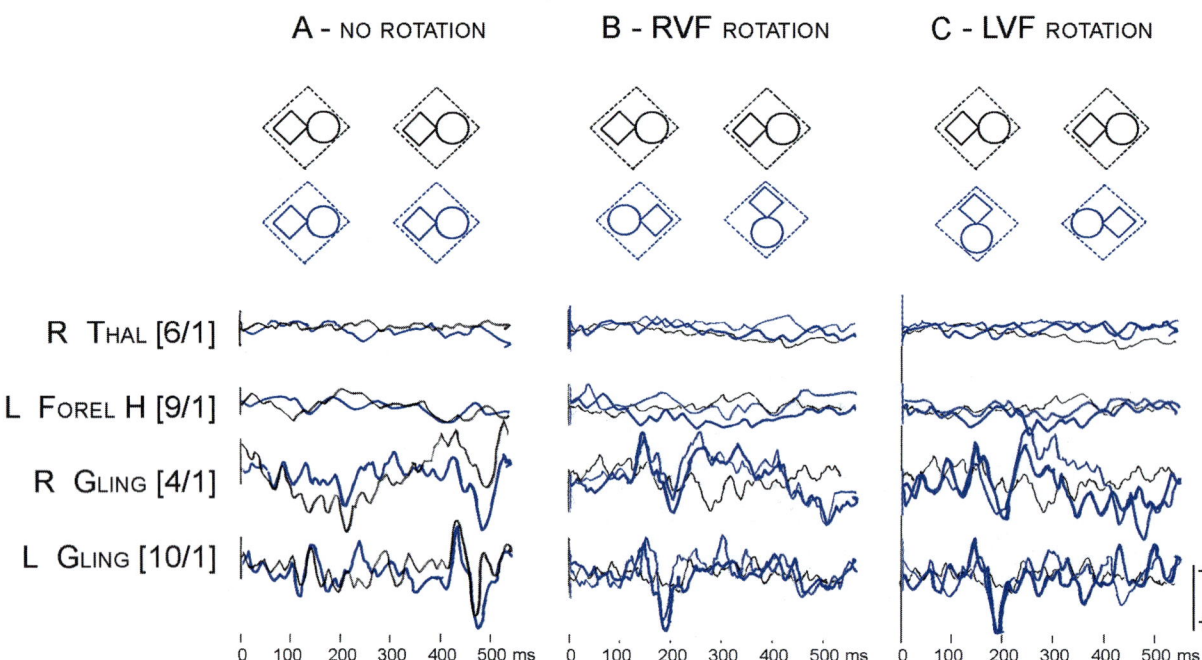

Figure 87. Cognitive evoked potentials following tachistoscopic presentation of geometric figures with or without rotation (blue lines; single run in A, double run in B and C) compared with baseline average (black lines).

Note the marked cognitive evoked potentials in the right [4/1] and left [10/1] lingual gyrus following rotation of the geometric figures (B, C) but not with the non-rotation paradigm (A). No cognitive evoked potentials were found in the right thalamus [6/1] and the left subthalamic area [9/1]. Recording is against a common reference fed by selected "inactive" depth electrode contacts situated in the white matter.

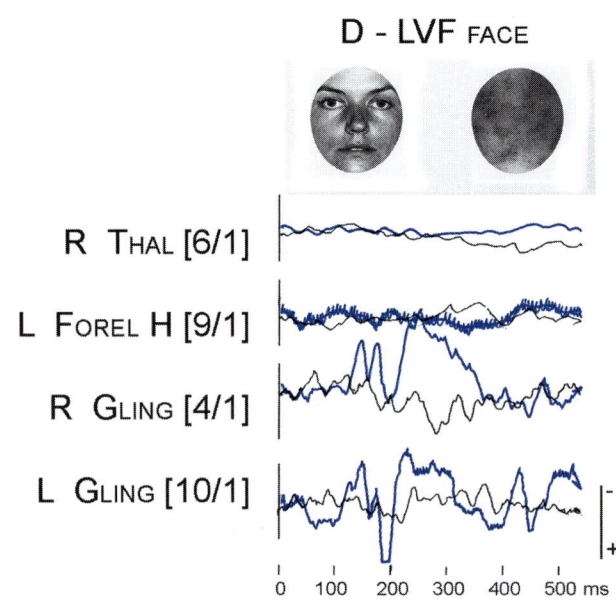

Figure 88. Cognitive evoked potentials following tachistoscopic presentation of faces vs. potato (blue lines) compared with baseline average (black lines).

Note the marked cognitive evoked potentials in the right [4/1] and left [10/1] lingual gyrus, but neither in the right thalamus [6/1] nor in the left subthalamic area [9/1].

Case 6

Patient History

This 27 year-old woman had a progressive encephalopathy and intractable epilepsy since age 6. Pregnancy, delivery, neonatal and childhood development were normal. There was no history of epilepsy in the family. At age 5, she had sustained a mild head injury. At age 6, she experienced absences for the first time, occurring with increasing frequency thereafter. She also had generalized seizures that were frequently followed by stuporous states lasting for hours or even days since age 9. A progressive mental and psychosocial decline was witnessed. At the time of admission at age 27, she had a verbal IQ of 61 (left hemisphere language dominance) and showed extreme slowing of thinking, "débilité motrice", and fearful behavior. Her neurological examination revealed a mild pupillary asymmetry (right wider than left), exaggerated tendon reflexes, and a positive plantar response on the right. Her head X-ray and scintigraphy were normal. The examination of her cerebrospinal fluid showed a moderate increase of protein. Her scalp EEG showed a marked rhythmic slowing of the background activity (with a predominance of 4 Hz theta rhythms) and a petit mal variant pattern.

SEEG Exploration

Chronic SEEG with 12 depth electrodes was carried out at age 27, with electrodes 6 and 12 located in the medial nuclei of both thalami (Fig. 89). Both frontal lobes and thalamic nuclei were explored with the aim to prove or refute a frontal interhemispheric seizure onset. The ulterior motives were the collection of eventual arguments towards a palliative intervention such as an anterior callosotomy or a Forel H-tomy. The electrographic recordings showed the characteristics of a so called petit mal variant and ictal findings suggesting a leading role of the left frontal interhemispheric cortex including the supplementary sensorimotor area (SSMA).

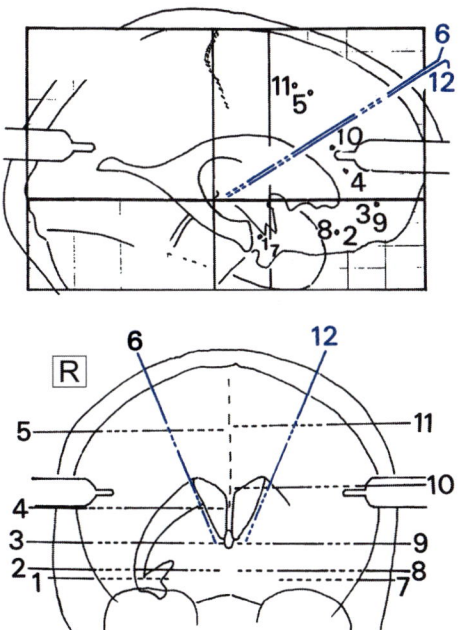

Figure 89. Location of depth electrodes in the proportional Talairach system, with electrodes 6 (right) and 12 (left) located in the medial thalamic nuclei, their deepest contacts [6/1-2 and 12/1-2] in the dorsomedial nuclei.

The remaining electrodes sampled both frontal (electrodes 2-5 and 8-11) and temporal lobes (electrodes 1 and 7).

Modified from: Wieser HG, Siegel AM. Relations between the EEG of the cortex, thalamus and periaqueductal gray in patients suffering from epilepsy and pain syndromes. In: Zschocke S, Speckmann EJ eds. *Basic Mechanisms of the EEG*. Boston: Birkhäuser 1993: 145-182 (Fig. 11.4).

Surgery

An anterior callosotomy was suggested but not agreed upon.

Interictal Activity

The EEG activity during waking state consisted of a marked slowing with 3 Hz delta rhythms showing a clear right frontal predominance (Fig. 90). The scalp EEG-recorded delta activity best correlated with intracerebral recordings from right basal frontal [2/6-7 and 3/7-8] and supplementary sensorimotor [5/2-3] cortical areas. With respect to the slow activity, there was no clear involvement of the dorsomedial nuclei [6/1-2 and 12/1-2]. Occasional high voltage spikes or spike-waves recorded over the right paramedian frontal scalp region did not reliably match with discharges recorded from intracerebral electrodes (if at all, they best correlated with activity recorded from the right SSMA [5/2-3]). There was definitely no clear involvement of the right dorsomedial nucleus [6/1-2] during epileptic discharges.

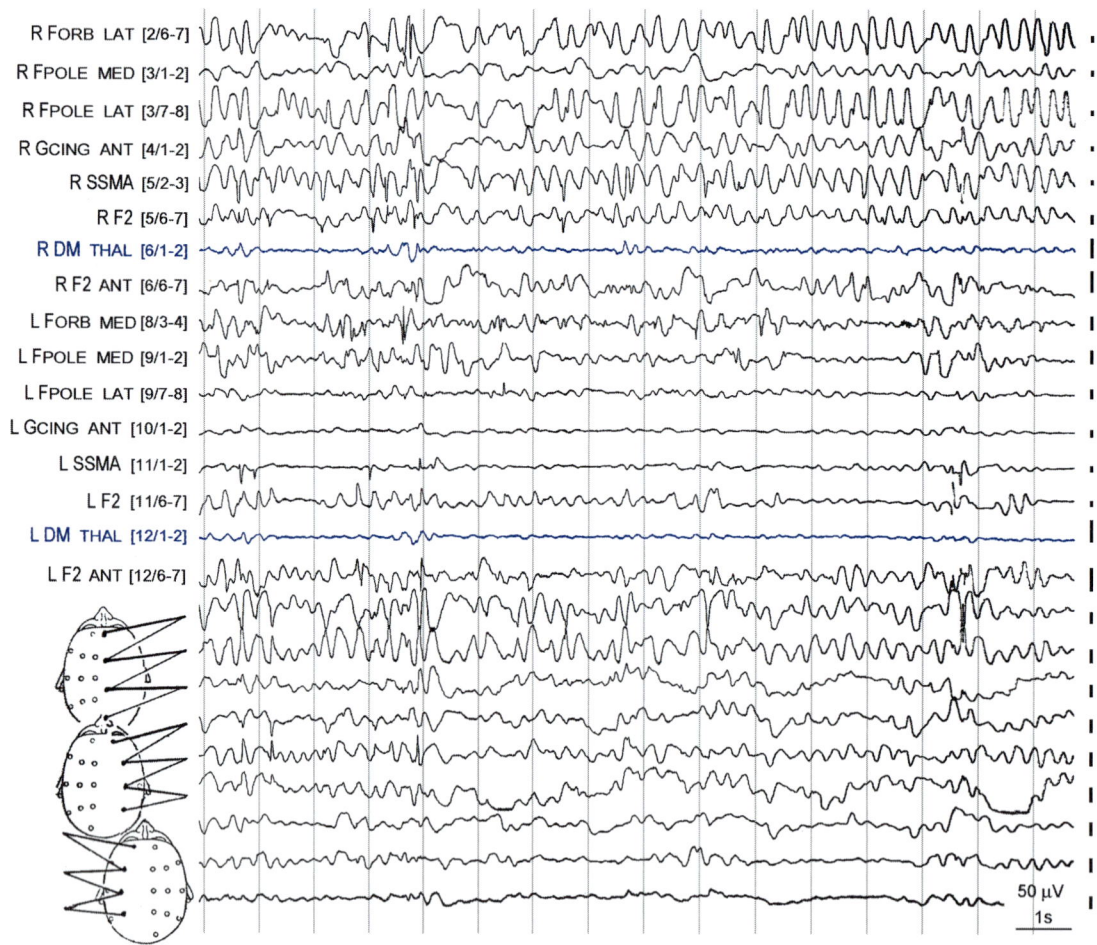

Figure 90. Interictal combined intracerebral (upper traces, channels 1-16) and scalp EEG (lower traces, channels 17-25) during waking state with little epileptic activity.

Note the increased gain of the thalamic recordings in comparison to other intracerebral recording sites (see black bars to the right). The higher voltage of the first two scalp channels (17 and 18) is best explained by breach rhythm activity (the frontal midline electrodes Fz and Cz were located next to the frontal burr holes). The electrode sites recorded from are indicated left to the traces by anatomical designations (based on the Talairach atlas) and numbers (electrode/contacts).
FORB, frontoorbital; **F**POLE, frontal pole; **G**CING, cingulate gyrus; **SSMA**, supplementary sensorimotor area; **F2**, middle frontal gyrus; **DM THAL**, dorsomedial thalamic nucleus; **LAT**, lateral; **MED**, medial; **ANT**, anterior; **R**, right; **L**, left.

Epileptic activity was clearly enhanced during night sleep (Fig. 91), and was periodically (every 25-30 seconds) interrupted by generalized electrical decremental periods of a duration of about 2 to 3 s. These decremental periods consisted of crescendo-like high frequency spike bursts that were best recorded from the right anterior cingulate gyrus [4/1-2]. The dorsomedial nuclei were only involved at the very end of these spike bursts [6/1-2 and 12/1-2]. Of note is the flattening of respiration clearly associated with decremental periods.

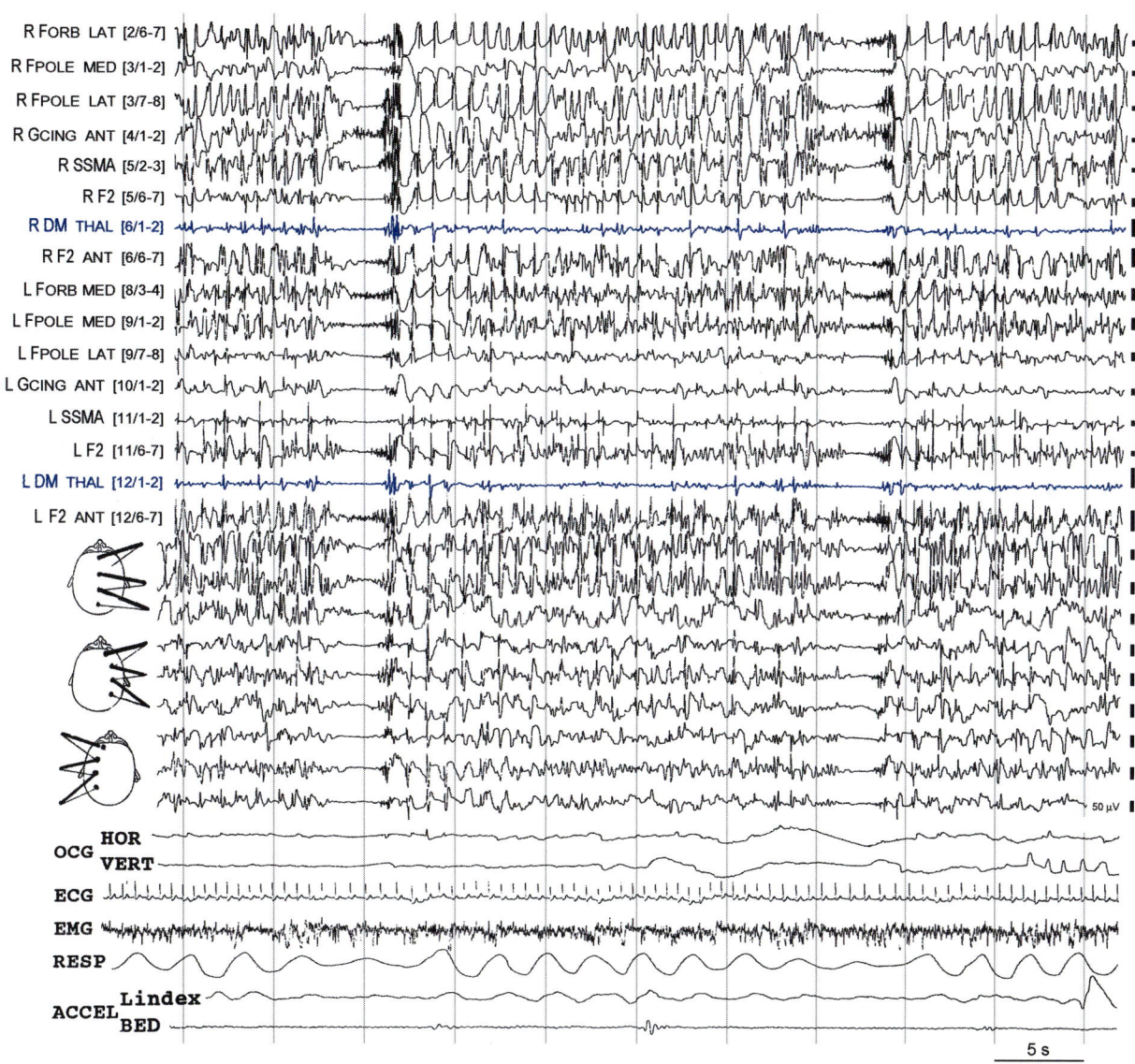

Figure 91. Polygraphic sleep recording with marked epileptic activity and periodic decremental periods.

Note the compressed time scale and the presumable breach rhythm of the first two scalp channels. – The electrode sites recorded from are indicated left to the traces by anatomical designations (based on the Talairach atlas) and numbers (electrode/contacts). Intracerebral electrode sites and assignments are identical to those of Fig. 90, with the exception of channel 16, where electrode 12 was now recording from contacts 6-7 instead of 7-8.
EOG, electrooculogram, **HOR**, horizontal; **VERT**, vertical; **ECG**, electrocardiogram; **EMG**, electromyogram; **RESP**, respiration; **ACCEL**, accelerometry; **Lindex**, left index finger; **BED**, bed movement.

Modified from: Wieser HG, Siegel AM. Relations between the EEG of the cortex, thalamus and periaqueductal gray in patients suffering from epilepsy and pain syndromes. In: Zschocke S, Speckmann EJ eds. *Basic Mechanisms of the EEG*. Boston: Birkhäuser 1993: 145-182 (Fig. 11.6).

Fig. 92 depicts an EEG segment during waking state with pronounced epileptic activity, which appeared to be most impressive in left mesial frontal cortical areas (particularly in the left

SSMA [11/1-2]), but was also observed in electrodes recording from left lateral frontal areas [12/7-8], right mesial [5/2-3] and right lateral [6/6-7] frontal cortical areas.

Occasionally, the dorsomedial thalamic nuclei of both sides [6/1-2 and 12/-2] were also involved, although these thalamic discharges were of much lower amplitude and of less "spiky" appearance. The corticocortical and corticothalamic relationships of these epileptic discharges were quite complex.

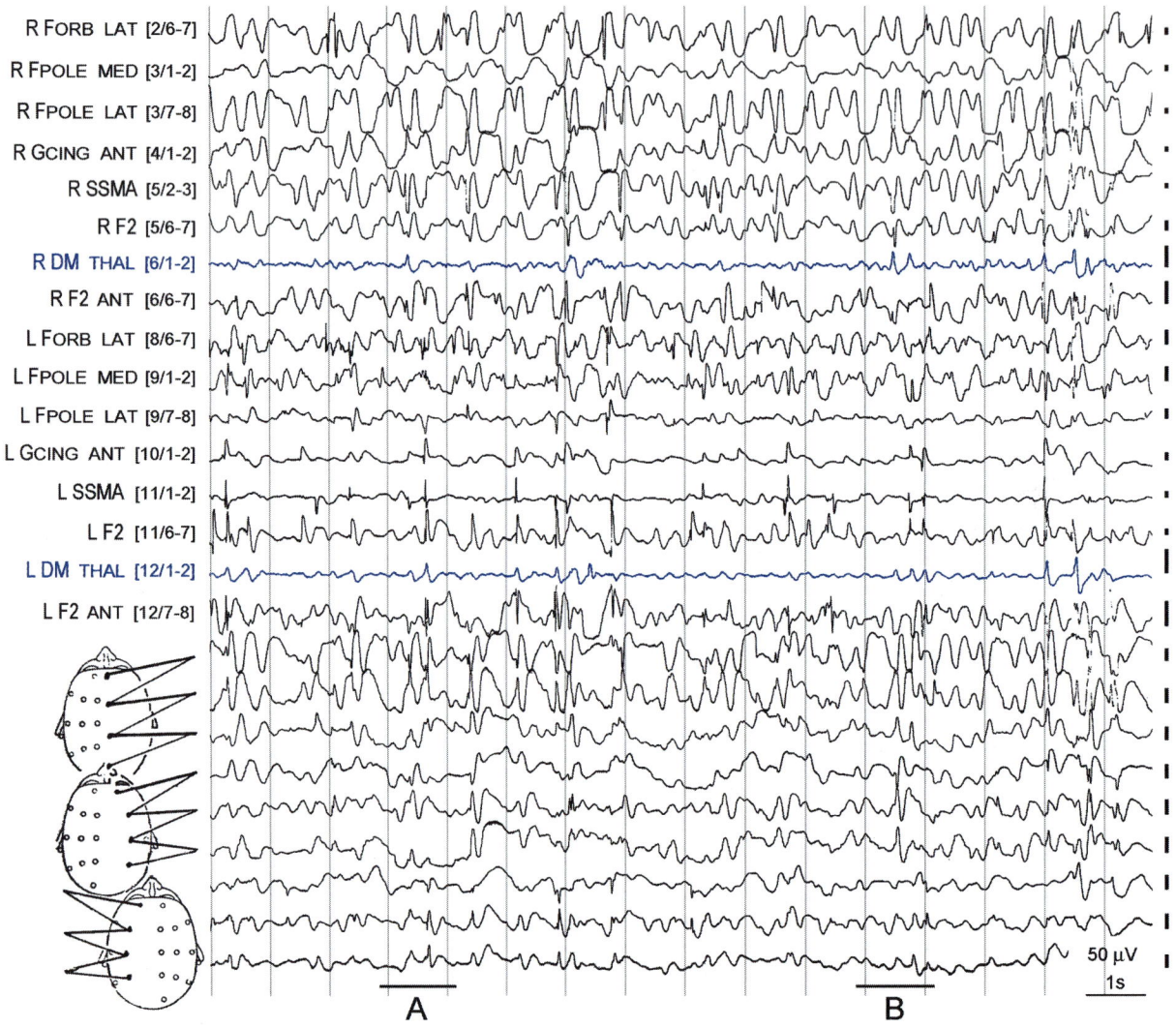

Figure 92. Interictal combined intracerebral (upper traces, channels 1-16) and scalp EEG (lower traces, channels 17-25) during waking state with pronounced epileptic activity.

Selected channels of epoch A and B are shown in Figs. 93 and 94 in greater detail. Note the increased sensitivity of the thalamic recordings in comparison to other intracerebral recording sites (see black bars to the right). Electrode sites were identical to those given in Fig. 90.

Fig. 93 shows nine selected left sided recording channels of a representative epoch (A) of the electrographic recording depicted in Fig. 92 in greater detail.

This epileptic discharge had widespread cortical sources involving mesial [10/1-2 and 11/1-2] and lateral frontal [11/6-7 and 12/7-8] cortical areas.

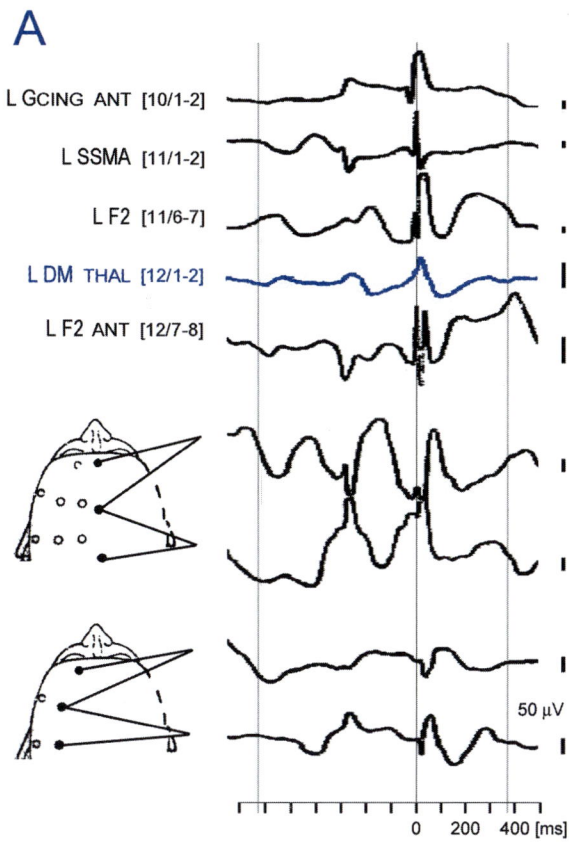

Figure 93. Enlargement of nine selected left sided intracerebral and scalp EEG channels during epoch A of the electrographic recording shown in Fig. 92.

The electrode sites recorded from are identical to those of figure 92 and are indicated left to the traces by anatomical designations (based on the Talairach atlas) and numbers (electrode/contacts).

Although the time resolution and accuracy of this paper recorded EEG may have hampered advanced spatiotemporal analysis, there was nevertheless a clear lag of about 30 ms with respect to the component recorded from the left dorsomedial thalamic nucleus [12/1-2]. Note that the epileptic discharge was also apparent in the scalp EEG recording, where it was discernible as a simultaneous tiny spike in Fz (as expected with a mesial generator) and a more complex deflection with a short lag over the precentral region. The epileptic discharges on the right side were presumably independent and generally of lower amplitude in comparison to the left side. Fig. 94 depicts an enlargement of nine right sided selected recording channels during a representative right hemispheric epileptic discharge (epoch B in Fig. 92). The selected spike was first discernible in the electrode recording from the right SSMA [5/2-3], and subsequently propagated towards lateral frontal cortical areas (peaking in [6/6-7] with a latency of about 30 ms and in [5/6-7] with a latency of about 50 ms) as well as to the ipsilateral dorsomedial thalamic nucleus with a latency of about 50 ms. Note that this medio-lateral delay was also noticed in the scalp EEG recording.

Spontaneous Seizure Activity

Fig. 95 depicts the EEG recording during an absence status epilepticus (formerly known as petit mal status). Clinically, the patient was in a stuporous state. The scalp EEG showed rhythmic spike waves occurring at a rate of about 1.5/s and revealing a bifrontal distribution with a slight predominance of the left side. The intracerebral recordings sites revealed a widespread bifrontal rhythmic epileptic spike wave activity without showing a clear predominance of either hemisphere. It is obvious that the dorsomedial nuclei [6/1-3 and 12/2-3]

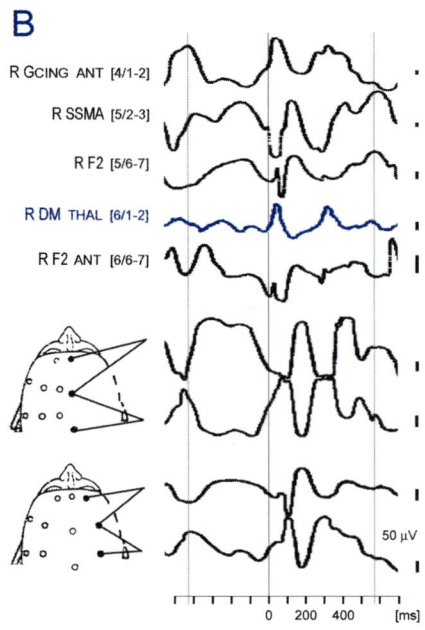

Figure 94. Enlargement of nine selected right sided intracerebral and scalp EEG channels during epoch B of the EEG in Fig. 92.

The electrode sites recorded from are identical to those of Fig. 92 and are indicated left to the traces by anatomical designations (based on the Talairach atlas) and numbers (electrode/contacts).

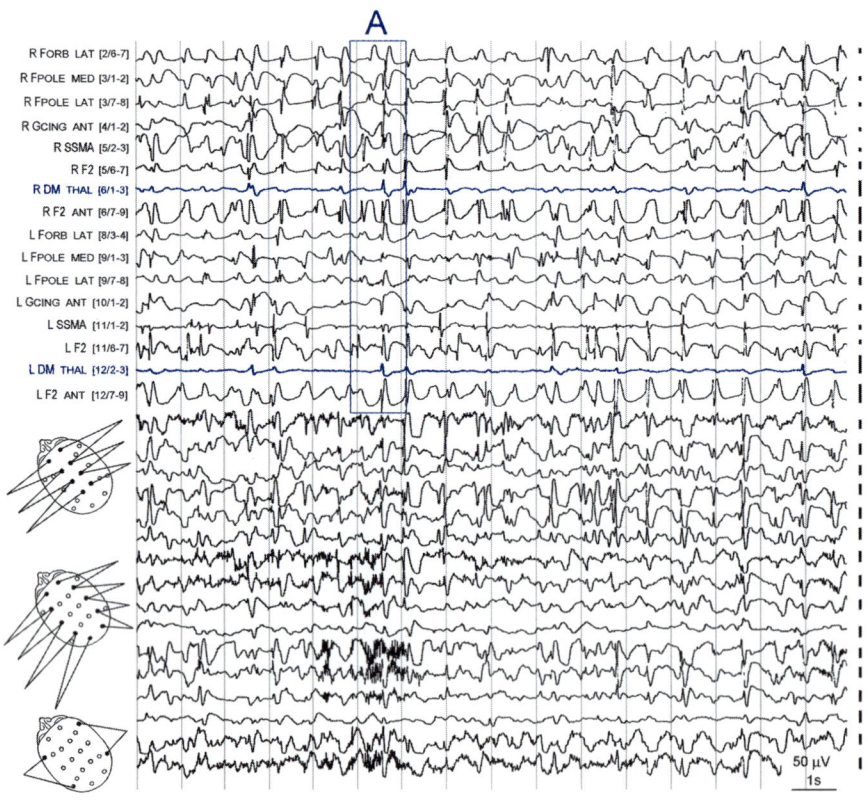

Figure 95. Combined intracerebral and scalp EEG of a petit mal variant status epilepticus. Inlay A is depicted in greater detail in Fig. 96.

Intracerebral electrode sites and assignments are identical to those of Fig. 92, with the exception of channel 16 where electrode 12 was now recording from contacts 7-9 instead of 7-8.

Modified from: Wieser HG, Siegel AM. Relations between the EEG of the cortex, thalamus and periaqueductal gray in patients suffering from epilepsy and pain syndromes. In: Zschocke S, Speckmann EJ eds. *Basic Mechanisms of the EEG*. Boston: Birkhäuser 1993: 145-182 (Fig. 11.5).

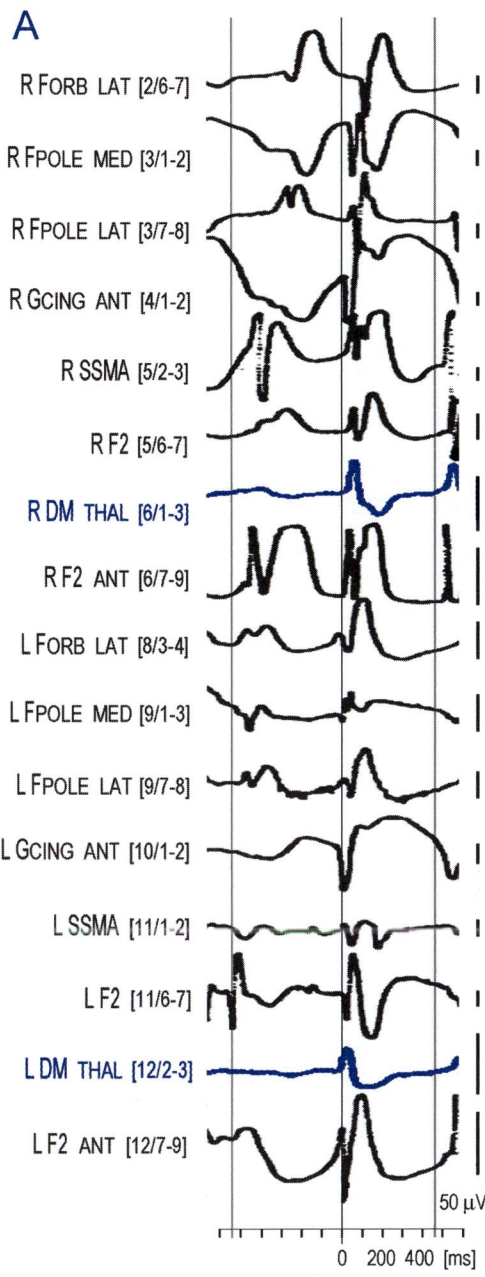

Figure 96. Enlargement of all intracerebral channels during epoch A of the EEG shown in Fig. 95. The electrode sites recorded from are identical to those of Fig. 95.

Modified from: Wieser HG, Siegel AM. Relations between the EEG of the cortex, thalamus and periaqueductal gray in patients suffering from epilepsy and pain syndromes. In: Zschocke S, Speckmann EJ eds. *Basic Mechanisms of the EEG*. Boston: Birkhäuser 1993: 145-182 (Fig. 11.5).

were not directly involved in this seizure activity, but showed interspersed bisynchronous discharges best correlating with the positive deflections recorded from the anterior cingulate gyri [4/1-2 and 10/1-2]. However, it is pertinent to note that this hemispheric bisynchrony was imperfect, as can be seen in the enlargement of epoch A depicted in Fig. 96. With respect to the 1.5/s spike wave seizure activity, the left hemisphere [11/6-7 and 12/7-9] apparently led the right hemisphere [6/7-9 and 5/2-3] by at least 10 to 20 ms. With respect to the thalamic discharges, the initial positive deflection recorded from the left anterior cingulate gyrus [10/1-2] was followed by biphasic potentials in the thalamus, again with the left side leading the right side.

Figs. 97 and 98 depict the EEG recording of a spontaneous habitual tonic seizure with head version to the right and slightly asymmetric tonic posturing.

Case studies

About four seconds before the clinical onset of the seizure, the intracerebral electrode contacts recording from left mesial frontal [10/1-2], left SSMA [11/1-2] and both thalamic sites [6/1-3 and 12/2-3] showed a distinct electrographic flattening. The initial complex consisted of a sharp-slow wave in the left SSMA [11/1-2] that was then followed by a positive deflection in the left anterior cingulate gyrus [10/1-2], biphasic potentials in both dorsomedial thalamic nuclei [12/2-3 and 6/1-3], and, finally, rhythmic 18 Hz spike trains maximally recorded from left anterolateral frontal electrode contacts [11/6-7 and 12/7-9]. The EEG activity subsequently evolved into a generalized seizure pattern of about 53 seconds duration, characterized by progressively increasing amplitudes and decreasing frequencies.

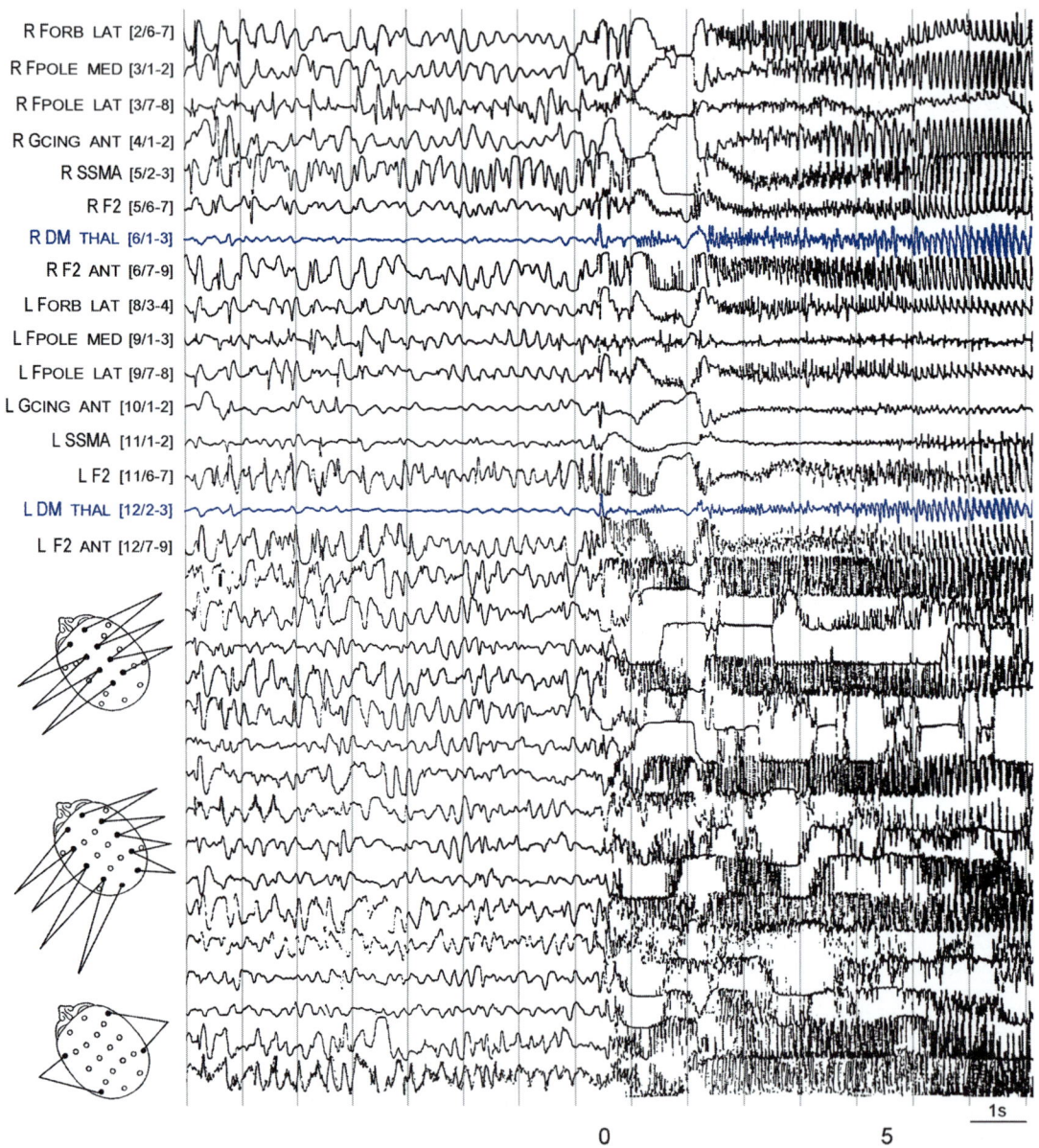

Figure 97. Combined intracerebral (upper traces, channels 1-16) and scalp EEG (lower traces, channels 13-32) recording of a spontaneous habitual tonic seizure. The seizure is continued on the next page (Fig. 98).

Note the increased sensitivity of the thalamic recordings in comparison to other intracerebral recording sites. Electrode sites were identical to those given in Fig. 92, with the exception of channel 16, where electrode 12 was recording from contacts 7-9 instead of 7-8.

Modified from: Wieser HG, Siegel AM. Relations between the EEG of the cortex, thalamus and periaqueductal gray in patients suffering from epilepsy and pain syndromes. In: Zschocke S, Speckmann EJ eds. *Basic Mechanisms of the EEG*. Boston: Birkhäuser 1993: 145-182 (Fig. 11.7).

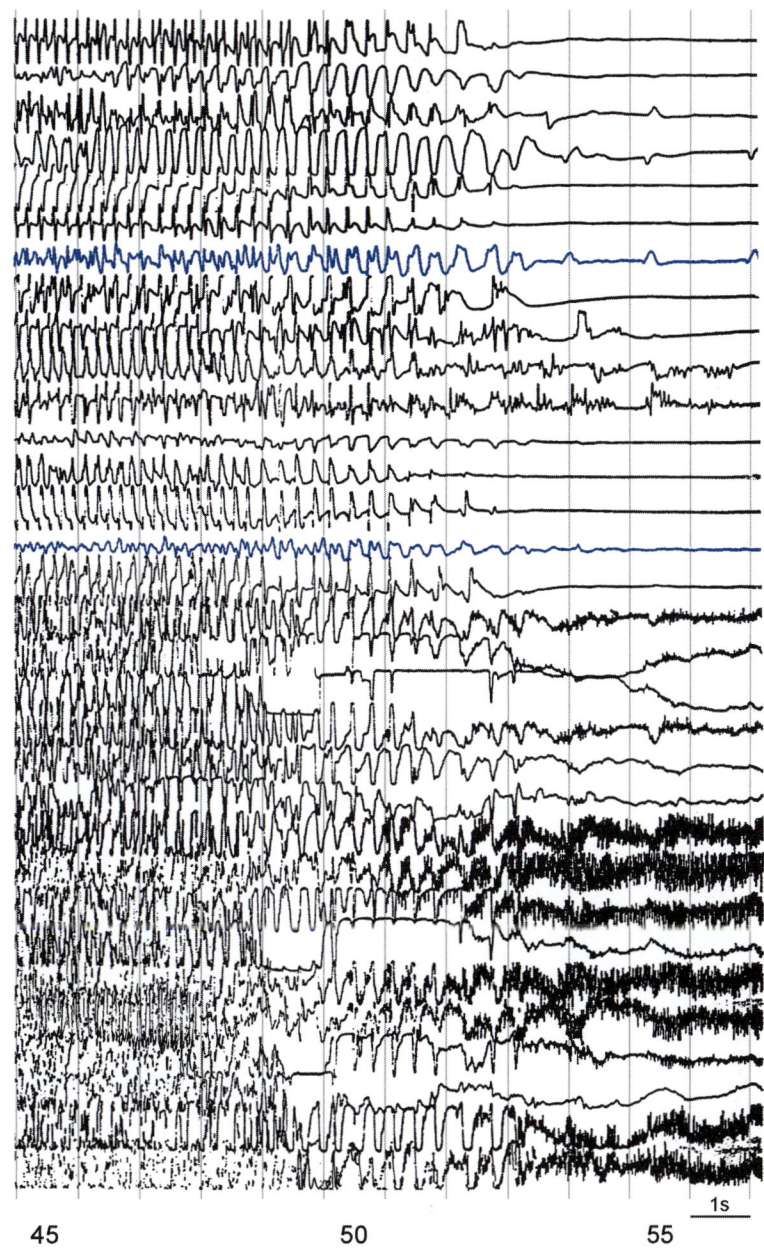

Figure 98. Continuation of the seizure shown in Fig. 97 (note the omission of 38 seconds between the two EEG segments shown in Figs. 97 and 98).
Electrode sites were identical to Fig. 97.
Modified from: Wieser HG, Siegel AM. Relations between the EEG of the cortex, thalamus and periaqueductal gray in patients suffering from epilepsy and pain syndromes. In: Zschocke S, Speckmann EJ eds. *Basic Mechanisms of the EEG*. Boston: Birkhäuser 1993: 145-182 (Fig. 11.7).

Single Pulse Stimulation

ERs following electrical 1 Hz single pulse stimulation have been extensively studied in this patient. Special emphasis was put on the functional relationship between the SSMA and other cortical or subcortical areas. Fig. 99 presents an overview of all stimulations applied in this patient. Figs. 100 to 103 depict selected ERs in greater detail. Following stimulation of the left dorsomedial thalamic nucleus [12/2-3], the ERs recorded from orbitofrontal cortical areas were most impressive (Fig. 100, left). The electrode recording from an area corresponding to Brodmann area 11 [8/3-4] revealed two early negative peaks with latencies of 20 and 50 ms, followed by a broader negative component peaking at about 190 ms post stimulus. The early

Case studies

negative deflections recorded from the lateral orbital region (corresponding to the lateral parts of Brodmann area 11 or 47) were of lower amplitude and showed latencies of 15, 30 and 80 ms. The ensuing slow potential was peaking at about 195 ms post stimulus. ERs recorded from other sites, including the anterior cingulate gryus [10/1-2] or more rostral mesial frontal areas [9/1-3], were less distinctive (Fig. 101). The ERs recorded from the SSMA following

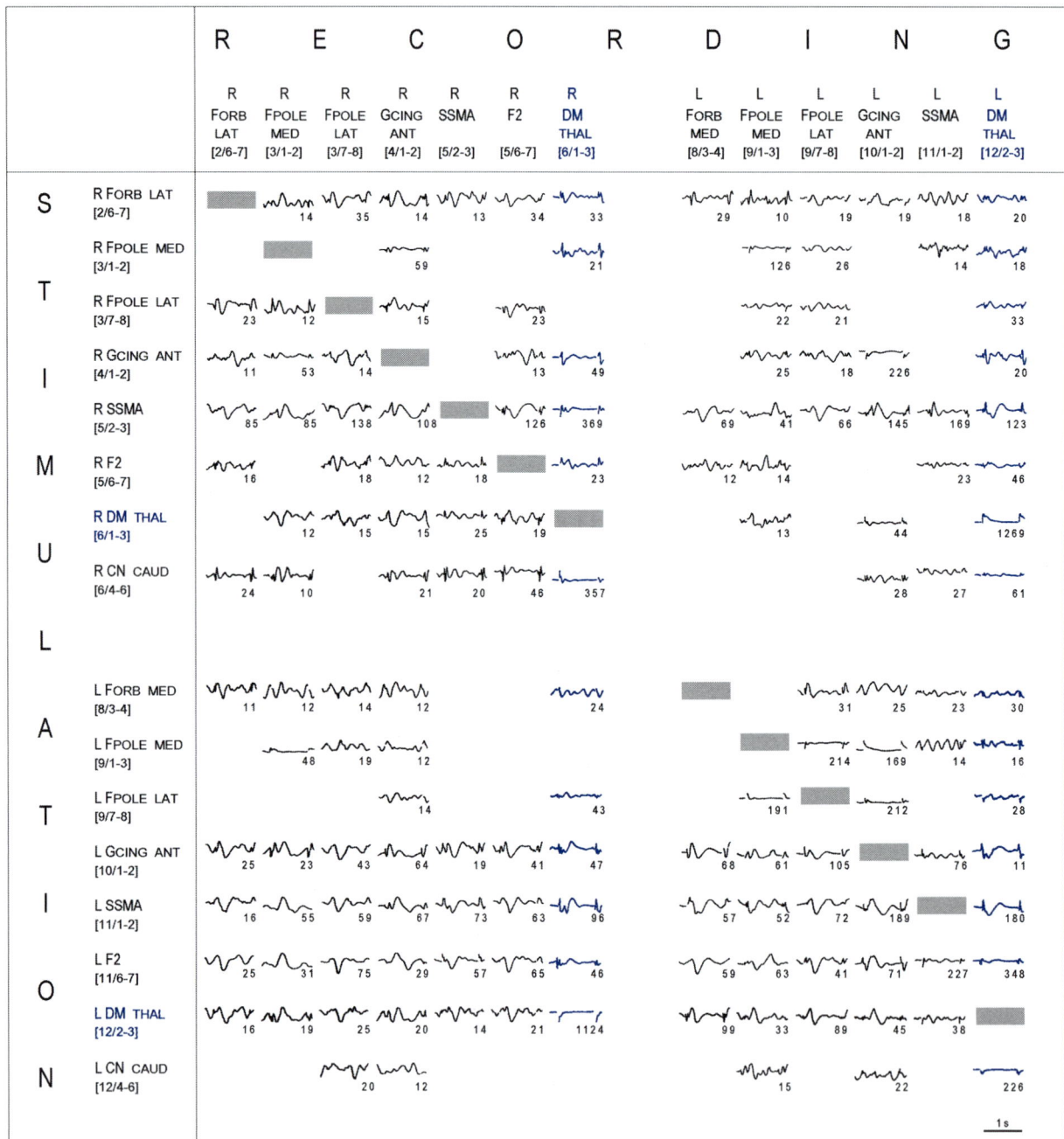

Figure 99. Overview of averaged cortical and subcortical ERs following intracerebral stimulation of various sites.

Sequential stimulation sites are listed vertically, and recording sites are indicated horizontally. Stimuli consisted of 1 Hz single pulses (10 V, 0.7 ms). All ERs in this figure are averages of 117 individual ERs. The ERs are depicted using a time window going from − 192 ms to + 1,136 ms. The small numbers next to the ERs represent the amplitude quotient, indicating the ratio between the amplitude of the ER and the amplitude of the averaged EEG multiplied by factor 10. Empty cells denote no recording or artifactual recordings.

Forb, frontoorbital; **Fpole**, frontal pole; **Gcing**, cingulate gyrus; **SSMA**, supplementary sensorimotor area; **F2**, middle frontal gyrus; **DM thal**, dorsomedial thalamic nucleus; **lat**, lateral; **med**, medial; **ant**, anterior; **R**, right; **L**, left.

thalamic stimulation were quite small, too (Fig. 102). In contrast, stimulation of the SSMA [5/2-3 and 11/1-2] caused marked ERs in the dorsomedial thalamic nuclei (Figs. 100 (right) and 103). The amplitudes of these ERs were about 5 to 10 times higher, if compared to the ERs discussed above. The ipsilateral ER consisted of a marked triphasic potential with a positive component peaking at about 30 ms, a negative component peaking at about 60 ms, and a broader W-shaped positive deflection peaking at about 250 ms post stimulus.

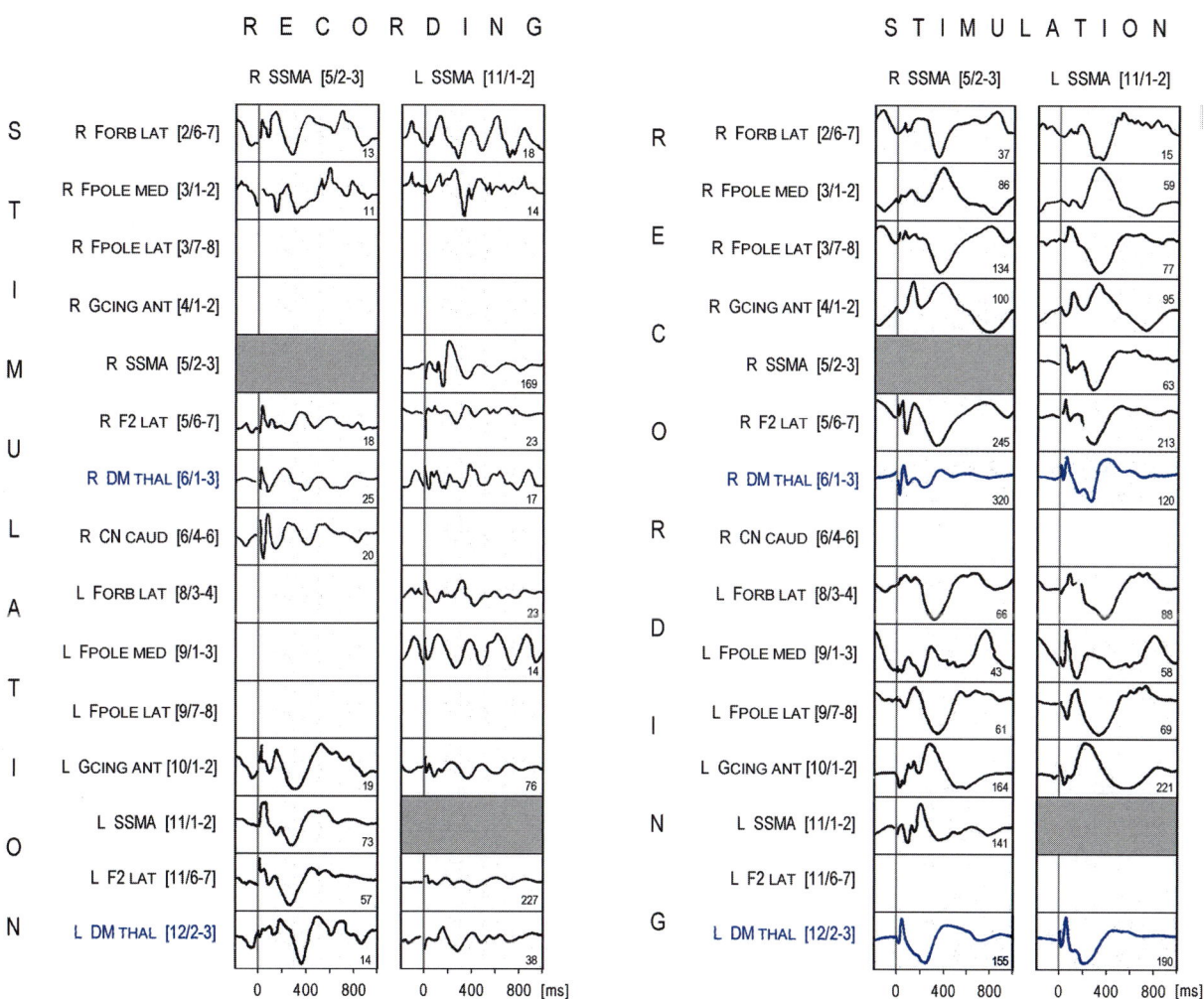

Figure 100. Averaged cortical and subcortical ERs following intracerebral stimulation of various sites.

Sequential stimulation sites are listed vertically, and recording sites are indicated horizontally (left part of the figure) and vice versa (right part of the figure). Stimuli consisted of 1 Hz single pulses (10 V, 0.7 ms). All ERs in this figure are averages of 117 individual ERs. The ERs are shown using a time window going from − 192 ms to + 1,136 ms. The small numbers next to the ERs represent the amplitude quotient, indicating the ratio between the amplitude of the ER and the amplitude of the averaged EEG multiplied by factor 10. Empty cells denote no recording or artifactual recordings.

Forb, frontoorbital; **Fpole**, frontal pole; **Gcing**, cingulate gyrus; **SSMA**, supplementary sensorimotor area; **F2**, middle frontal gyrus; **DM thal**, dorsomedial thalamic nucleus; **lat**, lateral; **med**, medial; **ant**, anterior; **R**, right; **L**, left.

The right part of the figure is modified from: Wieser HG, Siegel AM. Relations between the EEG of the cortex, thalamus and periaqueductal gray in patients suffering from epilepsy and pain syndromes. In: Zschocke S, Speckmann EJ eds. *Basic Mechanisms of the EEG.* Boston: Birkhäuser 1993: 145-182 (Fig. 11.9).

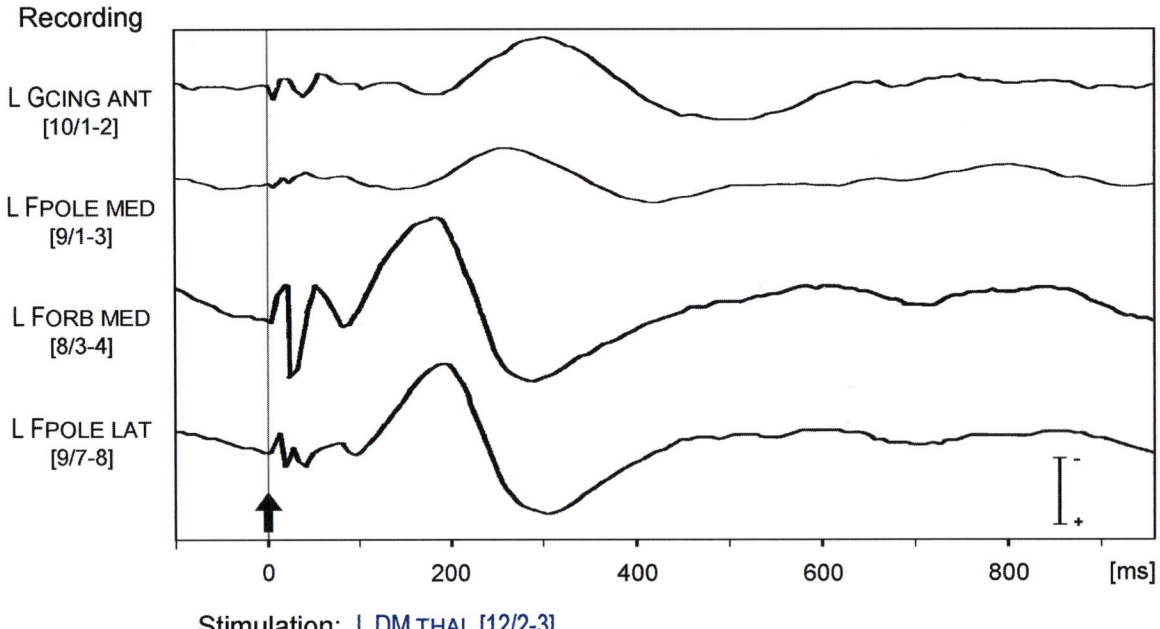

Figure 101. Averaged ERs (n = 122) following intracerebral stimulation of the left dorsomedial thalamic nucleus [12/2-3].

Stimuli were 1 Hz single pulses (10 V, 0.7 ms). The amplitude scales of the ERs were equally adjusted for all traces. GCING, cingulate gyrus; FPOLE, frontal pole; FORB, frontoorbital; ANT, anterior; MED, medial; LAT, lateral; L, left.

Modified from: Wieser HG, Siegel AM. Relations between the EEG of the cortex, thalamus and periaqueductal gray in patients suffering from epilepsy and pain syndromes. In: Zschocke S, Speckmann EJ eds. *Basic Mechanisms of the EEG*. Boston: Birkhäuser 1993: 145-182 (Fig. 11.8).

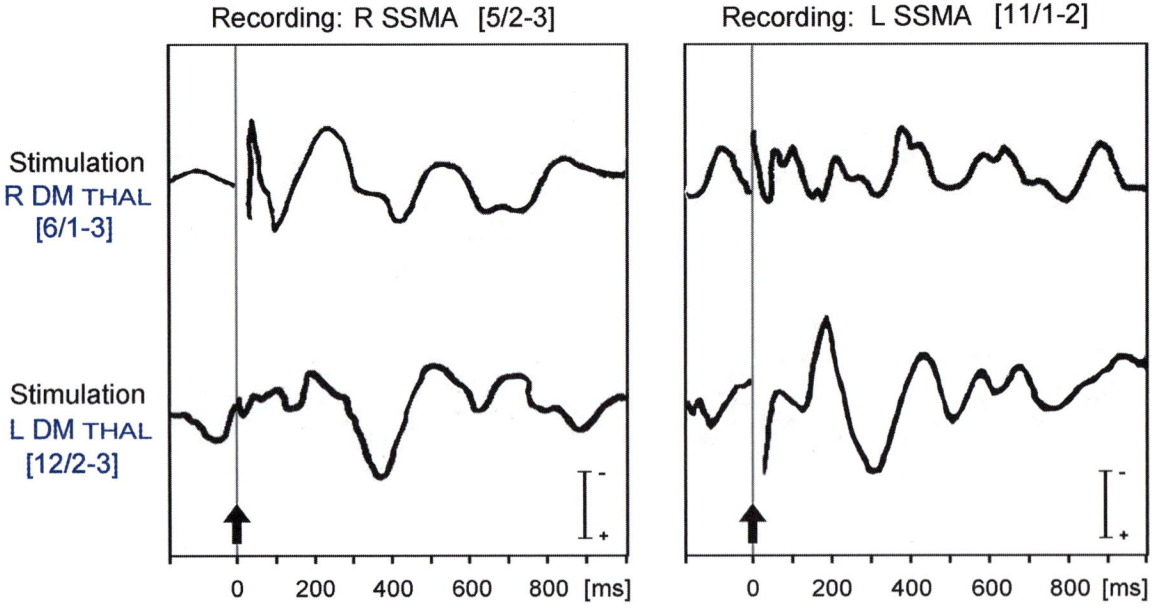

Figure 102. Averaged ERs (n = 122) recording from both SSMA [5/2-3 and 11/1-2] following sequential subcortical stimulation of the dorsomedial thalamic nuclei (DM THAL) [6/1-3, 12/2-3].

Stimuli were 1 Hz single pulses (10 V, 0.7 ms). The amplitude scales of the ERs were equally adjusted for all traces. Note that these ERs were of much lower amplitude and also appeared to be less reproducible in comparison to the ERs shown in Fig. 103. R, right; L, left.

Modified from: Wieser HG, Siegel AM. Relations between the EEG of the cortex, thalamus and periaqueductal gray in patients suffering from epilepsy and pain syndromes. In: Zschocke S, Speckmann EJ eds. *Basic Mechanisms of the EEG*. Boston: Birkhäuser 1993: 145-182 (Fig. 11.9).

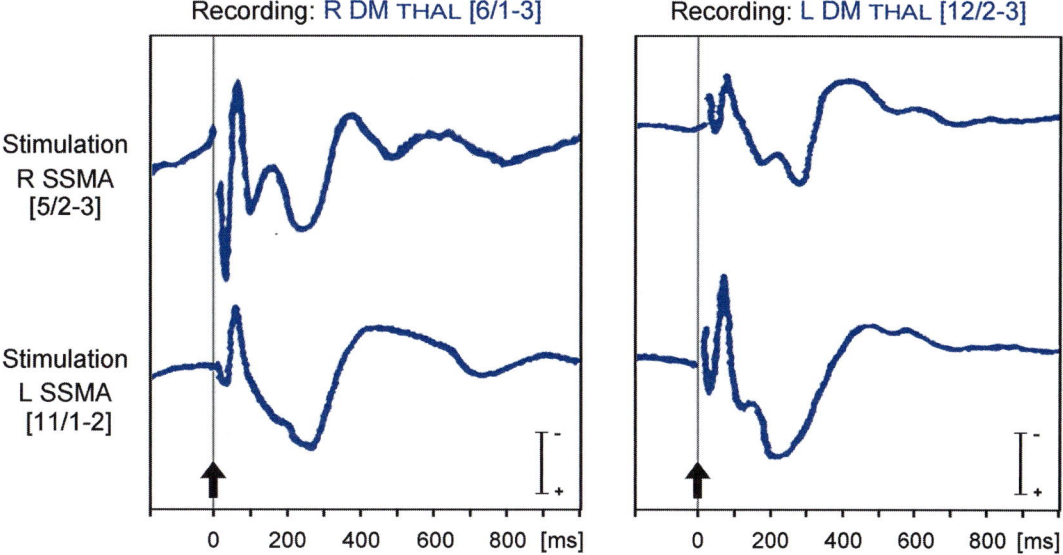

Figure 103. Averaged ERs (n=122) recorded from both dorsomedial thalamic nuclei (DM THAL) [6/1-3 and 12/2-3] following sequential cortical stimulation of the right and left SSMA [5/2-3 and 11/1-2].

Stimuli were 1 Hz single pulses (10 V, 0.7 ms). The amplitude scales of the ERs were equally adjusted for all traces. Note that these ERs were of much higher amplitude than the ERs shown in Fig. 102. **R**, right; **L**, left.

Modified from: Wieser H, Siegel AM. Relations between the EEG of the cortex, thalamus and periaqueductal gray in patients suffering from epilepsy and pain syndromes. In: Zschocke S, Speckmann EJ eds. *Basic Mechanisms of the EEG*. Boston: Birkhäuser 1993: 145-182 (Fig. 11.9).

Summary

This case illustrates bilateral recordings and stimulations of the DM in a patient with tonic seizures originating in (or propagating early to) the left SSMA. During the waking state, occasional interictal epileptic discharges were independently recorded from the DM of both sides. These discharges best corresponded with discharges recorded from the anterior cingulate gyri, with the cortical sites generally leading the thalamic nuclei by about 30 to 50 ms, and with the left side obviously leading the right side. During night sleep, epileptic activity was slightly enhanced, both within thalamic and cortical structures. During an absence status epilepticus, the DM remained virtually unaffected, although the synchrony between the left and right side of the DM might have been enhanced to some extent. In contrast, the dorsomedial nuclei became obviously involved during a spontaneous habitual tonic seizure, by clearly revealing a flattening of EEG activity that occurred several seconds before the clinical onset of the seizure, and by progressively and synchronously participating in the emerging generalized seizure activity. With repetitive 1 Hz single pulse stimulation of the dorsomedial nuclei, we could demonstrate clear cut ERs in cortical areas that are well known to be reciprocally connected with the DM, namely in Brodmann areas 11 and 47 (these areas are virtually "hardwired", with the posterior aspects of the DM; area 11 with the medial part and area 47 with the lateral part, according to Hassler [1982]). The largest ERs in the DM could be recorded with repetitive 1 Hz single pulse stimulation of the ipsilateral SSMA.

Case 7

Patient History

This 20 year-old man with intractable epilepsy had frequent convulsive ("grand mal") and nonconvulsive ("absences") seizures since age 6, occurring with ever increasing frequency of up to 25 per day despite medical treatment with various AEDs including phenobarbital, levopropylhexedrine (Maliasin®), valproic acid and diazepam. Pregnancy was uneventful but his birth was complicated by fetal distress requiring forceps delivery. Neonatal and childhood development were normal, with the exception of several febrile seizures during early childhood. There was no history of epilepsy in the family. The EEG during absence seizures showed a typical petit mal variant pattern (that is, 2.5 to 3 Hz sharp slow wave or spike wave) with a predominance over the left frontoparietal region. The neuropsychological examination revealed a left frontal lobe dysfunction. The neuroradiological examination under stereotactic conditions revealed no abnormality.

SEEG Exploration

Based on the hypothesis of a left frontal seizure origin, chronic SEEG was carried out with 14 depth electrodes at age 20, with electrodes 7 and 14 located in the dorsomedial nuclei of both thalami (Fig. 104). The exploration revealed multiple, badly delineated regional maxima of epileptogenicity with a left frontal predominance. The epileptiform discharges recorded from intracerebral frontal sites correlated with the slow waves in scalp and thalamic EEG recordings. During slow wave sleep, the activity of the DM was highly correlated and displayed activity resembling K-complexes with superposed slow (6.5 Hz) spindle-like activity.

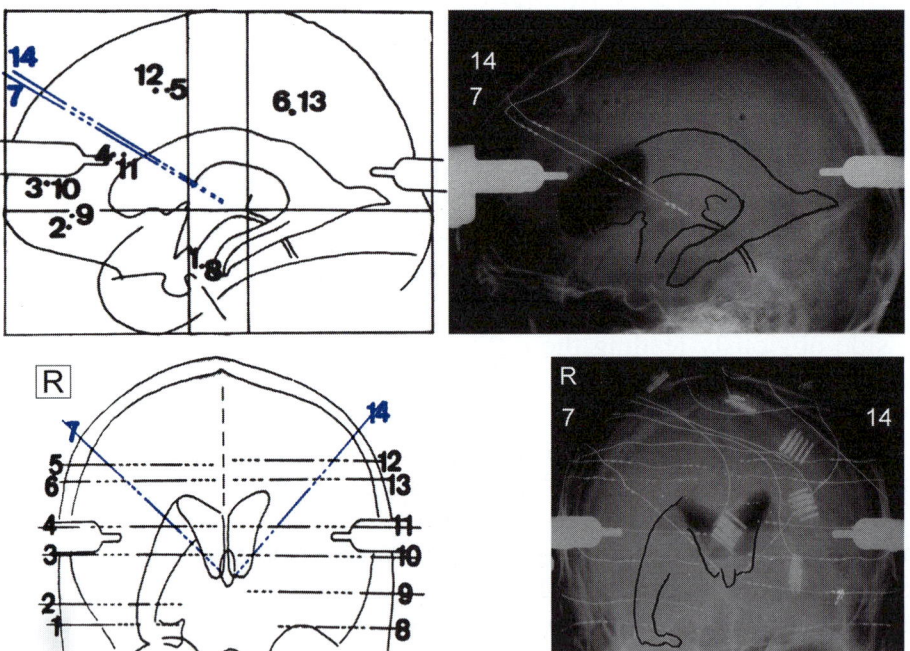

Figure 104. Location of depth electrodes and corresponding x-ray (repérage) in the proportional Talairach system.

The deepest contacts of electrodes 7 and 14 (contacts 1-2) were in the dorsomedial nuclei of the thalami. Note that electrodes 7 and 14 have differently grouped contacts, with larger intercontact spacing between contacts 3 and 4 and contacts 5 and 6.

Surgery

The performance of an anterior callosotomy was considered but rejected.

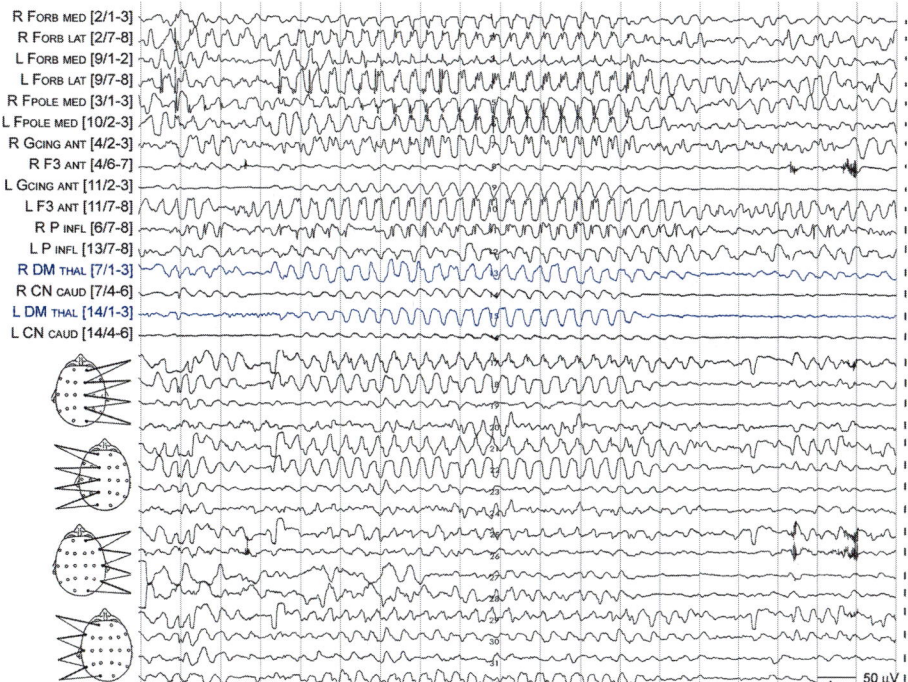

Figure 105. Petit mal variant like pattern, recorded simultaneously from frontal and parietal cortical areas (channels 1-12), dorsomedial nuclei of the thalami [7/1-3 and 14/1-3], caput nuclei caudati [7/4-6 and 14/4-6], and the scalp (channels 17-32).

Scalp electrodes were located according to the Hess system, as indicated in the sketches. The electrode sites recorded from are indicated left to the traces by anatomical designations (based on the Talairach atlas) and numbers (electrode/contacts, cf. Fig. 104).
Forb, frontal orbital; **Fpole**, frontal pole; **Gcing**, cingulate gyrus; **F3**, inferior frontal gyrus; **P infl**, parietal inferior lobule; **DM thal**, dorsomedial nucleus of the thalamus; **CN caud**, head of the caudate nucleus; **ANT**, anterior; **MED**, medial; **LAT**, lateral; **R**, right; **L**, left.

Modified from: Wieser HG, Siegel AM. Relations between the EEG of the cortex, thalamus and periaqueductal gray in patients suffering from epilepsy and pain syndromes. In: Zschocke S, Speckmann EJ eds. *Basic Mechanisms of the EEG*. Boston: Birkhäuser 1993: 145-182 (Fig. 11-2).

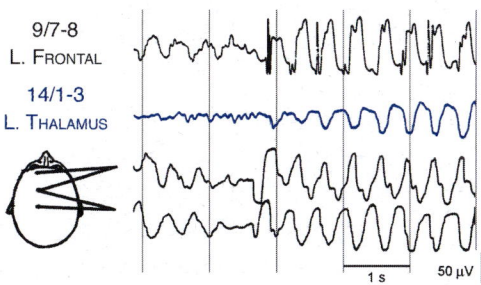

Figure 106. Enlarged detail of Fig. 105 showing the left frontal recorded spike waves [9/7-8] correlating with slow waves of the scalp EEG and the recording from the left dorsomedial nucleus of the thalamus [14/1-3].

Note that the slow waves of the thalamus were of opposite polarity to the slow waves of the frontal cortex (most likely reflecting the positive ending of a cortically generated dipole) and exhibited a crescendo-like increase in amplitude.

Modified from: Wieser HG, Siegel AM. Relations between the EEG of the cortex, thalamus and periaqueductal gray in patients suffering from epilepsy and pain syndromes. In: Zschocke S, Speckmann EJ eds. *Basic Mechanisms of the EEG*. Boston: Birkhäuser 1993: 145-182 (Fig. 11-2).

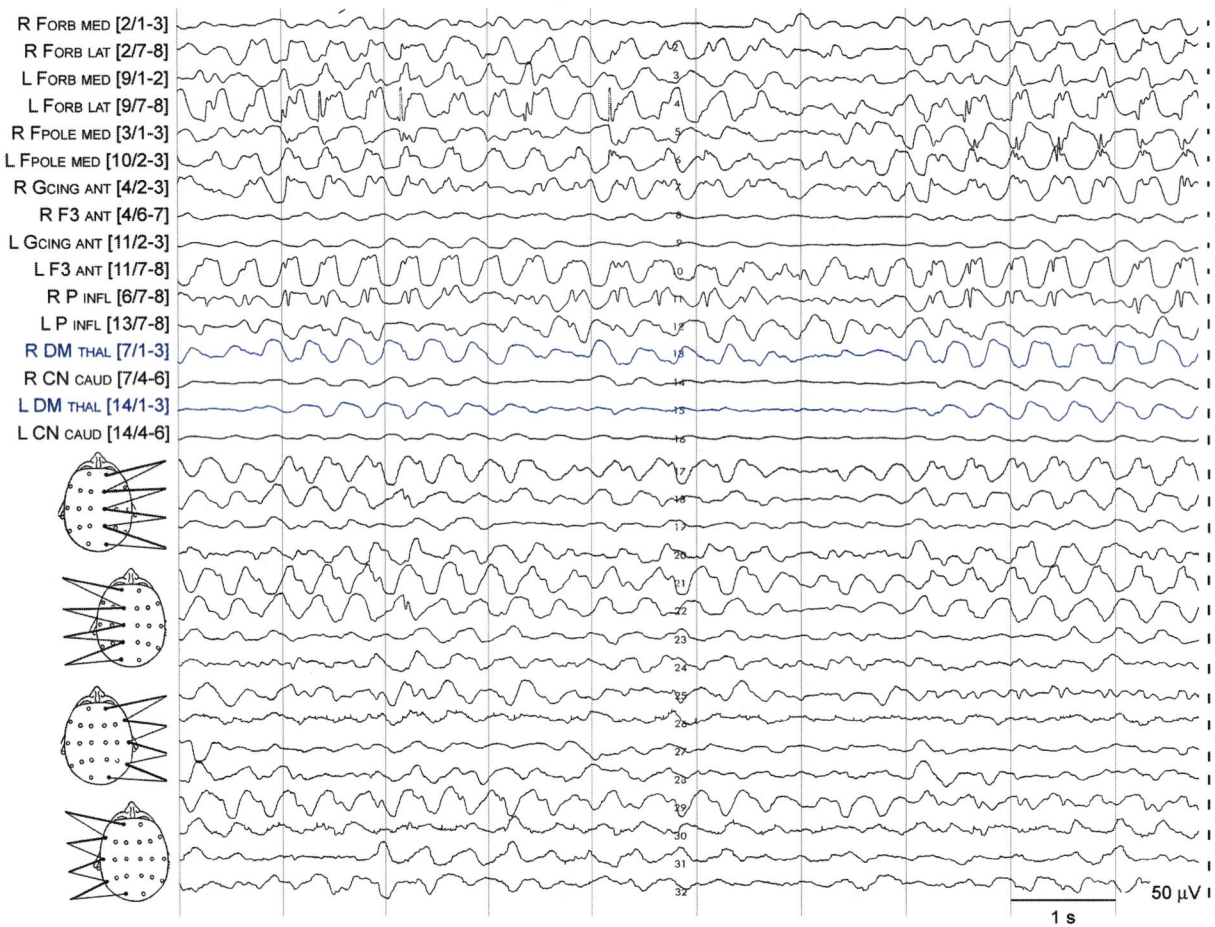

Figure 107. Another example of a petit mal variant like pattern, recorded simultaneously from frontal and parietal cortical areas (channels 1-12), dorsomedial nuclei of the thalami [7/1-3 and 14/1-3], caput nuclei caudati [7/4-6 and 14/4-6], and the scalp (channels 17-32).

Note the spike-waves and the notched waves in the frontal cortical areas [9/7-8], [6/7-8] and [11/7-8], together with the corresponding sinusoidal delta rhythms of opposite polarity in thalamic recordings [14/1-3]. Electrode sites were identical to Fig. 105.

Summary

The case of this patient with presumed frontal lobe epilepsy characterized by a petit mal variant EEG pattern with predominance over left frontal regions is interesting because of the bilateral depth electrode recordings from both dorsomedial thalamic nuclei. The SEEG exploration revealed multiple badly delineated regional maxima of epileptogenicity within frontal cortical areas, with a clear predominance of the left side. The left frontoorbital rhythmic spike wave complexes were in evident synchrony with slow waves recorded from thalamic sites with opposite polarity, but, unlike the frontoorbital discharges, the thalamic slow waves comprised no clear-cut spikes preceding the slow wave. We suggest that these thalamic slow waves may most likely be attributably to the positive ending of a cortically generated dipole. During slow wave sleep, the dorsomedial thalamic nuclei highly correlated to slow wave activity with superimposed 6.5 Hz spindle-like activity recorded in cortical areas, evidently resembling K-complexes.

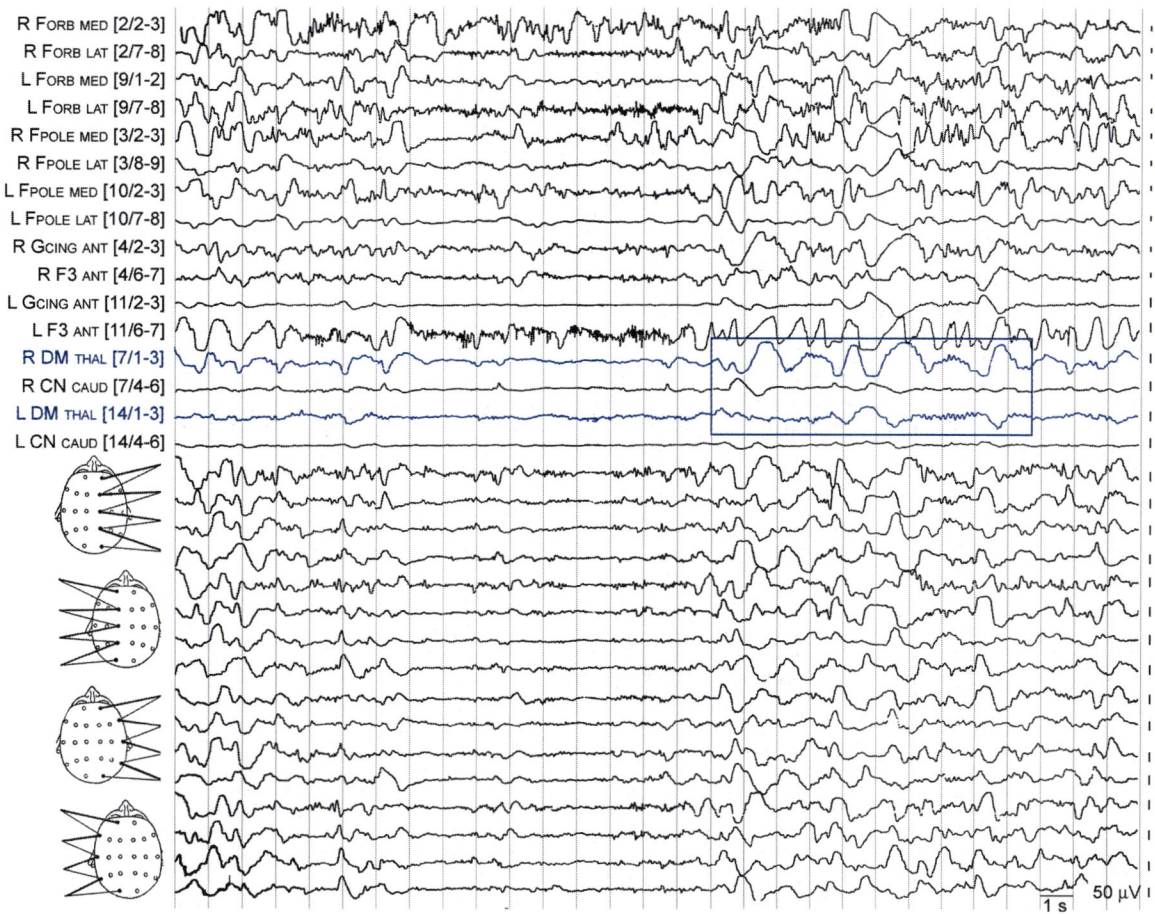

Figure 108. Simultaneous depth and scalp EEG recording during slow wave sleep.

Both dorsomedial thalamic nuclei showed high-amplitude slow waves (of more or less opposite polarity) with superimposed 6.5 Hz spindle-like activity (blue box). These complexes were also seen in the corresponding mesial frontal cortical areas with the same polarity (right and left anterior cingulate gyri, [4/2-3] and [11/2-3]). They evidently resembled K-complexes. Electrode sites were identical to Fig. 105.

Case 8

Patient History

This 13 year-old boy had epilepsia partialis continua (EPC) of the right side due to presumptive left Rasmussen's encephalitis. Pregnancy, birth, neonatal and childhood development were normal. He had no family history of epilepsy. At age 6, he suffered from recurrent tonsillitis and subsequently developed behavioral changes (reportedly "fearful" and "somewhat changed and less bright") and right clonic jerks starting at the face and evolving into the full clinical picture of EPC within days. Penicillin and diazepam were administered and a tonsillectomy was performed. After initiation of antiepileptic medical treatment with carbamazepine, phenytoin and primidone, there was a slight improvement but no cessation of EPC. At age 8, he had focal motor seizures of the Jacksonian type and frequent generalized seizures. The EEG showed a progressive slowing over the left anterior region. His neurological examination, cerebrospinal fluid and CT scan were normal. At age 13, he presented to our hospital with rhythmic cloni of the right periorbital and perioral muscles, and, to a lesser extent, also of the tongue, the oropharynx and the platysma. Neurological examination then demonstrated a mild right spastic hemiparesis with predominant paresis of the right hand. There was a left ventricular enlargement in the pneumencephalogram. Neuropsychological examination showed an

IQ of 85, with a verbal score of 76. The diagnosis of Rasmussen's encephalitis was made on electroclinical grounds (histology was not available).

SEEG

Chronic SEEG with 9 depth electrodes was carried out at age 13. At the end of the exploration (day 8), acute thalamic recordings were performed using a so called wing electrode ("Seitenelektrode") whose tip was located in the left ventrolateral thalamus (Fig. 109). The spontaneous seizures and interictal epileptiform activity of this patient originated in widespread left hemispheric cortical structures, predominantly from sensory and motor cortical areas of the face and hand region. Yet, acute thalamic recordings revealed no clear epileptiform discharges clearly related to spontaneous epileptic myclonus. Electrical 5 Hz train stimulation of the left ventrolateral thalamus elicited ERs in the left sensory and motor hand area. Stimulation of the left posterior ventro-oral nucleus in close proximity to the capsula interna produced positive motor effects clinically. Marked vegetative effects were elicited with thalamic stimulation when the stimulating electrode was referenced against the right ear.

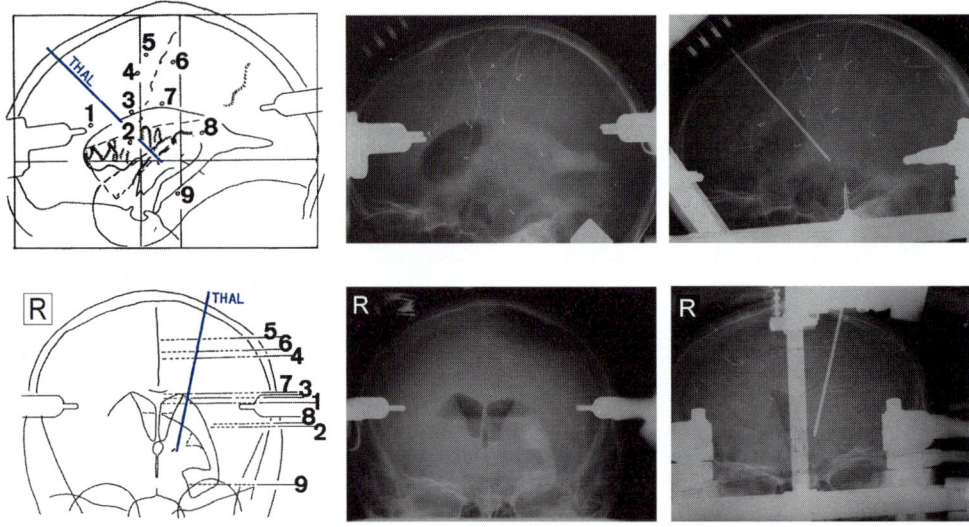

Figure 109. Location of depth electrodes and corresponding x-rays (repérage) in the proportional Talairach system.

Acute insertion of a bipolar stereotactic wing electrode ("Seitenelektrode") into the left ventrolateral thalamus, with its tip presumably located in or next to the anterior and posterior ventro-oral nucleus.

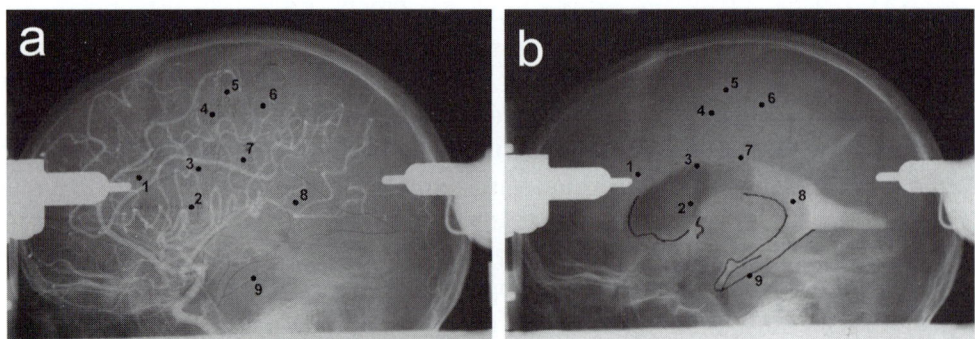

Figure 110. Lateral x-rays (repérage) showing the position of the 9 depth electrodes in relation to the left middle cerebral artery (a, arteriography) and the ventricle (b, ventriculography).

Note that the thalamic wing electrode ("Seitenelektrode") is not depicted, because it was not inserted before the end of the SEEG exploration.

Surgery

A stereotactic high frequency thermocoagulation was performed in the left ventrolateral thalamus (more specifically, in the anterior and posterior ventro-oral nucleus) before removal of all depth electrodes and the wing electrode. Hemispherectomy or other resective surgery was not performed. Therefore, histological examination was not obtainable.

Outcome

There was a transitory improvement of myoclonia and scalp EEG findings following thermocoagulation. The further course of the disease was characterized by a slowly progressive stepwise neurological deterioration of right sided motor function. At age 39, seizure exacerbation with status-like clusters of partial motor seizures of the right side resulted in admission to the intensive care unit. Neurological examination demonstrated a severe right hemiparesis, a right homonymous hemianopsia, dysarthria and dysnomia.

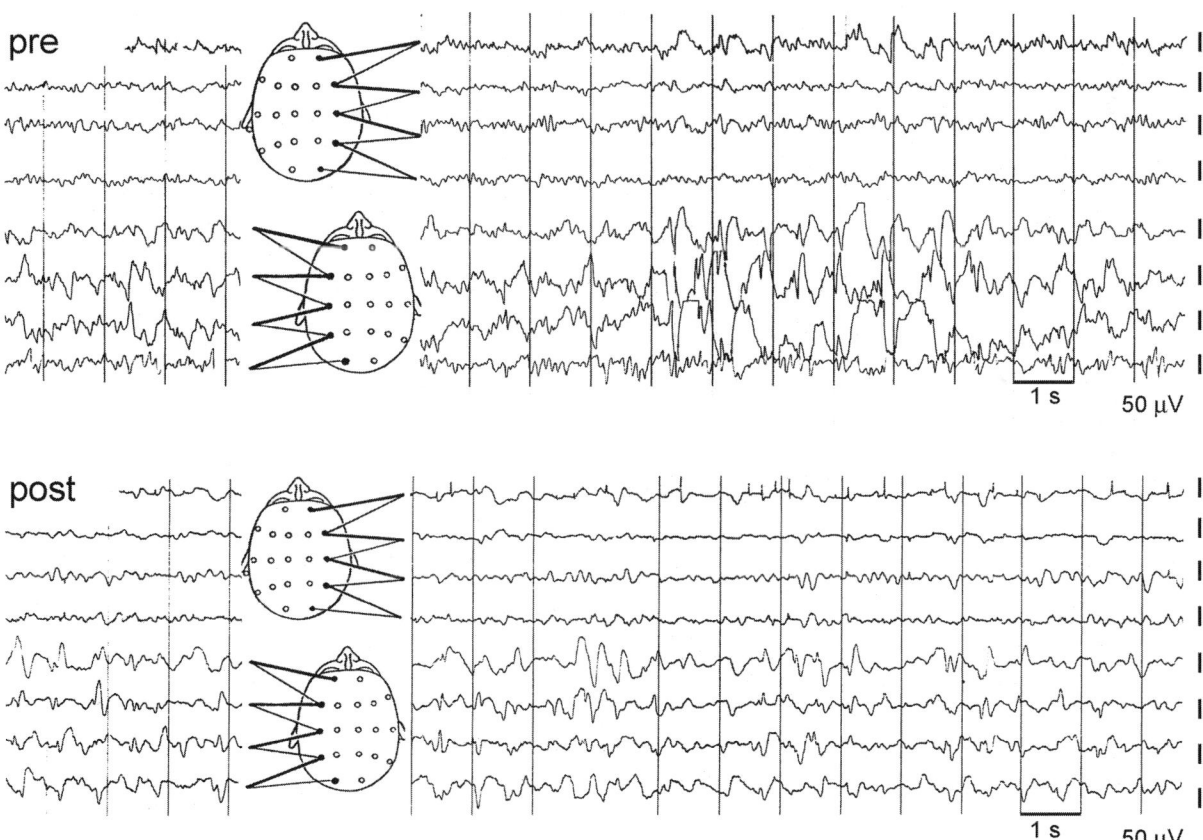

Figure 111. Comparison of scalp EEG before and after thermocoagulation in the left ventrolateral thalamus.

PRE: The scalp EEG recording (electrodes placed according to the Hess scheme) 4 months before the performance of a thermocoagulation in the left ventrolateral thalamus showed a left frontocentral slowing with intermingled spike waves and sharp-slow waves.

POST: Representative scalp EEG recording 3 days after thermocoagulation, showing a reduction of epileptiform activity, in concordance with the transitory clinical improvement of the patient.

Modified from: Wieser HG, Siegel AM. Relations between the EEG of the cortex, thalamus and periaqueductal gray in patients suffering from epilepsy and pain syndromes. In: Zschocke S, Speckmann EJ eds. Basic Mechanisms of the EEG. Boston: Birkhäuser 1993: 145-182 (Fig. 11.16).

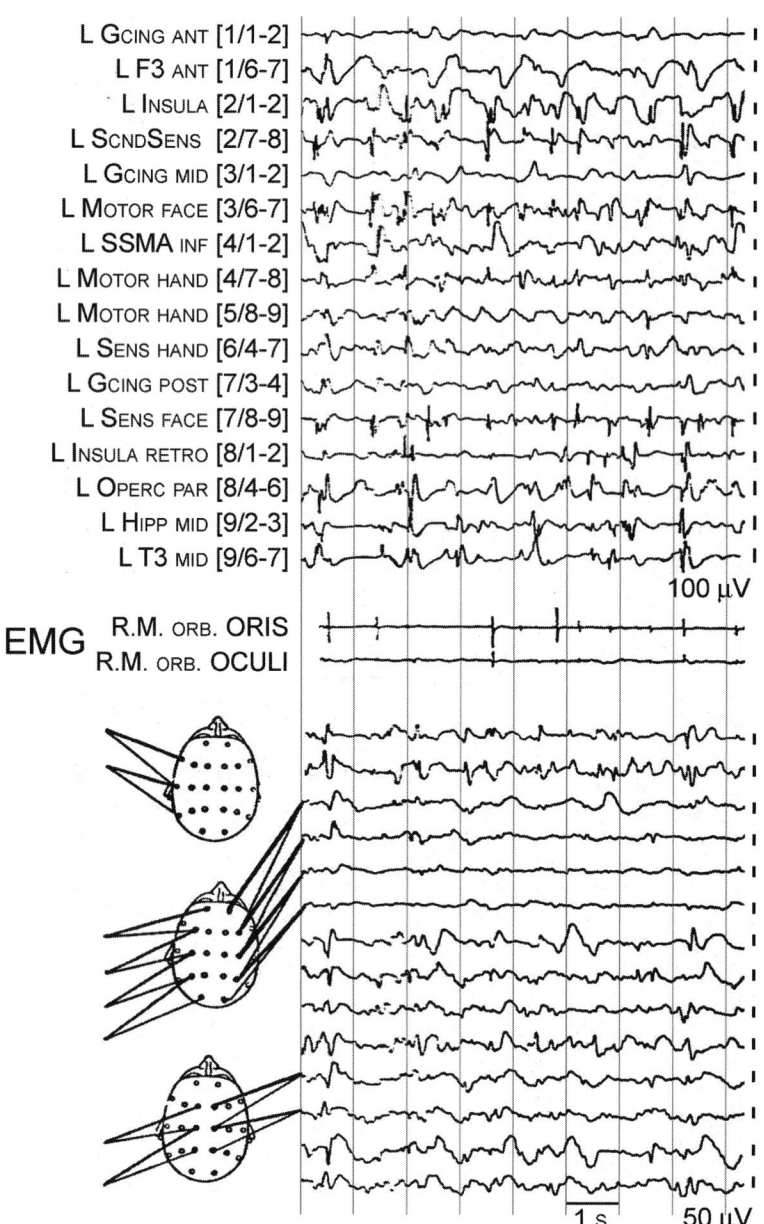

Figure 112. Combined depth/scalp EEG and electromyographic (EMG) recording showing the correlation between depth EEG spikes and myoclonic jerks of the right face.

A selection of relevant recording sites is depicted in Fig. 113 in greater detail. The electrode sites recorded from are indicated left to the traces by anatomical designations (based on the Talairach atlas) and numbers (electrode/contacts, cf. Fig. 109).

GCING, cingulate gyrus; **F3**, inferior frontal gyrus; **SCNDSENS**, secondary sensory area, **MOTOR FACE**, motor face area; **SSMA**, supplementary sensorimotor area; **MOTOR HAND**, motor hand area; **SENS HAND**, sensory hand area; **SENS FACE**, sensory face area; **INSULA RETRO**, retroinsular region; **OPERC PAR**, parietal opercular area; **HIPP**, hippocampus; **T3**, inferior temporal gyrus; **ANT**, anterior, **MID**, medial; **L**, left; **R.M. ORB. ORIS**, right oral muscle; **R.M. ORB. OCULI**, right ocular orbicular muscle.

Modified from: Wieser HG. Stereoelectroencephalographic correlates of focal motor seizures. In: Speckmann EJ, Elger CE eds. *Epilepsy and Motor System*. Baltimore: Urban and Schwarzenberg 1983b: 287-309 (Fig. 3) and from: Wieser HG, Siegel AM. Relations between the EEG of the cortex, thalamus and periaqueductal gray in patients suffering from epilepsy and pain syndromes. In: Zschocke S, Speckmann EJ eds. *Basic Mechanisms of the EEG*. Boston: Birkhäuser 1993: 145-182 (Fig. 11.15).

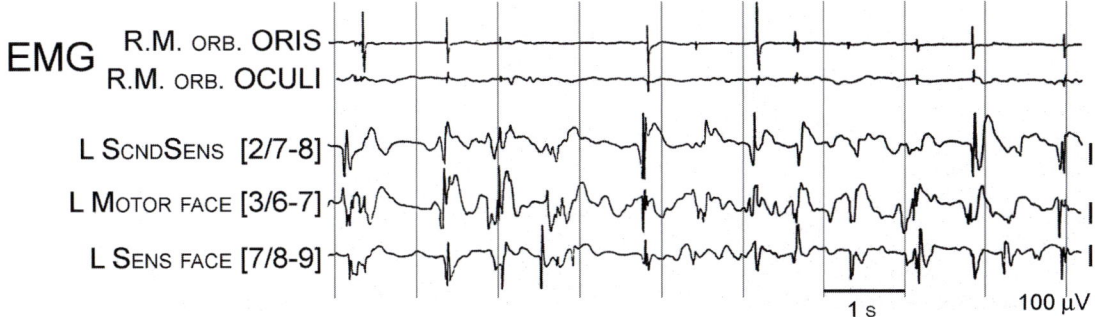

Figure 113. Combined EMG and depth/scalp EEG recording (selected recording sites of Fig. 112) showing the good correlation between depth EEG spikes and myoclonic jerks of the right face.

L Scndsens, left secondary sensory area; **L Sens face**, left sensory face area and motor cortical areas of the face; **L Motor face**, left motor face area; **R.M. orb. oris/oculi**, right oral/ocular orbicular muscle.

Modified from: Wieser HG. Stereoelectroencephalographic correlates of focal motor seizures. In: Speckmann EJ, Elger CE eds. *Epilepsy and Motor System*. Baltimore: Urban and Schwarzenberg 1983b: 287-309 (Fig. 3) and from: Wieser HG, Siegel AM. Relations between the EEG of the cortex, thalamus and periaqueductal gray in patients suffering from epilepsy and pain syndromes. In: Zschocke S, Speckmann EJ eds. *Basic Mechanisms of the EEG*. Boston: Birkhäuser 1993: 145-182 (Fig. 11.15).

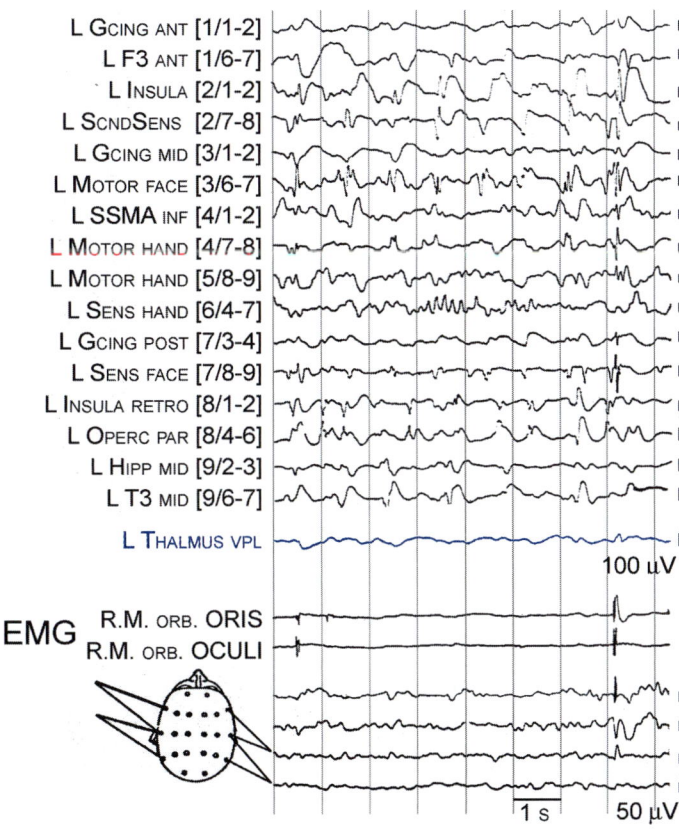

Figure 114. Combined depth/scalp EEG (including the acute left thalamic wing electrode) and electromyographic (EMG) recordings showing the correlation between depth EEG spikes and myoclonic jerks of the right face.

Note that there were no clear discharges in the electrographic recording of the left ventrolateral thalamus undoubtedly attributable to the spontaneous epileptic myoclonus of the face, with the exception maybe of small sharp transients that were associated with violent myoclonia. Electrode sites were identical to Fig. 112, with the exception of the thalamic electrode (L Thalamus vpl).

Modified from: Wieser HG. Stereoelectroencephalographic correlates of focal motor seizures. In: Speckmann EJ, Elger CE eds. *Epilepsy and Motor System*. Baltimore: Urban and Schwarzenberg 1983b: 287-309 (Fig. 3) and from: Wieser HG, Siegel AM. Relations between the EEG of the cortex, thalamus and periaqueductal gray in patients suffering from epilepsy and pain syndromes. In: Zschocke S, Speckmann EJ eds. *Basic Mechanisms of the EEG*. Boston: Birkhäuser 1993: 145-182 (Fig. 11.15).

Extensive stimulation of the thalamic wing electrode ("Seitenelektrode") produced both positive and negative motor phenomena. The topography of the negative motor phenomena was mapped and projected to the Schaltenbrand-Wahren atlas (Fig. 115).

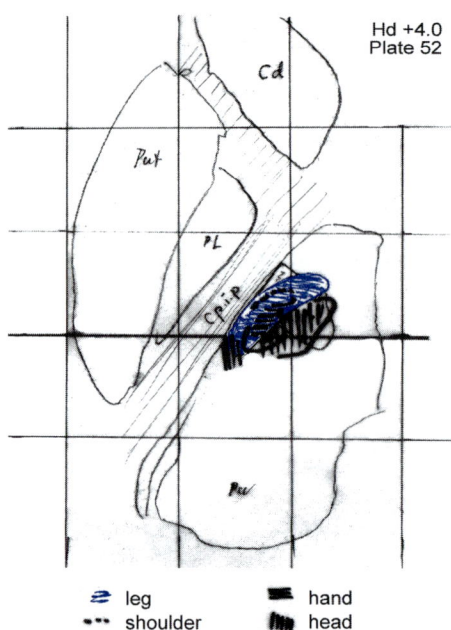

Figure 115. Topographical map of the inhibitory motor areas in the left ventrolataral thalamus, projected on the map of the Schaltenbrand-Wahren atlas.

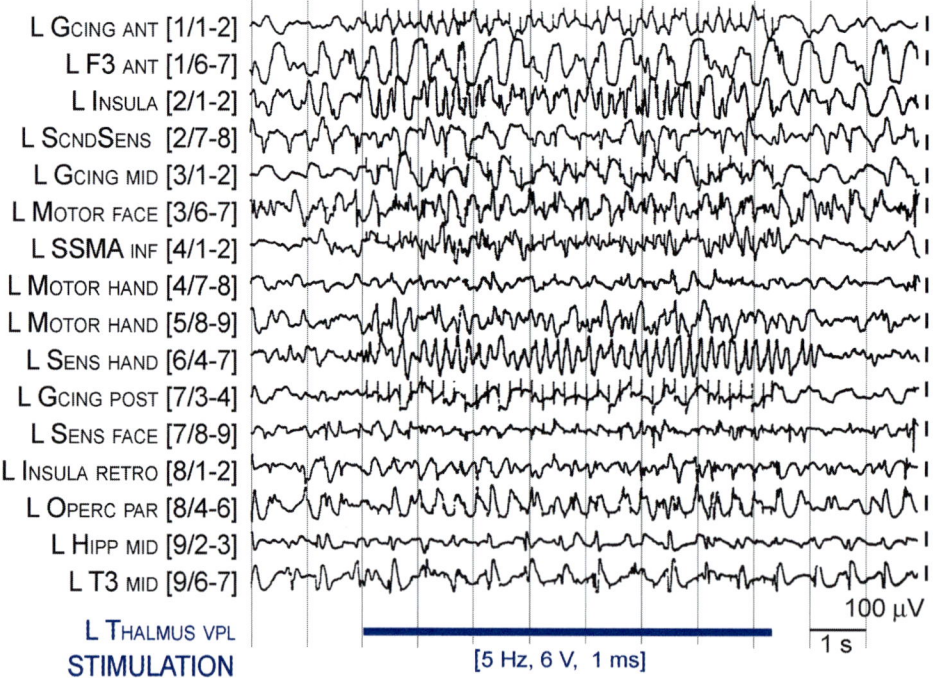

Figure 116. Repetitive 5 Hz train stimulation of the left ventrolateral thalamus (indicated by a blue bar) elicited ERs that were best seen at electrodes sites recording from the left sensory hand area (L Sens hand [6/4-7]) and left motor hand area (L Motor hand [5/8-9]) of the cortex. Electrode sites were identical to Fig. 112.

Modified from: Wieser HG. Stereoelectroencephalographic correlates of focal motor seizures. In: Speckmann EJ, Elger CE eds. *Epilepsy and Motor System*. Baltimore: Urban and Schwarzenberg 1983b: 287-309 (Fig. 3) and from: Wieser HG, Siegel AM. Relations between the EEG of the cortex, thalamus and periaqueductal gray in patients suffering from epilepsy and pain syndromes. In: Zschocke S, Speckmann EJ eds. *Basic Mechanisms of the EEG*. Boston: Birkhäuser 1993: 145-182 (Fig. 11.15).

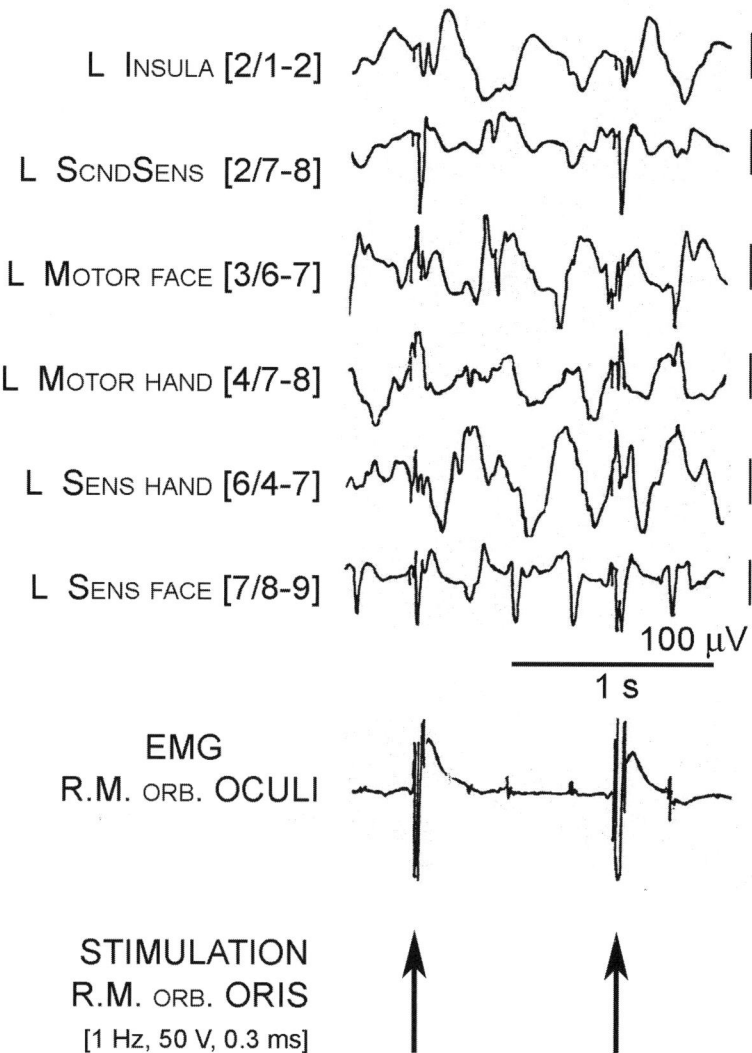

Figure 117. Suprathreshold electrical stimulation of the right corner of the mouth elicited ERs in a considerably wide area of the contralateral epileptogenic cortex.

SCNDSENS, secondary sensory area, MOTOR FACE, motor face area; MOTOR HAND, motor hand area; SENS HAND, sensory hand area; SENS FACE, sensory face area; EMG, electromyography; R.M. ORB. OCULI, right ocular orbicular muscle; R.M. ORB. ORIS, right oral orbicular muscle; L, left; R, right.

Modified from: Wieser HG. Stereoelectroencephalographic correlates of focal motor seizures. In: Speckmann EJ, Elger CE eds. *Epilepsy and Motor System*. Baltimore: Urban and Schwarzenberg 1983b: 287-309 (Fig. 3) and from: Wieser HG, Siegel AM. Relations between the EEG of the cortex, thalamus and periaqueductal gray in patients suffering from epilepsy and pain syndromes. In: Zschocke S, Speckmann EJ eds. *Basic Mechanisms of the EEG*. Boston: Birkhäuser 1993: 145-182 (Fig. 11.15).

Summary

The case of this patient with EPC of the right side due to presumptive left Rasmussen's encephalitis is interesting because the combined EMG and depth/scalp EEG recordings showed a clear correlation between depth EEG spikes of left sensory and motor cortical areas and myoclonic jerks in the right face and extremities. The wing electrode located in the left ventrolateral thalamus (more specifically, in the anterior and posterior ventro-oral nucleus) showed no clear discharges undoubtly attributable to the spontaneously occurring epileptic myclonus, with the exception of fairly small sharp transients occurring with more violent myoclonia only. Repetitive 5 Hz train stimulation of the left ventrolateral thalamus elicited ERs that were best seen at electrodes sites recording from the left sensory and motor cortical hand area. There was no more than a transient improvement of myocloni following stereotactic high frequency thermocoagulation in the left ventrolateral thalamus.

Case 9

Patient History

This 14 year-old girl had EPC of the right side due to presumptive left Rasmussen's encephalitis. Pregnancy, birth, neonatal and childhood development were normal. She had no family history of epilepsy. Her first partial seizure ("absences") occurred at age 6, the first generalized seizure at age 9. Involuntary jerks of the left hand occurred at age 10 for the first time. At age 11, she had three generalized tonic clonic seizures, subsequently leading into the development of intractable EPC with continuous clonic jerking of varying intensity of the right hand and forearm, and subsequent propagation to the right face. AED treatment with various drugs including primidone, ethosuximide, phenytoin and sulthiame showed no effect. At the time of admission to our hospital at age 14, EPC was characterized by rhythmic clonic jerking of the right periorbital and perioral muscles, but also involving the oropharynx and the uvula. Neurological examination demonstrated a mild right hemiparesis. Neuropsychological examination revealed a shift of handedness to the left (originally right) and oligophrenia. The diagnosis of Rasmussen's encephalitis was made on electroclinical grounds (histology was not available).

SEEG

Chronic SEEG with 7 depth electrodes within the left hemisphere was carried out at age 14. Acute thalamic SEEG was performed using a rigid 15-contact electrode with a diameter of 2.5 mm, inserted in the ventrolateral thalamus using a left frontal approach. The tip of this electrode was located in or next to the anterior ventro-oral nucleus (Fig. 118). In this fashion, the source of the interictal epileptiform discharges corresponding to the myclonic jerks could be localized to the left motor cortical area [Wieser et al., 1978].

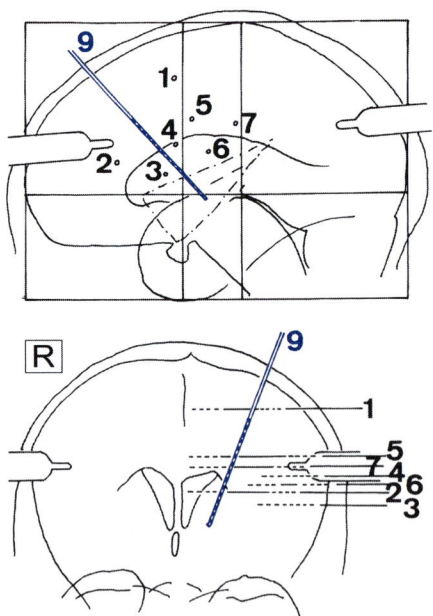

Figure 118. Location of depth electrodes in the proportional Talairach system.
Electrodes 1-7 (gold, flexible, diameter of 800 µm, 8 contacts) were chronically implanted. Electrode 9 (Ag/AgCl, rigid, diameter 2.5 mm, 15 contacts) was used for acute exploration of the left ventrolateral thalamus (the tip of the electrode was presumably located in or next to the anterior ventro-oral nuclei).

Modified from: Wieser HG, Graf HP, Bernoulli C, Siegfried J. Quantitative analysis of intracerebral recordings in epilepsia partialis continua. *Electroenceph Clin Neuropysiol* 1978; 44: 14-22 (Figs. 1 and 2) and from: Wieser HG, Siegel AM. Relations between the EEG of the cortex, thalamus and periaqueductal gray in patients suffering from epilepsy and pain syndromes. In: Zschocke S, Speckmann EJ eds. *Basic Mechanisms of the EEG*. Boston: Birkhäuser 1993: 145-182 (Fig. 11.10).

Surgery

A stereotactic high frequency thermocoagulation was performed in the left ventrolateral thalamus (more specifically, in the anterior and posterior ventro-oral nucleus) before removal of all depth electrodes. Hemispherectomy or other resective surgery was not performed. Therefore, histological examination was not obtainable.

Outcome

There was a long lasting improvement of myoclonia and scalp EEG findings following thermocoagulation, despite persistence of some myoclonia and "absence-like spells". Generalized seizures no longer occurred. The patient married at age 21 and gave birth to two healthy girls. At age 34, she suffered a cerebral hematoma, from which she never recovered. She remained comatose for 1 year and died at age 35. No autopsy was performed.

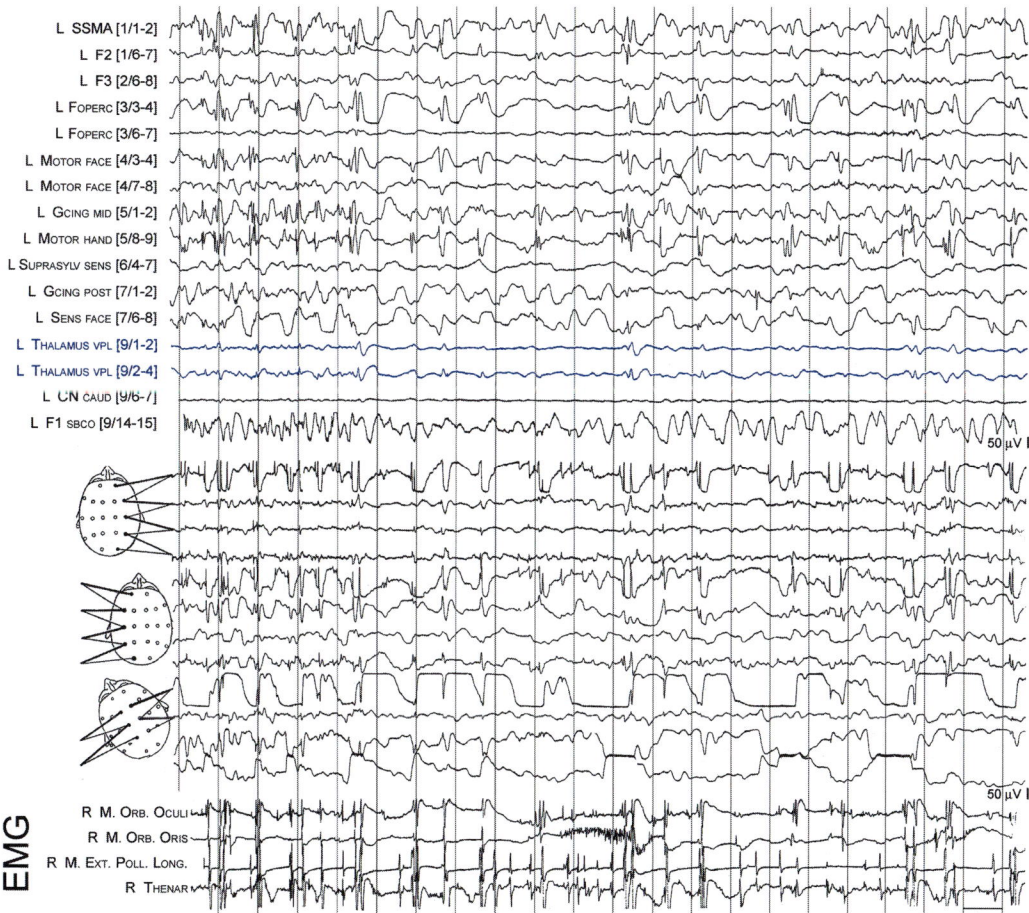

Figure 119. Combined depth/scalp EEG and EMG recording showing the correlation between depth EEG spikes and myoclonic jerks of the right face and hand.

A selection of relevant recording sites is depicted in Fig. 120 in greater detail. The electrode sites recorded from are indicated left to the traces by anatomical designations (based on the Talairach atlas) and numbers (electrode/contacts, *cf.* Fig. 118).

SSMA, supplementary sensorimotor area; **F2**, middle frontal gyrus; **F3**, inferior frontal gyrus; **Foperc**, frontal operculum; **Suprasylv sens**, suprasylvian sensory area; **Motor face**, motor face area; **Gcing**, cingulate gyrus; **Motor hand**, motor hand area; **Sens face**, sensory face area; **Thalamus vpl**, ventrolateral nucleus of the thalamus; **CN caud**, head of the caudate nucleus; **F1**, superior frontal gyrus; **ant**, anterior, **mid**, middle; **post**, posterior; **sbco**, subcortical; **L**, left; **R.M. orb. oculi**, right ocular orbicular muscle; **R.M. orb. oris**, right oral orbicular muscle; **R.M. ext. poll. long**, right long extensor muscle of the thumb; **R Thenar**, right thenar muscles.

Modified from: Wieser HG, Graf HP, Bernoulli C, Siegfried J. Quantitative analysis of intracerebral recordings in epilepsia partialis continua. *Electroenceph Clin Neuropysiol* 1978; 44: 14-22 (Fig. 2).

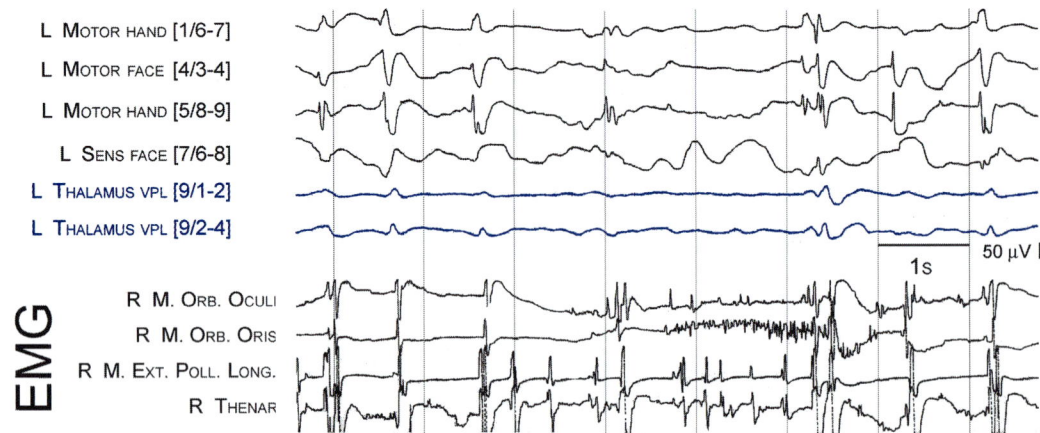

Figure 120. Combined EMG and depth/scalp EEG recording (selected recording sites of Fig. 119) showing the correlation between depth EEG spikes in motor (L MOTOR FACE, left motor face area; L MOTOR HAND, left motor hand area;), to a lesser extent, sensory cortical areas (L SENS FACE, left sensory face area) and myoclonic jerks of the right face (R.M. ORB. OCULI/ORIS, right ocular/oral orbicular muscle) and right hand (R.M. EXT. POLL. LONG., right long extensor muscle of the thumb; R THENAR, right thenar muscles).

Note the small sharp waves in the left ventrolateral thalamic nucleus (L THALAMUS VPL) obviously corresponding to the myoclonic jerks.

Modified from: Wieser HG, Graf HP, Bernoulli C, Siegfried J. Quantitative analysis of intracerebral recordings in epilepsia partialis continua. *Electroenceph Clin Neuropysiol* 1978; 44: 14-22 (Fig. 2).

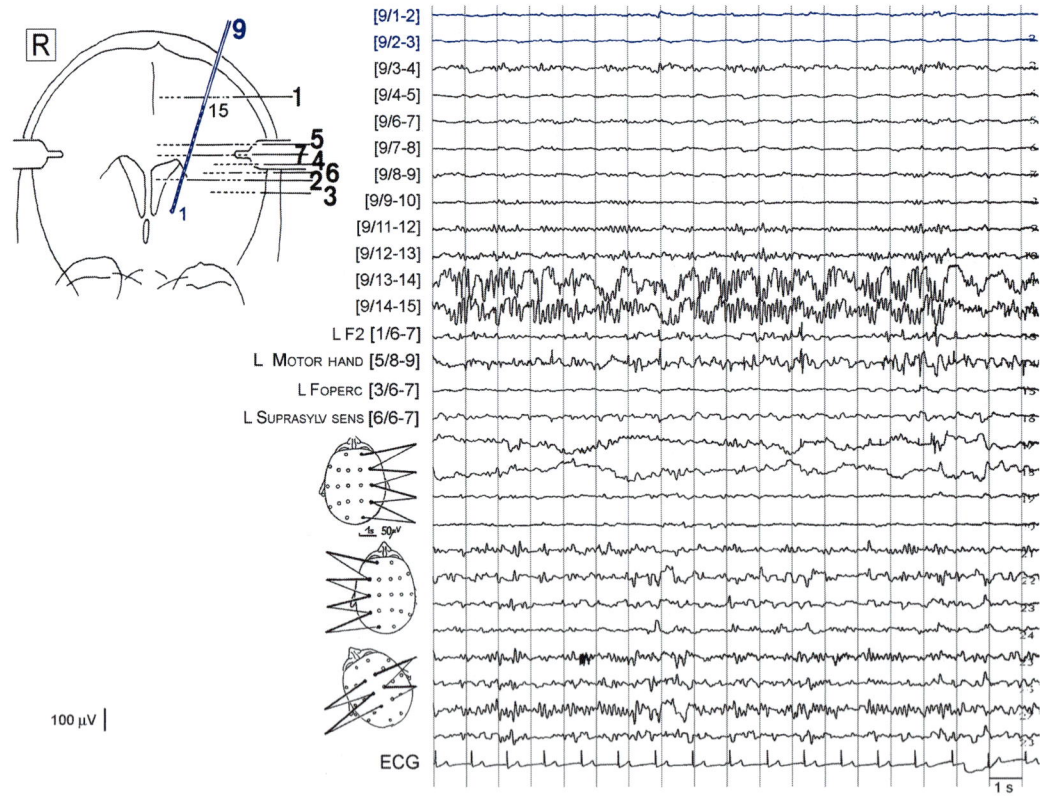

Figure 121. Combined scalp and depth EEG recording along the thalamic electrode number 9 (bipolar montage) and selected depth contacts.

Note that the thalamic activity as well as the activity of the caudate nucleus (contacts 6-7 of electrode 9) showed only low amplitude background activity compared to the cortical contacts (contacts 14-15 of electrode 9).

Modified from: Wieser HG, Siegel AM. Relations between the EEG of the cortex, thalamus and periaqueductal gray in patients suffering from epilepsy and pain syndromes. In: Zschocke S, Speckmann EJ eds. *Basic Mechanisms of the EEG*. Boston: Birkhäuser 1993: 145-182 (Fig. 11.11).

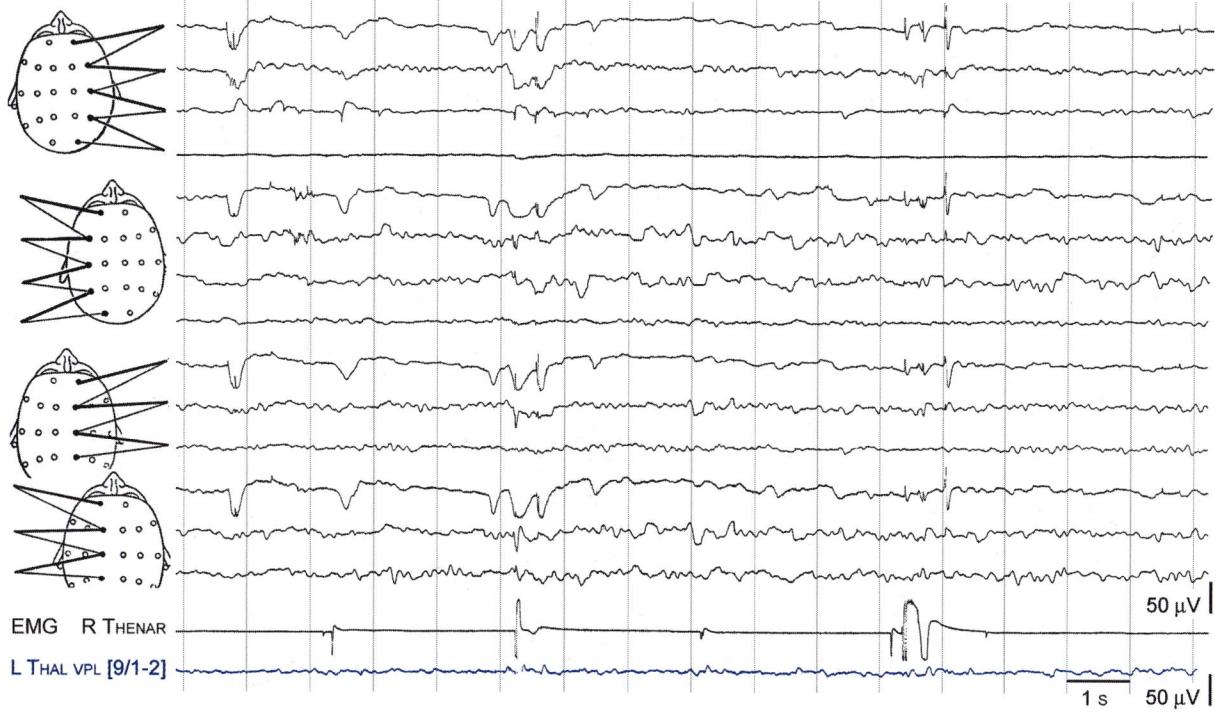

Figure 122. Combined scalp EEG, left thalamic depth EEG (L Thal vpl) and electromyogram of the right thenar (EMG R THENAR).

The myoclonic jerks of the right hand were associated with eye blinks and face twitching, and obviously corresponded with small sharp waves in the left ventrolateral thalamic recording.

Summary

The findings in this patient with EPC of the right side due to presumptive left Rasmussen's encephalitis were very similar to the findings of the patient illustrated in the previous case No 8. The combined EMG and depth/scalp EEG recordings showed a good correlation between depth EEG spikes in the left sensory and motor cortical areas and myoclonic jerks of the right face and extremities, as recorded electromyographically. In this patient, we also performed averaging of intracortical activity time locked to the EMG signal attributable to the myclonus [Wieser et al., 1978]. In this fashion, we were able to show clear cut cortical generator potentials with different maxima and latencies with respect to the facial and hand muscles: The generator potential of the right M. orbicularis oculi myoclonia was located in the left precentral gyrus and preceded the muscle action potential by 17 ms, whereas the generator potential of the right thenar muscle myoclonia first appeared in left premotor cortical areas with a latency of 24 ms, subsequently propagating to the left corona radiata and capsula interna. Stimulation of the lateral aspects of the left primary motor area (corresponding to Brodmann area 4) elicited right sided myoclonic jerks that, with respect to distribution and latency, were very similar to those occurring spontaneously. In contrast, direct electrical stimulation of the left ventrolateral thalamic nucleus had no motor effect. The frequency of the myoclonia was diminished during slow wave sleep, while REM sleep periods were obviously preceded and followed by a clear increase of myoclonic jerking. The electrographic recordings from depth electrode contacts located in the left ventrolateral thalamic nucleus (more specifically, in the anterior and posterior ventro-oral nuclei) showed small but clear sharp waves occurring synchronously to the spontaneous epileptic myoclonia. The generator of these sharp waves was not entirely clear, although the near field characteristics of these discharges (as evidenced by phase reversals in bipolar thalamic recordings, see Fig. 121) might emphasize a thalamic generator rather than reflect simple volume conduction of cortically generated activity. In contrast to the patient illustrated in the previous case No 8, the performance of a

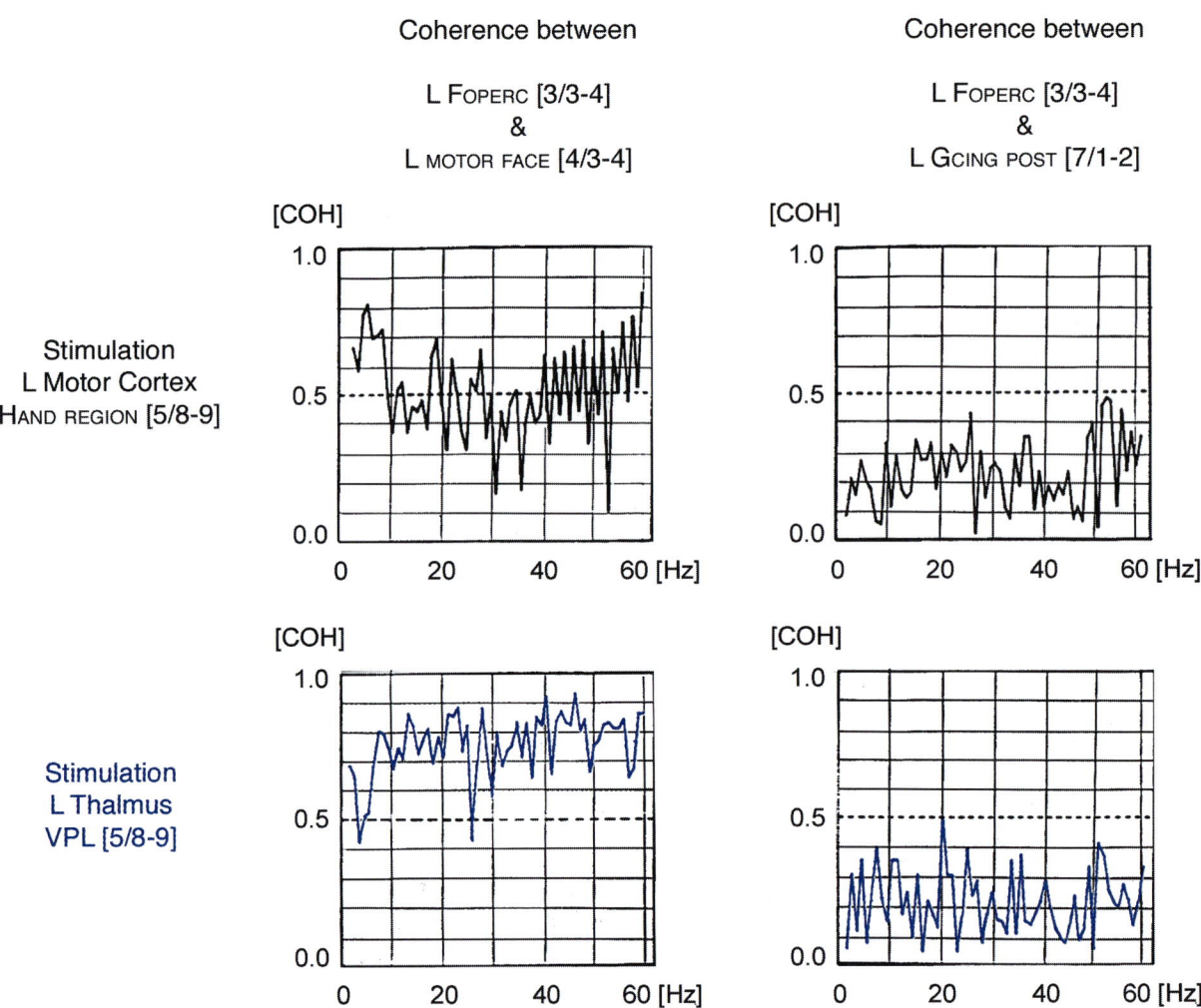

Figure 123. Frequency dependent coherence (COH, values ranging from 0 to 1) between the signals recorded from two neighboring left cortical sites (frontal opercular [3/3-4] and motor face area [4/3-4]; left charts) and between signals recorded from left frontal opercular [3/3-4] and left posterior cingulate [7/1-2] sites (right charts) during stimulation of the ipsilateral motor cortex ([5/8-9]; upper charts) and the ipsilateral ventrolateral thalamus ([5/8-9]; lower charts).

Note the influence of left thalamic stimulation on the coherence of the left frontal opercular and motor face sites (left charts): Coherence in the theta range appeared to be decreased during stimulation, whereas coherence in the beta and gamma range was clearly augmented.

Modified from: Wieser HG, Siegel AM. Relations between the EEG of the cortex, thalamus and periaqueductal gray in patients suffering from epilepsy and pain syndromes. In: Zschocke S, Speckmann EJ eds. *Basic Mechanisms of the EEG*. Boston: Birkhäuser 1993: 145-182 (Fig. 11.14).

stereotactic high frequency thermocoagulation in the left ventrolateral thalamus here was followed by a long lasting improvement of the epileptic condition. This finding might emphasize a greater role of the thalamus with respect to the generation of the myoclonia in this patient.

Case 10

Patient History

This 21 year-old man with intractable epilepsy of presumptive left occipital or temporo-occipital onset since age 14 had frequent psychomotor seizures (about 30 per month) as well as seizures that were associated with falls (about 15 per month). Pregnancy was uneventful

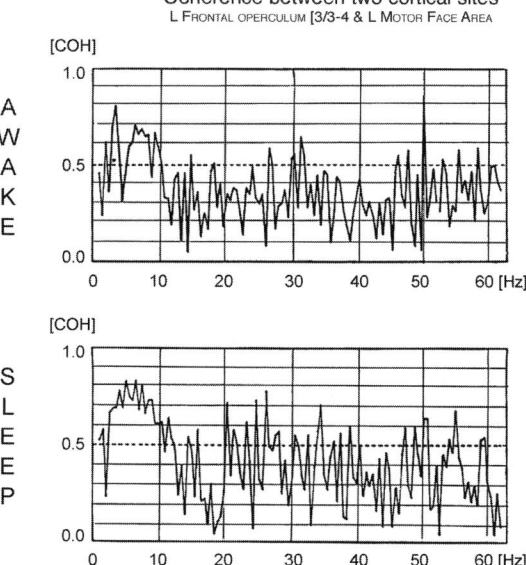

Figure 124. Frequency dependent coherence (COH, values ranging from 0 to1) between the signals recorded from two neighboring left cortical sites (frontal operculum [3/3-4] and motor face area [4/3-4]) during wakefulness and sleep.

Note the increase of COH for lower frequencies (theta range) and the decrease of COH for faster frequencies (15-20 Hz beta range) during sleep.

but delivery was preterm and complicated requiring forceps delivery. Subsequent neonatal and childhood development was normal. He had no family history of epilepsy. His habitual psychomotor seizures were characterized by teleopsia, micropsia, difficulties to recognize numbers, right visual field restriction, motor arrest, clouding of consciousness, automatisms, facultative head version to the right and a Gerstmann like syndrome postictally. Neurological examination demonstrated right homonymous hemianopsia and right hypacusis. Neuropsychological examination of this left handed man revealed a Waxman-Geschwind personality syndrome with marked circumstantiality. Neuroradiological examination showed a substantial enlargement of the left trigonum.

SEEG

Acute SEEG was carried out using 9 depth electrodes at age 21, with electrode 3 located in the left pulvinar of the thalamus (Fig. 125). Three spontaneous seizures were recorded, all of which showing a left occipital onset with subsequent propagation to the left lingual gyrus and left lateral temporal lobe. Seizures induced by electrical stimulation of the left pulvinar showed spread to the ipsilateral mesial temporal lobe including the amygdala. Electrical 1 Hz single pulse stimulation of the left pulvinar elicited ERs in the ipsilateral amygdala. Administration of diazepam induced beta spindles in pulvinar recordings.

Surgery

A left occipital resection was performed at age 22. The site of resection is depicted in Fig. 125 (dashed area), and the resected specimen is shown in Fig. 126. Histological examination of the resected specimen revealed gliosis.

Outcome

The postsurgical outcome was excellent (Engel class IA), allowing for the cessation of AED treatment within 15 years post surgery. The patient partially resumed his work as an office clerk.

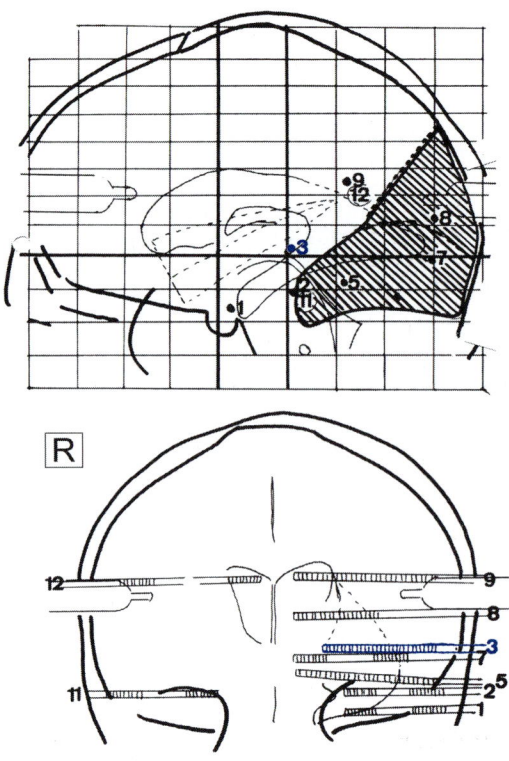

Figure 125. Location of depth electrodes in the proportional Talairach system, with electrode 3 located in the left pulvinar of the thalamus.

The remaining electrodes covered the left temporo-occipital region (electrodes 5, 7 and 8), both temporal lobes (electrodes 1, 2 and 11) and the posterior cingulate gyri bilaterally (electrodes 9 and 12).

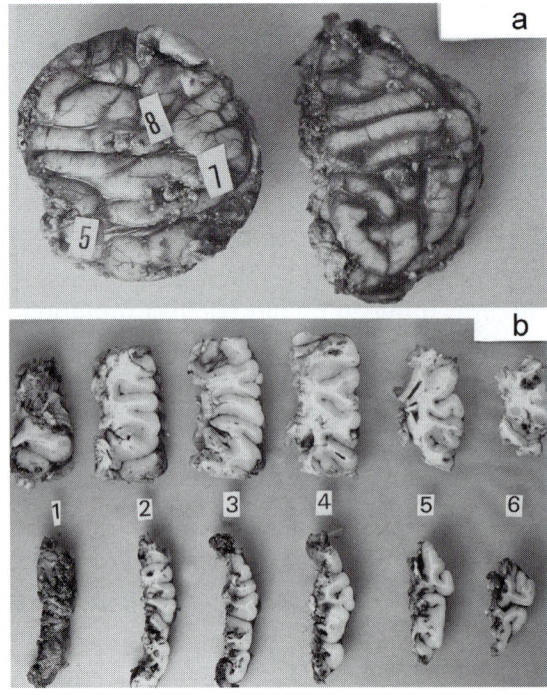

Figure 126. Resected brain specimen as outlined in Fig. 125 (dashed area).

a) in toto (the numbers 5, 7 and 8 corresponded to the sites of the depth electrodes). **b)** transsections of the specimen that revealed gliosis on histological examination.

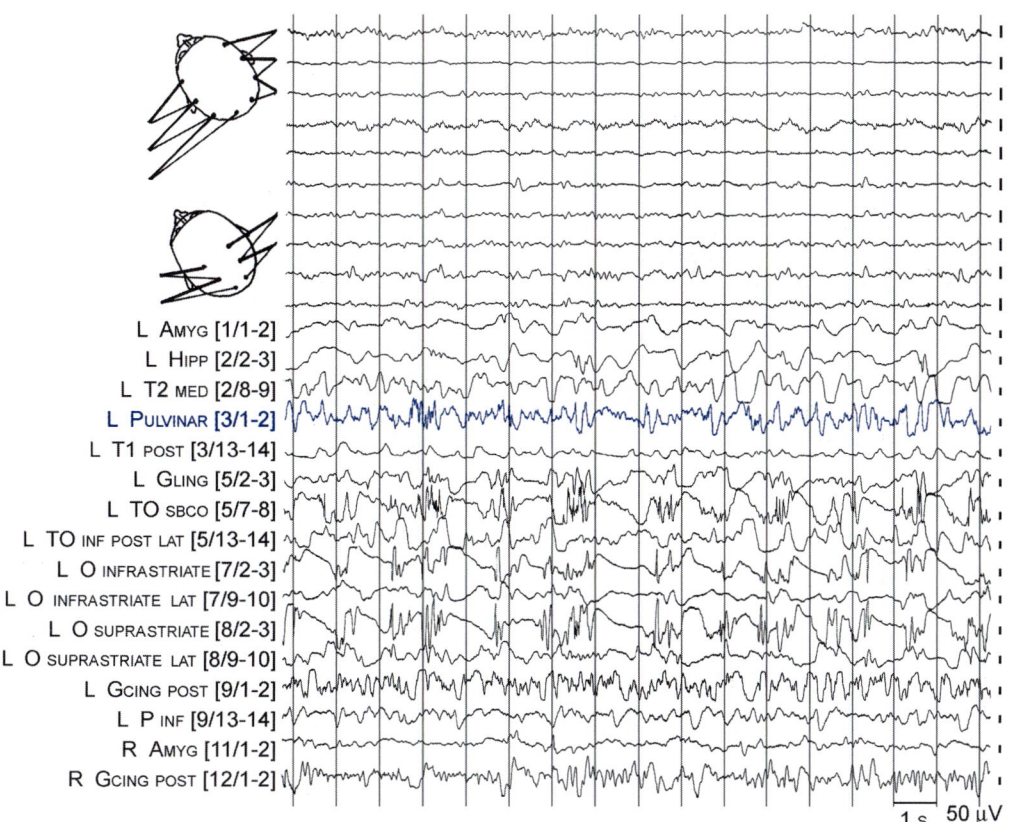

Figure 127. Spontaneous semi-ictal discharges in the left temporal and occipital (medial aspect of the infra- and supracalcarine cortex) areas showing projection into the pulvinar.

The electrode sites recorded from are indicated left to the traces by anatomical designations (based on the Talairach atlas) and numbers (electrode/contacts, *cf.* Fig. 125).
AMYG, amygdala; HIPP, hippocampus; T2, middle temporal gyrus; T1, superior temporal gyrus; GLING, lingual gyrus; TO, temporo-occipital area, O, occipital area; GCING, cingulate gyrus; PINF, parietal inferior lobule; MED, medial; LAT, lateral; INF, inferior; POST, posterior; SBCO, subcortical; R, right; L, left.

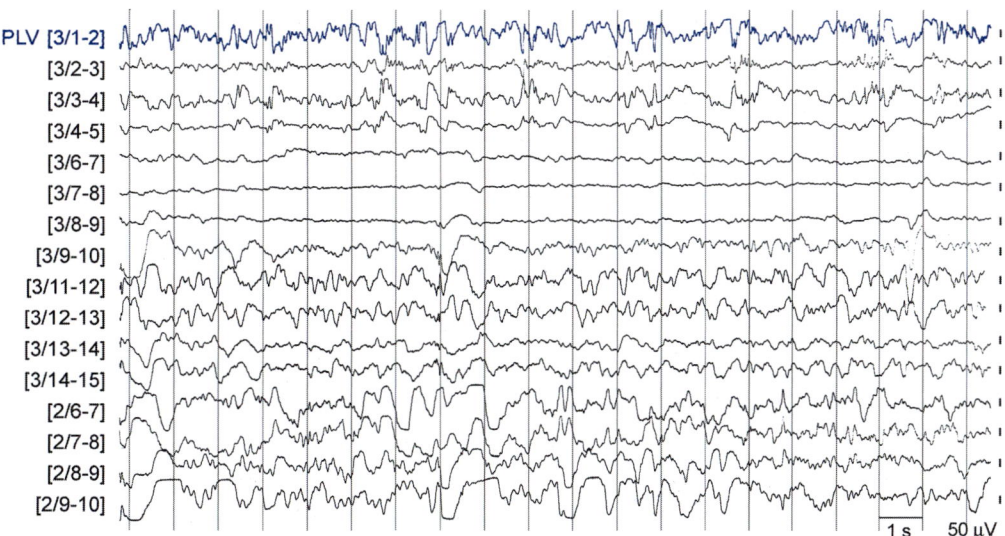

Figure 128. Interictal depth recordings from electrode 3 and the outer contacts of electrode 2 (see Fig. 125).

The tip of electrode 3 (contact 1, blue) was located in the left pulvinar. Note the near-field sharp wave potentials recorded from or close to the pulvinar thalamic nucleus.
Modified from: Wieser HG, Kausel W. Limbic seizures. In: Wieser HG, Elger CE eds. *Presurgical Evaluation of Epileptics.* Berlin, Heidelberg, New York: Springer 1987: 227-248 (left part of Fig. 9).

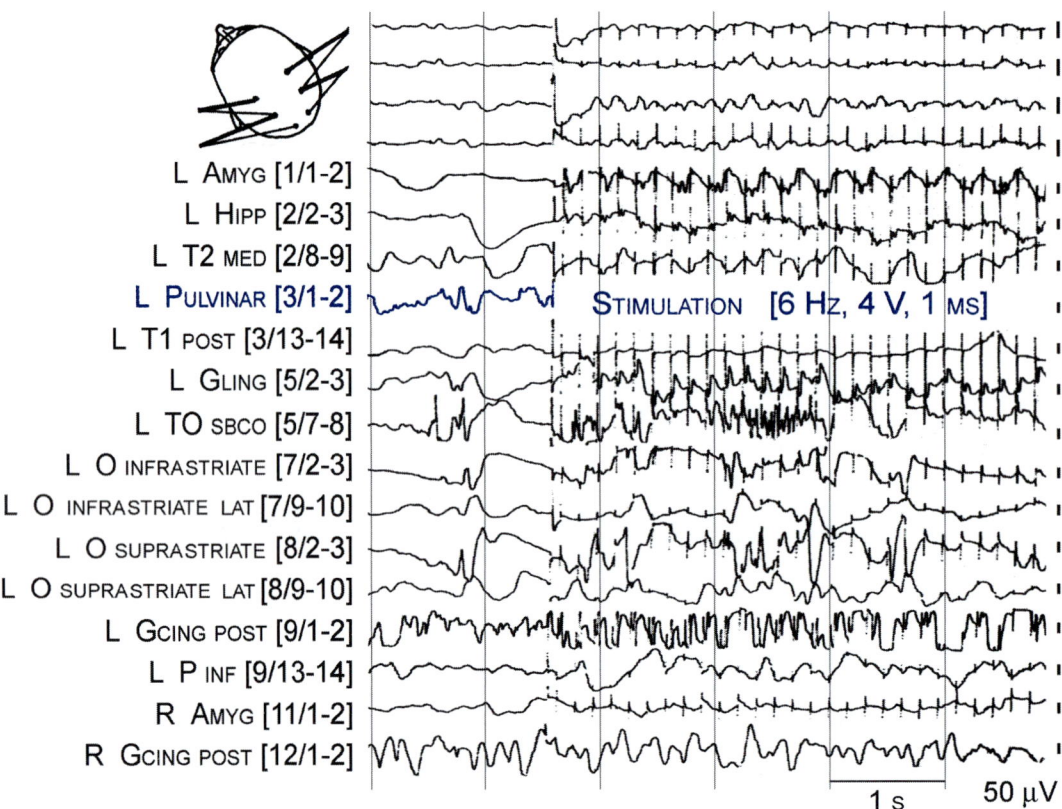

Figure 129. Electrical 6 Hz train stimulation (4 V, 1 ms pulse width) of the left pulvinar elicited ERs in the ipsilateral amygdala [1/1-2], the left lingual gyrus [5/2-3] and the ipsilateral posterior cingulate gyrus [9/1-2].

Electrode sites were identical to Fig. 127.

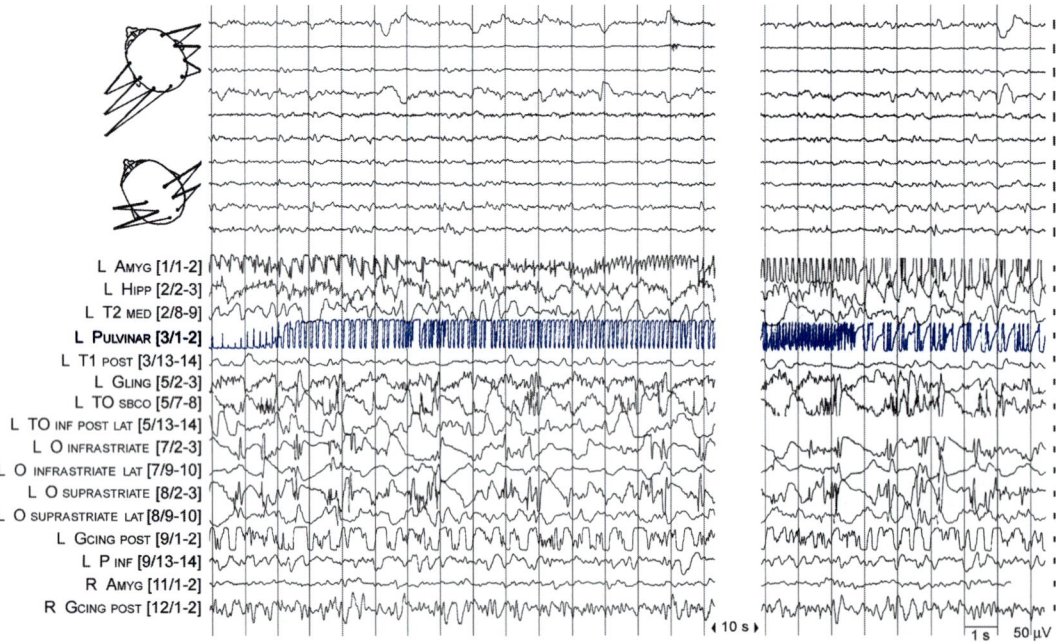

Figure 130. Electrically induced seizure following 6 Hz train stimulation of the left pulvinar [3/1-2] with early propagation to the left amygdala [1/1-2].

Note that the spontaneous epileptiform discharges in the left temporal and occipital areas (medial aspect of the infra- and suprastriate cortex, [7/2-3] and [8/2-3]) remained virtually unaffected by the electrically induced seizure in the pulvinar and the amygdala. Electrode sites were identical to Fig. 127.

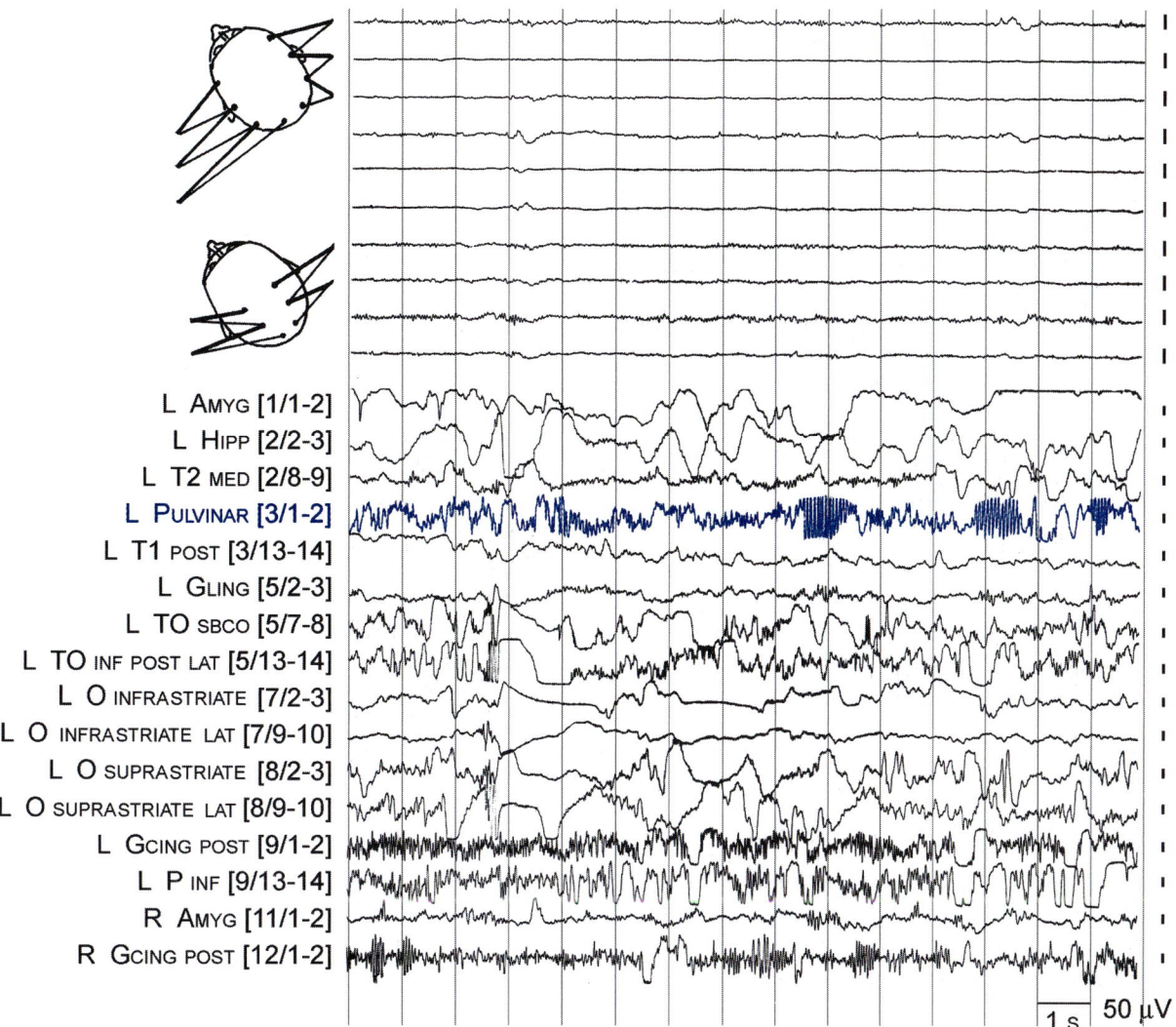

Figure 131. Drug induced beta activity (spindles) in the posterior cingulate gyri bilaterally ([9/1-2] and [12/1-2]) as well as the left pulvinar [3/1-2] following administration of diazepam. Electrode sites were identical to Fig. 127.

Summary

The case of this patient with a left occipital (or temporo-occipital) epilepsy and excellent outcome following occipital lobe resection is interesting because of the pulvinar exploration evidently revealing projection of epileptiform potentials from the primary epileptogenic parastriate and lateral occipital cortex to the pulvinar. It is particularly interesting to note that the electrically induced pulvinar seizure discharge spread to the ipsilateral amygdala, but did not cause alteration of the interictal parastriate and lateral occipital cortical activity. Finally, it is remarkable that diazepam induced beta spindle activity that was most prominent in the pulvinar and in posterior cingulate cortical areas.

Case 11

Patient History

This 21 year-old woman had no family history of epilepsy. Her birth and development were uneventful. She had her first focal motor seizure associated with left dominant clonic activity at age 4. The seizures later evolved with gradually increasing frequency and intractability despite various AED regimens including valproic acid, phenobarbital, phenytoin and clonazepam. Generalized convulsive seizures occurred since age 5. At age 21, she presented to our hospital with a mild left spastic hemiparesis, corresponding to a right hemispheric atrophy. At that time, she had four types of seizures: (1) left motor seizures that were commonly associated with falls; (2) psychomotor seizures with autonomic signs and symptoms such as flushing, mydriasis, hyperventilation and, occasionally, motor arrest; (3) seizures with staring, conjugate rapid eye movements with a clear predominance to the right and tachycardia, followed by "deep sleep" for about three hours or, rarely, by confusion with wandering or other semipurposeful gestual and verbal automatisms; and (4), since age 18, episodic EPC with left-sided fairly regular 1/s motor jerks lasting two to three weeks. Repeated CT scans and MRIs showed a progressive atrophy of the right hemisphere, as well as a marked signal alteration of the right mesial anterior temporal lobe. Rasmussen's encephalitis was suspected. She did not qualify for hemispherectomy at this stage, and a SEEG exploration was thus performed.

SEEG

Chronic SEEG exploration with 10 depth electrodes of the right hemisphere together with a left sided 1 contact FO electrode was carried out at age 21. The tip of electrode 10 targeted to the right Forel H field was located in the right mesencephalon in close proximity (slightly posterior) to the red nucleus (Figs. 132 and 133). Her seizures causing staring, conjugate rapid eye movements to the right, tachycardia and sleep induction (type 3, as described above) were characterized by rhythmic EEG discharges (often spike trains) in the right mesencephalic contacts 1-2 of electrode 10 and a concomitant, widespread EEG attenuation at the remaining temporal and frontal depth-EEG recording sites, except in those electrodes recording from the right rolandic areas (that is, electrodes 3 and 4, Fig. 134). In contrast, her psychomotor seizures with autonomic signs and symptoms (type 2, as described above) were characterized by stereotyped amygdalar [8/2-3] and hippocampal [9/1-2] EEG discharges, frequently associated with rhythmic right mesencephalic [10/1-2] discharges.

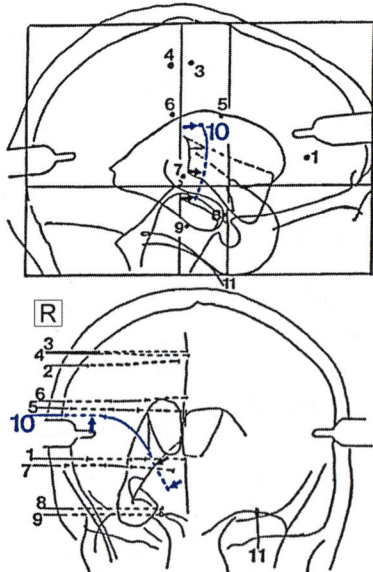

Figure 132. Location of the 10 depth electrodes in the proportional Talairach system, with the tip of electrode 10 located in the right brainstem area close to the red nucleus (Fig. 133).

The remaining electrodes covered the right Rolandic cortex (electrodes 3, 4, 5 and 6), the right temporal lobe (electrode 8 with its tip in the amygdala, electrode 9 with its tip in the hippocampus) and the right frontal lobe (electrode 1). Electrode 11 was a unipolar FO electrode inserted contralaterally, with its tip located in the ambient cistern.

Surgery and Outcome

Following SEEG exploration, a hemispherectomy was suggested but rejected. Based on the occurrence of frequent psychomotor seizures, a decision was then made to combine a diagnostic brain biopsy with a "palliative" right sided selective AHE. Histology of the resected tissue and of a biopsy taken from the frontal right neocortex revealed perivascular lymphocytic cuffs and glial nodules with marked neuronal fallout and gliosis but without evidence of inflammatory elements, which was consistent with Rasmussen's encephalitis. Selective AHE led to a cessation of psychomotor seizures (type 2, as described above) and, quite surprisingly, also to a transitory improvement with regard to EPC (type 4). The patient was classified to outcome class III, but within 2 years the further course was characterized by a steadily progressive worsening with frequent episodes of status epilepticus, atonic generalized seizures with severe falls, and unilateral focal motor seizures resulting in marked left hemiparesis. Immunosuppressive therapy was without effect. She was then reevaluated with the goal to detect GluR3 autoantibodies [Rogers et al., 1994; Twyman et al., 1995], but our search for the presence of anti-GluR3 antibodies in sera and cerebral spinal fluid was negative [Tönnes et al., 1998]. As a consequence, plasmapheresis was not suggested (an option, which had been proposed in anti-GluR3 positive Rasmussen's encephalitis patients by Andrews et al. [1996] and Wieser [1996]). After extensive studies on the localization of the motor functions of the left leg [Wieser et al., 1999], a partial anterior right hemispherectomy with undercutting of the remaining posterior occipito-parietal cortex was performed at age 37. The patient was completely seizure and aura free following this procedure (outcome class IA). Unfortunately, shunt insufficiency with subsequent tentorial herniation occurred 7 months after hemispherectomy, leading to brain stem infarction with persisting oculomotor, motor and sensory deficits despite urgent surgery.

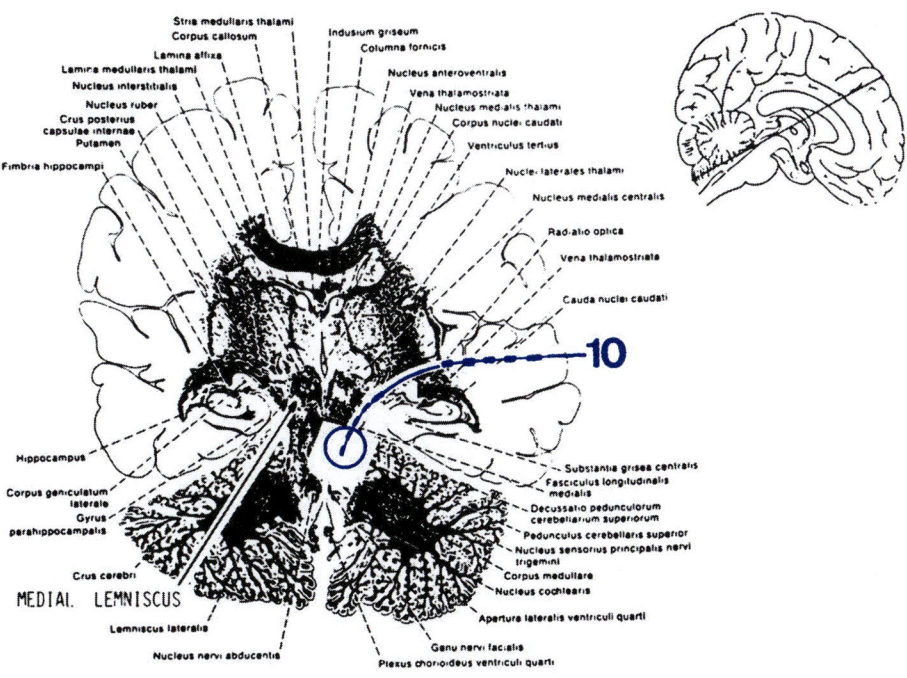

Figure 133. Reconstruction of the location of electrode 10 in the right midbrain area close to the red nucleus.

Modified from Wieser HG. The phenomenology of limbic seizures. In: Wieser HG, Speckmann EJ, Engel J Jr eds. *The Epileptic Focus*. London: John Libbey 1987c: 113-136 (Fig. 8), and from: Wieser HG. Stereo-EEG, intraoperative monitoring and anaesthesia. In: Halliday AM, Butler SR, Paul R eds. *A Textbook of Clinical Neurophysiology*. London: John Wiley & Sons Ltd. 1987b: 269-304 (Fig. 7).

Summary

The case of this patient with Rasmussen's encephalitis is interesting because of the recording of a "paroxysmal sleep attack" reflecting an uncommon and poorly understood ictal phenomenon. The seizure onset was characterized by rhythmic spike trains in right mesencephalic structures next to the red nucleus that were preceded and followed by amygdalar discharges and that were accompanied by a widespread attenuation of the other temporal and frontal depth EEG electrode sites. The phenomenon of ictal widespread EEG attenuation is poorly understood. The data of this patient may provide support for the assumption that widespread EEG attenuation might be related to some sort of "arousal reaction", mediated by ictal activation of mesencephalic structures such as the ascending reticular activating system (ARAS) [Penfield and Jasper 1954]. The finding that these seizures were commonly followed by "deep sleep" might be regarded as additional evidence for the participation of sleep regulatory centers during the seizures of this patient.

The recordings of this patient are also interesting with respect to the recording of lemniscal SEP components following median nerve stimulation: A conduction velocity of ~ 15 m/s could be determined along the course of the medial lemniscus in the brain stem. Otherwise, this case illustrates the classical clinical and electroencephalographic features of a patient with Rasmussen encephalitis.

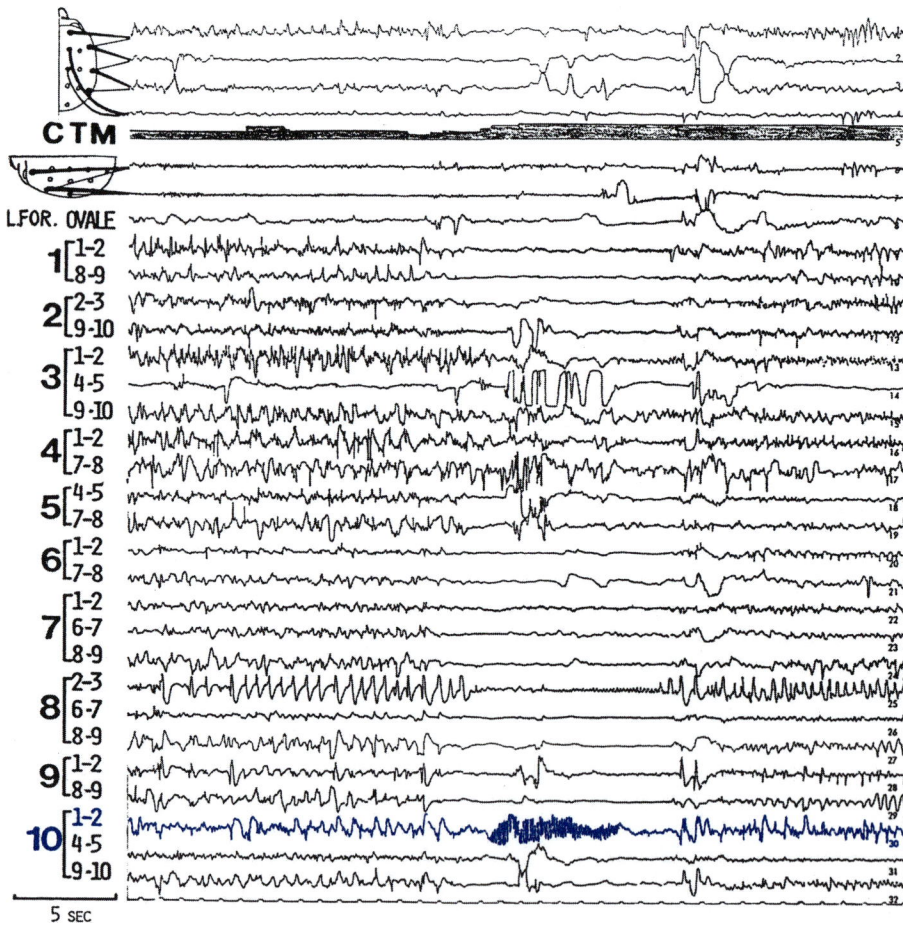

Figure 134. Combined surface and depth recordings of the onset of a "paroxysmal sleep attack" (type 3, as described in the text).

Note the EEG attenuation with appearance of a spike train of about 14 Hz in the tegmental mesencephalon [10/1-2], preceded and followed by a spike train in the amygdala [8/2-3]. The EEG attenuation was accompanied by an increase of the heart frequency of initially 60/min (left margin) to 120/min (right margin).
L.FOR.OVALE, left FO electrode (electrode #11 in Fig. 132); **CTM**, cardiotachymeter (heart frequency).

Modified from Wieser HG. The phenomenology of limbic seizures. In: Wieser HG, Speckmann EJ, Engel J Jr eds. *The Epileptic Focus*. London: John Libbey 1987c: 113-136 (Fig. 8).

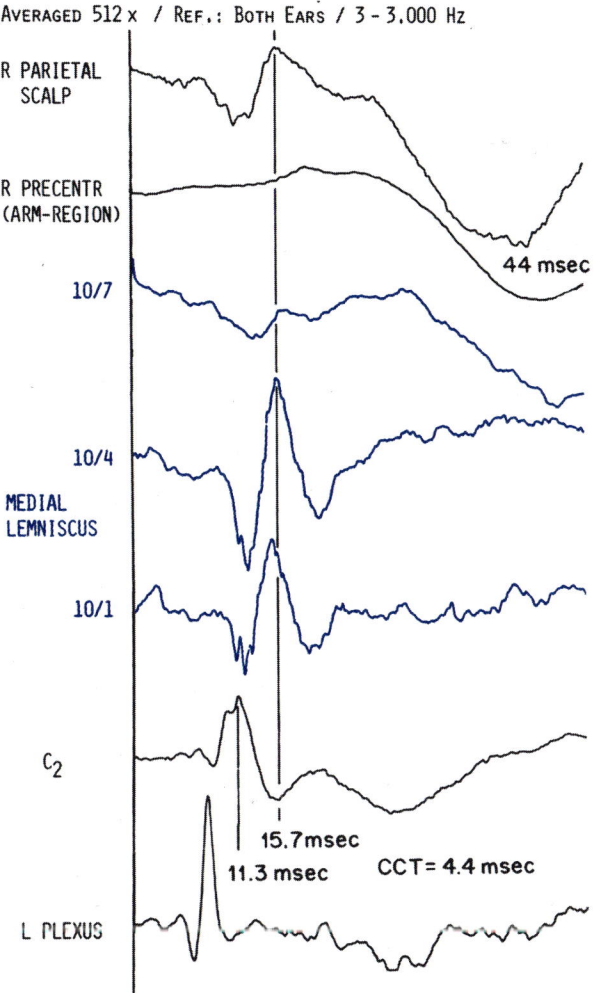

Figure 135. Somatosensory evoked potentials following left median nerve stimulation (n = 512; random 3 Hz; 0.2 ms, referenced to linked ears; filtered at 3-3,000 Hz) revealing a normal medial lemniscal N18 response and a pathologically deformed cortical response with a low amplitude N20 component.

The tip of electrode 10 was located in the vicinity of the right medial lemniscus (Fig. 133). Note the peak difference between the recording sites 10/1 and 10/4 (0.8 ms = 6 mm distance), which corresponds to a conduction velocity of 15 m/s.

Modified from: Wieser HG. Stereo-EEG, intraoperative monitoring and anaesthesia. In: Halliday AM, Butler SR, Paul R eds. *A Textbook of Clinical Neurophysiology*. London: John Wiley & Sons Ltd. 1987b: 269-304 (Fig. 6).

Case 12

Patient History

This 69 year-old woman had severe myoclonus due to definite (that is, neuropathologically confirmed) sporadic Creutzfeldt-Jakob disease (CJD). The exploration of this patient unfortunately caused iatrogenic CJD in two patients at our center, as previously reported [Bernoulli *et al.*, 1977, Wieser *et al.*, 2004]. At this time (1974), CJD was not generally known to be a transmissible prion disease, but was considered by many to be a neurodegenerative spongiform encephalopathy. Following implantation, the depth electrodes were cleaned and sterilized for reuse in 70% alcohol and formaldehyde vapor (comp. polyoxymethyani 1.0) in preautoclaved boxes for at least 48 hours. The type of the electrodes used at this time ("electrodes de type aigu" [Buser and Bancaud, 1967]) prevented steam autoclaving at 134° C for 18 minutes, as now recommended for prion decontamination of instruments [McDonnel and Burke, 2003; Ironside, 2003].

SEEG Exploration

Chronic SEEG was carried out using two depth electrodes inserted into the right ventrolateral thalamic nucleus and the right prefrontal cortex (Fig. 136D). Depth electrode recordings from electrodes 1 and 2 showed typical generalized periodic sharp wave complexes (PSWC, Fig. 136A-C). There was a phase reversal of the thalamic deflection (Fig. 136C, upper traces) and a delay of about 4 ms with respect to the cortical discharge (Fig. 136C, lower traces).

Surgery

Following diagnostic cortical biopsy, a therapeutically motivated thermocoagulation was performed in the ventrolateral thalamic nucleus, with the aim to reduce her violent mycloni.

Outcome

The patient deceased 3 months after the intervention.

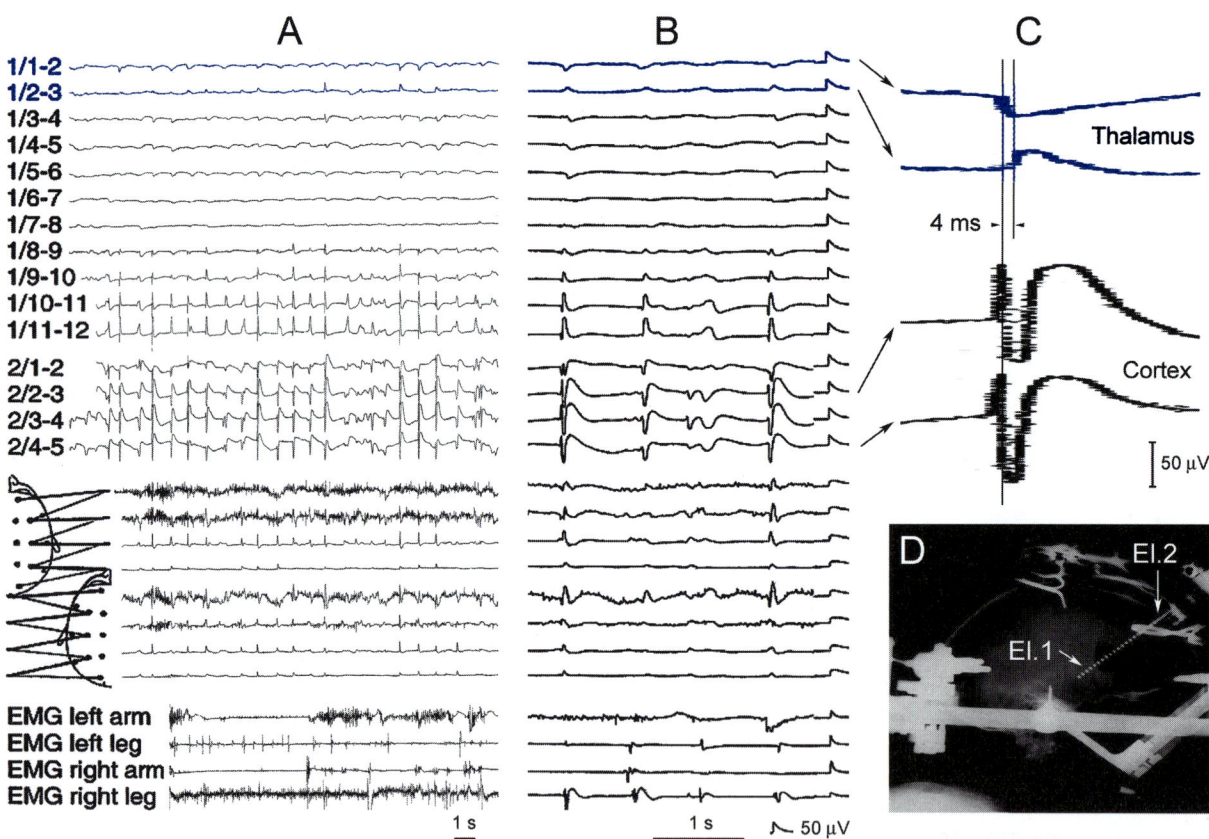

Figure 136. Depth electrode recording with two depth electrodes inserted into the right ventrolateral thalamic nucleus (electrode 1) and the right prefrontal cortex (electrode 2) in a patient with definite sporadic CJD.

The recording was performed during cortical biopsy and stereotactic electrocoagulation in the ventrolateral thalamus for treatment of violent myoclonus. Depth electrode recordings from electrodes 1 and 2 (contact 1 of electrode 1 denoting the deepest contact, located within the right ventrolateral thalamic nucleus) showed typical generalized PSWC, also depicted with a better time resolution in (B) and (C). Note the phase reversal of the thalamic deflection (C, upper traces) and its delay with respect to the cortical discharge (C, lower traces). D: Intraoperative radiography showing the position of the depth electrodes.

Modified from Wieser HG, Schwarz U, Blättler T, Bernoulli C, Sitzler M, Stoeck K, Glatzel M. Serial EEG findings in sporadic and iatrogenic Creutzfeldt-Jakob Disease. *Clin Neurophysiol* 2004; 115: 2467-2478, and from: Wieser HG, Schindler K, Zumsteg D. EEG in Creutzfeldt-Jakob disease. *Clin Neurophysiol* 2006; 117: 935-951.

Summary

The case of this patient with sporadic CJD is interesting because of the concomitant depth recordings of PSWC in ventrolateral thalamic and prefrontal cortical structures. PSWC were reported to occur in EEG recordings of about two thirds of patients with sporadic CJD (Levy et al., 1986; Steinhoff et al., 1996, Steinhoff et al., 2004) and the occurrence of PSWC was therefore included in the World Health Organization (1998) diagnostic classification criteria of sporadic CJD. Morphologically, typical PSWC consist of either simple sharp waves (including biphasic and triphasic waves) or complexes with mixed spikes, polyspikes and slower waves with a typical duration of 100 to 600 ms, recurring every 0.5 to 2 s [Gloor, 1980], while the intervening background usually consists of generalized low voltage slowing. Topographically, PSWC commonly reveal a bilateral voltage distribution with a fronto-precentral midline maximum. PSWC resemble generalized spike and wave absence seizures and, therefore, a thalamic pacemaker role has been hypothesized. However, there is no satisfactory model to explain the periodicity of the pattern. It has been suggested that bihemispherically synchronized discharges such as PSWC do not necessarily imply pacing from deep midline structures but might be synchronized by way of the corpus callosum [Traub and Pedley, 1981]. It has further been speculated that fusion of dendritic membranes of affected neurons could result in increased electrotonic coupling and pathologically synchronized bursting activity. The ventrolateral thalamic depth recordings of this patient revealed small near-field potentials that were clearly related to PSWC in the prefrontal right cortex and scalp EEG (since these thalamic deflections showed a thalamic phase reversal they are not volume conducted but must have a thalamic generator). These thalamic potentials apparently showed a delay of about 4 ms with respect to the cortical discharge, which may indicate a primary cortical generator of PSWC [Wieser et al., 2006].

Cases 13 to 17

Patient Histories

In the context of a functional treatment for intractable pain disorders we had the rare opportunity to record from chronically implanted electrodes located in the periaqueductal gray matter (PAG) and the thalamic nuclei in 5 patients.

Case 13: This 69 year-old man had anesthesia dolorosa of the left face following thermorhizotomy at age 67. Thermorhizotomy was performed for the relief of severe left postherpetiform trigeminal neuralgia (V3).

Case 14: This 62 year-old woman had an incomplete right thalamus syndrome (Déjerine-Roussy) comprising burning pain and slight spastic left hemiparesis following a thalamo-capsular hemorrhage at age 60.

Case 15: This 47 year-old man had severe causalgiform pain of both legs after a total traumatic transverse lesion of the spinal cord (and subsequent spinal surgeries) at the level of T11.

Case 16: This 67 year-old woman had left postherpetiform anesthesia dolorosa at the level of T1-4 following herpes zoster at age 61. The herpes zoster occurred during immunosuppressive therapy for the treatment of Hodgkin lymphoma stage IIIA, leading to a complete remission.

Case 17: This 26 year-old man had posttraumatic phantom pain of the left arm with a maximal intensity in digits II-IV after an almost complete traumatic avulsion of his left arm demanding amputation of the limb at age 20. A stereotactic thermocoagulation of the centromedian thalamic nucleus was performed at age 21, with no effect. A spinal cord stimulation using a "floating electrode" at the level of C4-6 was carried out at age 25, again with no benefit.

EEG Recordings

Fig. 137 shows the location of the depth electrodes in the appropriate sagittal sections of the Schaltenbrand-Wahren atlas in one of the five patients (case 13) with electrodes in the right PAG (deepest contacts 1-3) and the right thalamic nuclei (contacts 4-5).

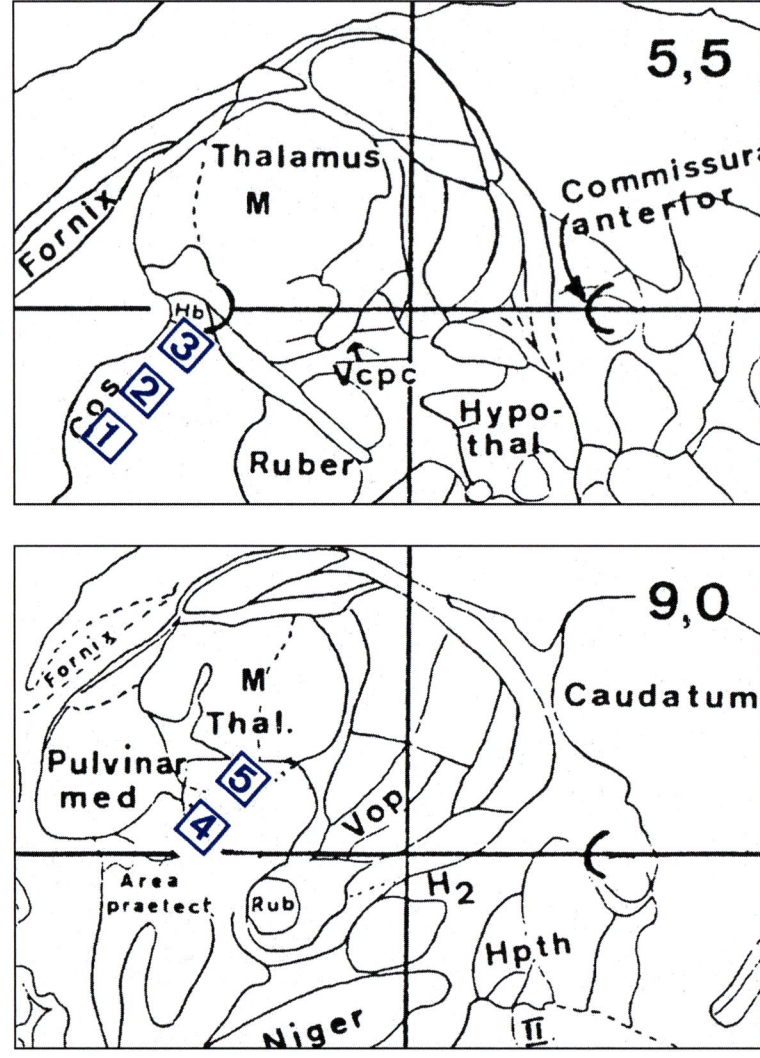

Figure 137. Representative location of depth electrodes in the appropriate sagittal sections (5.5. and 9.0 mm lateral from midline of the Schaltenbrand-Wahren atlas) in case 13.

The deepest contacts 1-3 in this patient were located in the right PAG, whereas contacts 4-5 recorded from right thalamic structures.

Modified from: Wieser HG, Siegfried J. Hirnstamm-Ableitungen (Makroelektroden) beim Menschen. 1. Elektrische Befunde im Wachzustand und Ganznachtschlaf. *Z EEG EMG* 1979a; 10: 8-19 (Fig. 1), and from: Wieser HG, Siegel AM. Relations between the EEG of the cortex, thalamus and periaqueductal gray in patients suffering from epilepsy and pain syndromes. In: Zschocke S, Speckmann EJ eds. *Basic Mechanisms of the EEG*. Boston: Birkhäuser 1993: 145-182 (Fig. 11.17).

The spontaneous activity of the PAG and the thalamus was analyzed and correlated to simultaneous scalp EEG recordings. The most conspicuous findings were structure specific differences between the activity of the PAG and the thalamus. There was a close functional relationship between the alpha activity of the PAG and the scalp EEG recording during waking state (not shown). Physiological sleep patterns recorded in the mesencephalon during slow wave sleep appeared to precede the scalp recorded sleep patterns (Fig. 138, A and B). During REM sleep, rhythmic theta trains preceding horizontal saccades to the right could be recorded from an area close to the right superior colliculus (Fig. 138, C). High spike bursts were seen in relation to

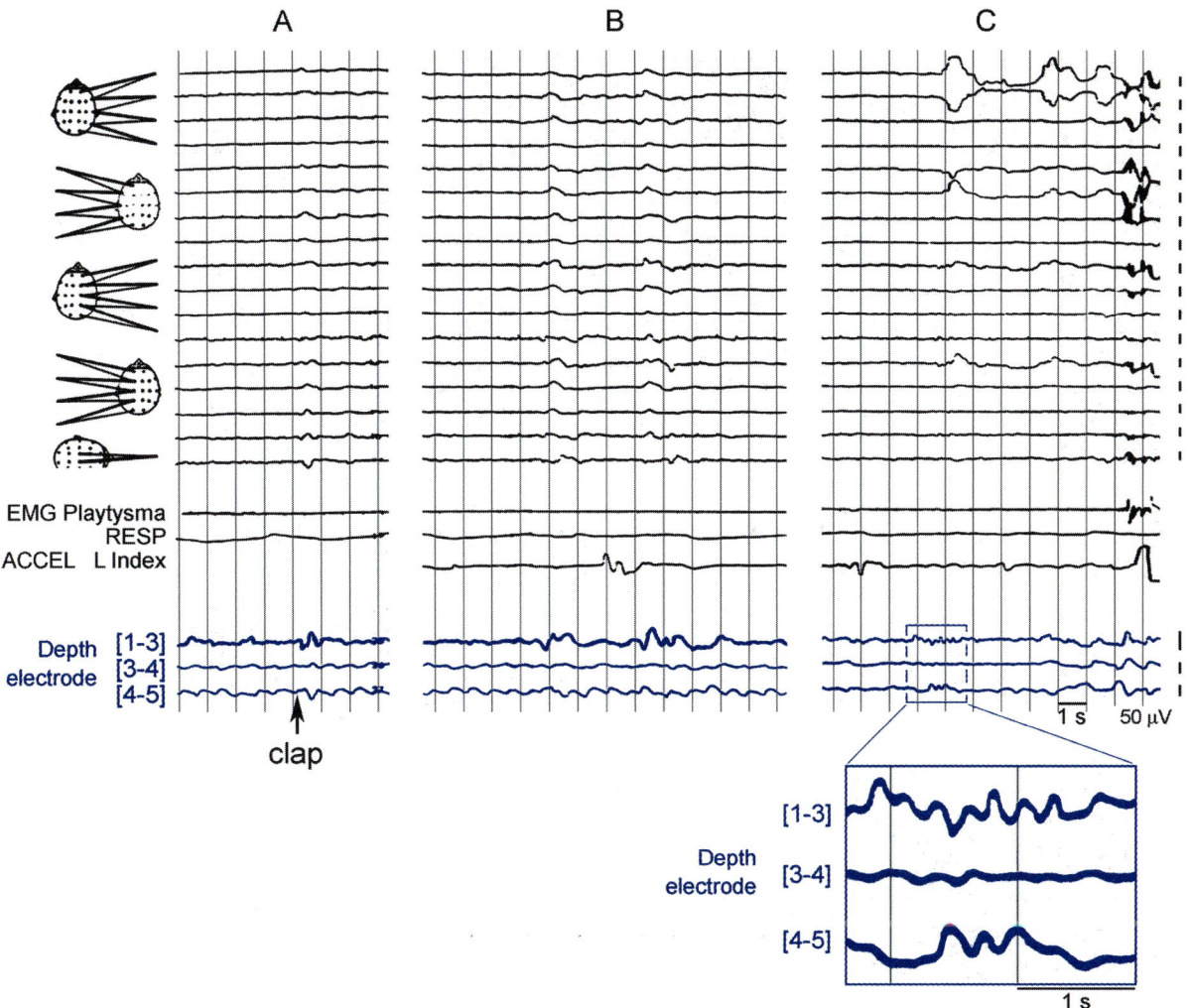

Figure 138. Combined scalp and depth EEG recordings during night sleep in a 69 year-old man with anesthesia dolorosa of the left face.

Two years prior to implantation of a right PAG electrode for the treatment of intractable pain, this patient had a thermorhizotomy because of severe left postherpetic trigeminal neuralgia (V3), with no clear benefit. The exact position of the depth electrode contacts 1-5 are shown in Fig. 137. **A**: EEG recording during stage 2 and 3 slow wave sleep, showing a physiological arousal pattern following an acoustical stimulus (clap). **B**: EEG recording during stage 2 and 3 slow wave sleep showing K-complex-like potentials (note that this potential was not due to a movement artifact, since the accelerometer attached to the left index finger (ACCEL) remained isopotential). **C**: EEG recording during REM sleep showing rhythmic theta trains at the level of the superior colliculus preceding a horizontal saccade to the right.

Modified from: Wieser HG, Siegfried J. Hirnstamm-Ableitungen (Makroelektroden) beim Menschen. 1. Elektrische Befunde im Wachzustand und Ganznachtschlaf. *Z EEG EMG* 1979a; 10: 8-19 (Figs. 8 and 9); from: Wieser HG. Temporal lobe epilepsy, sleep and arousal: Stereo-EEG findings. In: Degen R, Rodin EA eds. Epilepsy, Sleep and Sleep Deprivation. Amsterdam: Elsevier 1991: 137-167 (Fig. 12.8); and from: Wieser HG, Siegel AM. Relations between the EEG of the cortex, thalamus and periaqueductal gray in patients suffering from epilepsy and pain syndromes. In: Zschocke S, Speckmann EJ eds. *Basic Mechanisms of the EEG*. Boston: Birkhäuser 1993: 145-182 (Fig. 11.17).

Case studies

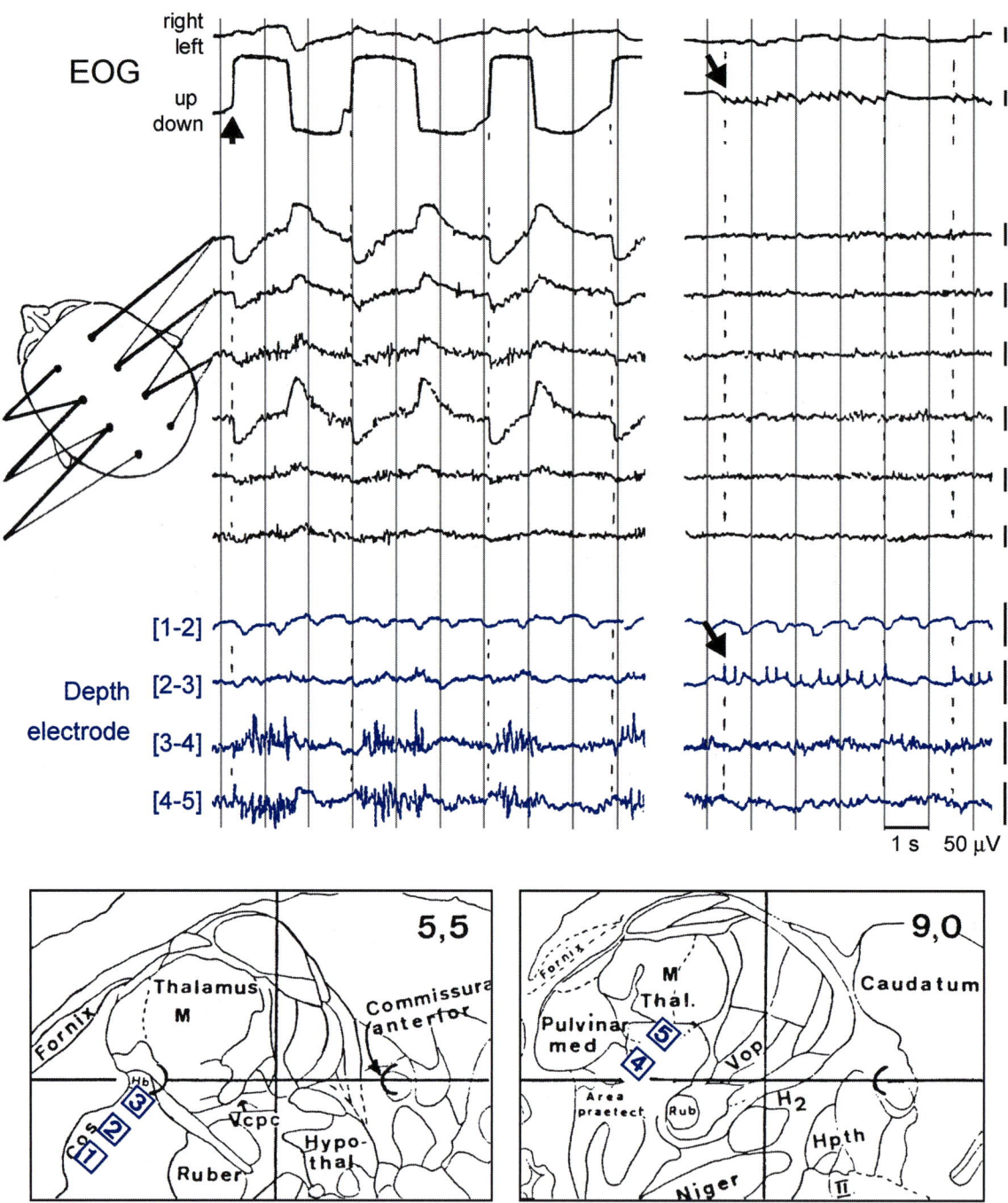

Figure 139. Combined scalp and depth EEG recordings in a 62 year-old woman with a burning pain of the left body and slight left spastic hemiparesis due to an incomplete thalamic syndrome (Déjerine-Roussy) following a right thalamocapsular hemorrhagic infarction at age 60.

The left section shows the grouped fast beta activity in the thalamus triggered by eye closure. The right section shows "eye movement premotor potentials" (lower arrow) concomitant with vertical optokinetic nystagmus (upper arrow). The exact position of the right depth electrode contacts 1-5 are shown in the scheme on the bottom. Train stimulation of the deepest contacts 1-2 situated at the level of right the superior colliculus close to the Edinger-Westphal nucleus of the oculomotor nerve produced a Parinaud syndrome [Siegfried and Wieser, 1978].

EOG, electrooculogram.

Modified from: Wieser HG, Siegfried J. Hirnstamm-Ableitungen (Makroelektroden) beim Menschen. 1. Elektrische Befunde im Wachzustand und Ganznachtschlaf. *Z EEG EMG* 1979a; 10: 8-19 (Fig. 5), from: Wieser HG, Siegfried J. Hirnstamm-Ableitungen (Makroelektroden) beim Menschen. 2. Klinische und elektrische Effekte bei Stimulation im periaquäduktalen Grau (PGM); Augenbewegungsabhängige Aktivität; visuelle und somatosensorische Reizantworten im PGM. *Z EEG EMG* 1979b; 10: 62-69 (Fig. 2); and from: Wieser HG, Siegel AM. Relations between the EEG of the cortex, thalamus and periaqueductal gray in patients suffering from epilepsy and pain syndromes. In: Zschocke S, Speckmann EJ eds. *Basic Mechanisms of the EEG*. Boston: Birkhäuser 1993: 152 (Fig. 11.18).

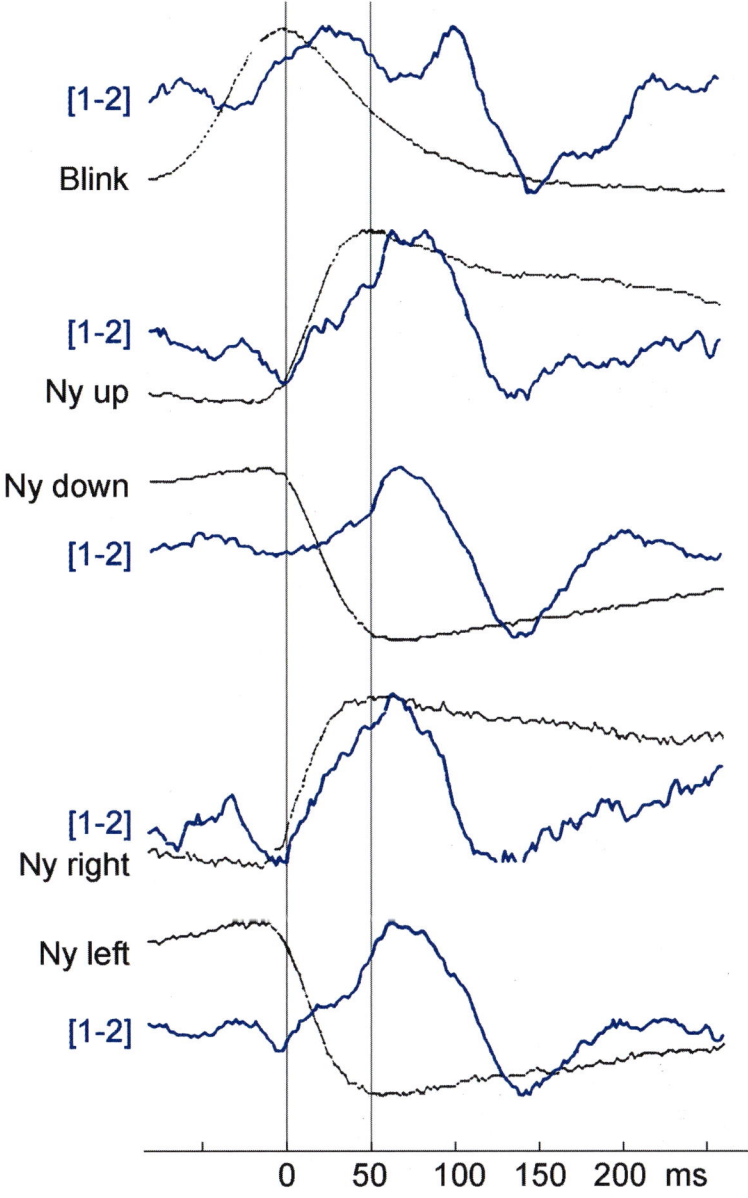

Figure 140. Averaged eye movement related potentials (blue lines, n = 12 to 29) recorded from the right PAG (depth electrode contacts 1-2, Fig. 137) following provoked blinks (Blink) and optokinetic nystagmus (Ny) in all four directions (the black lines denote the averaged oculographic recordings).

Modified from: Wieser HG, Siegfried J. Hirnstamm-Ableitungen (Makroelektroden) beim Menschen. 2. Klinische und elektrische Effekte bei Stimulation im periaquäduktalen Grau (PGM); Augenbewegungsabhängige Aktivität; visuelle und somatosensorische Reizantworten im PGM. *Z EEG-EMG* 1979b; 10: 62-69 (Fig. 4), and from: Wieser HG, Siegel AM. Relations between the EEG of the cortex, thalamus and periaqueductal gray in patients suffering from epilepsy and pain syndromes. In: Zschocke S, Speckmann EJ eds. *Basic Mechanisms of the EEG*. Boston: Birkhäuser 1993: 152 (Fig. 11.19).

rhythmic eye opening and closure in depth recordings from the thalamus (Fig. 139, left). Vertical optokinetic nystagmus induced "eye movement premotor potentials" in subcortical areas close to the superior colliculus (Fig. 139, right). These findings may indicate additional evidence for the functional role of the well known anatomical connections between mesencephalic, thalamic and temporo-occipital cortical structures, and may furthermore emphasize the role of ponto-mesencephalic structures in the generation of slow wave and REM sleep.

We have also analyzed the clinical and electrical effects of stimulation of the PAG and areas close to the superior colliculus. Train stimulation of deep contacts situated at the level of the right superior colliculus in close proximity to the Edinger-Westphal nucleus of the oculomotor nerve produced a Parinaud syndrome [Siegfried and Wieser, 1978]. Finally, we have also studied eye movement correlated activity following blinks and optokinetic nystagmus in all four directions. Evoked responses could be recorded from the PAG or from areas close to the superior colliculus and the Edinger-Westphal nucleus (Figs. 140 and 141). A more detailed description of these recordings has been published elsewhere [Wieser and Siegfried 1979a, b].

Summary

These findings illustrate spontaneous EEG activity in the PAG and the thalamus during waking state, slow wave sleep, REM sleep, intermittent photic stimulation, spontaneous blinks and optokinetic nystagmus in five non-epileptic patients undergoing PAG stimulation for the treatment of intractable central pain [Wieser and Siegfried, 1979a, b]. We analyzed the clinical effects of PAG stimulation and examined the effect of therapeutic PAG stimulation on evoked potentials after stimulation of the N. infraorbitalis [Siegfried and Wieser, 1978]. We found a close functional relationship between the alpha activity of the PAG and the scalp EEG re-

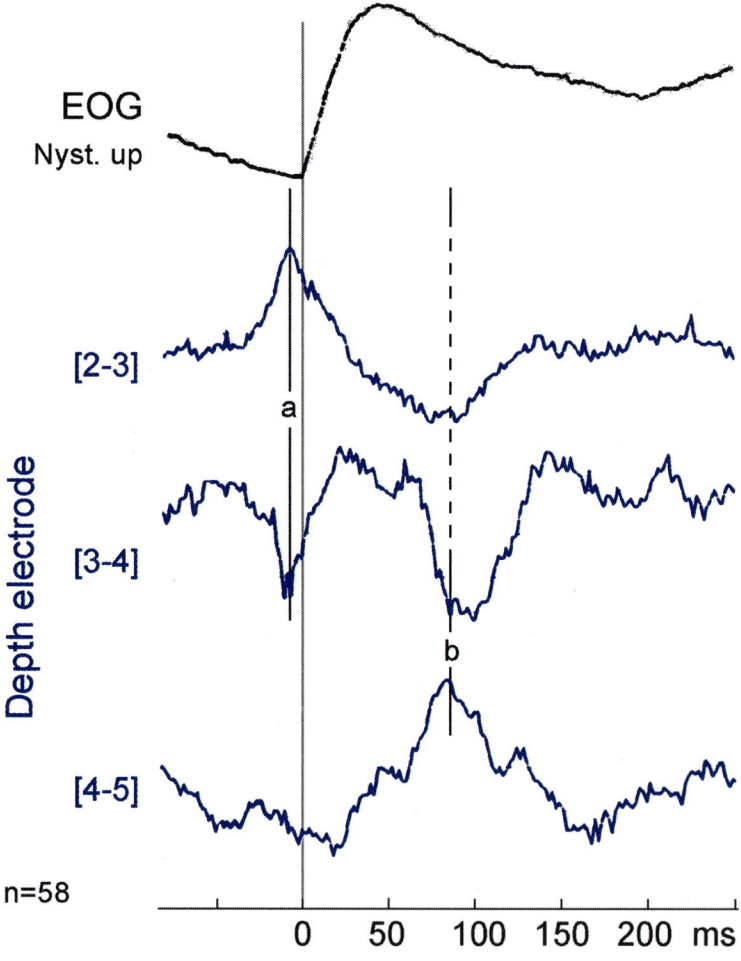

Figure 141. Averaged eye movement potentials (blue lines, n = 58) recorded from the right PAG (depth electrode contacts 2-3, 3-4, 4-5, see Fig. 137) occurring concomitantly with vertical optokinetic nystagmus (Nyst. up).

There was a positive premotor potential at contact 3 of the depth electrode peaking at about −8 ms (a) and a second negative component at contact 4 peaking at about 90 ms (b).

Modified from: Wieser HG, Siegfried J. Hirnstamm-Ableitungen (Makroelektroden) beim Menschen. 2. Klinische und elektrische Effekte bei Stimulation im periaquäduktalen Grau (PGM); Augenbewegungsabhängige Aktivität; visuelle und somatosensorische Reizantworten im PGM. *Z EEG EMG* 1979b; 10: 62-69 (Fig. 6), and from: Wieser HG, Siegel AM. Relations between the EEG of the cortex, thalamus and periaqueductal gray in patients suffering from epilepsy and pain syndromes. In: Zschocke S, Speckmann EJ eds. *Basic Mechanisms of the EEG.* Boston: Birkhäuser 1993: 152 (Fig. 11.20).

cording during waking state. Electrical train stimulation of the PAG produced a classical arousal with desynchronization of the alpha rhythm [Moruzzi and Magoun, 1949]. During slow wave sleep, periodic oscillating physiological sleep patterns could be recorded in the mesencephalon, which appeared to precede the scalp recorded sleep patterns. K-complex-like activity could be recorded in the PAG and thalamus following acoustic stimulation, but also in close temporal relationship with respiration. During REM sleep, rhythmic theta trains preceding horizontal saccades were recorded from an area close to the right superior colliculus. This activity resembled ponto-geniculo-occipital (PGO) waves, a phasic pattern related to pontine generators. Train stimulation of deep contacts located at the level of right the superior colliculus close to the Edinger-Westphal nucleus of the oculomotor nerve produced a Parinaud syndrome [Siegfried and Wieser, 1978]. High spike bursts were seen in relation to rhythmic eye opening and closure in depth recordings from the thalamus. Eye movement correlated activity following blinks and optokinetic nystagmus in all four directions could be recorded from the PAG or from areas close to the superior colliculus and the Edinger-Westphal nucleus. Vertical optokinetic nystagmus induced "eye movement premotor potentials" in areas close to the superior colliculus.

Discussion

Approximately 25% of patients with epilepsy remain poorly controlled despite various regimens of AEDs and are not eligible for resective surgery because the seizure focus cannot be identified, or the epilepsy is multifocal, or involves eloquent brain areas [Sillanpaa et al., 1998]. Novel therapeutic strategies are needed for this group of patients.

Old and New Treatment Options for Intractable Epilepsies

Older non-pharmacological and non-resective treatment options comprise behavioral management and dietetic measures such as ketogenic diet. A number of "experimental" therapeutic approaches or therapies "in evaluation" including VNS, DBS, radiosurgery (in particular, Gamma Knife surgery), transcranial magnetic stimulation (TMS) and cell transplantation have enriched this armamentarium in the last decade. For the sake of conciseness, the focus here will be limited to the various anatomical targets relevant to stereotactic epilepsy surgery. These anatomical targets are of renewed interest because of the emerging issue of DBS in patients with intractable epilepsy. VNS and cell transplantation will only be briefly mentioned. The important issues of behavioral management, dietetic measures, radiosurgery and TMS will not be discussed in this book.

Vagus Nerve Stimulation (VNS)

VNS was the first adjunctive treatment for epilepsy using electrical stimulation that has been approved by the US FDA in 1997 for the treatment of medically intractable epilepsy in patients over age 12 [Handforth et al., 1998; Morris et al., 1999]. The VNS device provides chronic intermittent stimulation to the left vagus nerve through a surgically implanted circumneural bipolar cuff electrode. Premarketing trials have shown that 30-40% of individuals with medically intractable partial seizures had a significant improvement, defined as a seizure reduction of at least 50% [The Vagus Nerve Stimulation Study Group, 1995]. Postmarketing experience suggests that the device may also be effective for the treatment of generalized seizures. Labar et al. [1999], for example, found a median seizure rate reduction of 46% with VNS in 24 patients with intractable generalized epilepsy. However, it is pertinent to note that the improvements in seizure control are modest, irrespective of the seizure type. Moreover, the mechanism by which VNS may exert its effects is unclear. It is our understanding that a true surgical sham control would have been necessary to truly ascertain how much of any benefit may have been related to placebo. Surgical sham control, however, is a priori precluded due to unavoidable though usually mild to moderate side effects with VNS, such as hoarseness, discomfort in the throat, cough or swallowing difficulties [Zumsteg et al., 2000; Uthman et al., 2004]. Furthermore, Wennberg [2004] commented on the intriguing findings of a study describing the effects of battery depletion in patients treated with VNS for epilepsy (these results can be found in the Cyberonics VNS Physician's Manual, but have not been formally published). A total of 72 battery depletions in 68 patients occurred over the course of follow up of patients in the E03 VNS trial [The Vagus Nerve Stimulation Study Group, 1995]. Of these, 42 patients (58%) had a greater than 25% decrease in seizures, whereas only 11 of 72 (15%) worsened, and 19 of 72 (26%) were unchanged. Wennberg reasoned that the large majority of patients improved after battery depletion and sarcastically noted that the effect of battery depletion was "the most significant finding of any statistical analysis performed in all of the VNS studies used to support licensing of the device as a treatment for epilepsy". Notwithstanding these limitations, recent reports on alerting effects and mood elevation with VNS have contributed to the growing use of this form of treatment [Rush et al., 2000; Shuchman, 2007]. However, it is our personal opinion that the efficacy of VNS for the treatment of intractable epilepsy in human is at best moderate.

Cell Transplantation

Animal studies have shown evidence that immature neural precursors may be capable of replacing lost neurons, restoring function and promoting brain self repair. The antiseizure effect of cell transplantation has been shown in a variety of epilepsy models; for example, in the rat kindling model, genetically epilepsy-prone rats, subcortically denervated hippocampus and administration of kainic acid or pilocarpine [Lindvall et al., 1994; Björklund and Lindvall, 2000].

Yet, the underlying mechanisms of graft action are not well understood. Huber et al. [2001] investigated the local release of adenosine from grafted cells as an ex vivo gene therapy approach to suppress synchronous discharges and epileptic seizures in electrically kindled rats. To this end, the authors engineered fibroblasts to release adenosine by inactivating the adenosine metabolizing enzymes adenosine kinase and adenosine deaminase. After encapsulation into semipermeable polymers, the cells were grafted into the brain ventricles of electrically kindled rats. This procedure provided a nearly complete protection from behavioral seizures and a near complete suppression of afterdischarges in EEG recordings, whereas the full tonic clonic convulsions in control rats remained unaltered. The authors concluded that the local release of adenosine resulting in adenosine concentrations < 25 nM at the site of action was sufficient to suppress seizure activity and, therefore, may provide a potential therapeutic principle for the treatment of human drug resistant partial epilepsies. However, it is pertinent to note that systemic administration of adenosine and its analogs may cause strong adverse effects ranging from sedation to hypothermia, leading to an almost complete cessation of spontaneous motor activity and to suppression of cardiovascular functions. These adverse effects may evidently prevent its therapeutic use. Shetty and Turner [2000] showed that fetal hippocampal grafts containing CA3 cells restore CA3 lesion induced depletions in hippocampal GAD interneurons, likely by reinnervation of GAD deficient interneurons. This specific graft mediated effect is considered beneficial because reactivation of interneurons could ameliorate both loss of functional inhibition and hyperexcitability in CA3-lesioned hippocampus. Transplants of embryonic serotoninergic, cholinergic or noradrenergic neurons have also been shown to be efficient in retarding seizure development induced by kindling stimulations. Clough et al. [1996] showed that transplantation of fetal raphe tissue into genetically epilepsy-prone rats promoted lasting reductions in increased seizure severity resulting from depletion of serotonin in the brain of genetically epilepsy-prone rats. Ferencz et al. [1998] demonstrated a marked seizure suppression in rats implanted with acetylcholine rich septal diagonal band tissue using a kindling model causing dramatic loss of the cholinergic innervation in cortical and hippocampal regions (this loss was induced by selective immunolesioning of the basal forebrain by 192 IgG saporin). Kokaia et al. [1994a] showed that fetal locus coeruleus grafts placed into a fimbria-fornix lesion cavity in 6-hydroxydopamine treated, noradrenaline denervated rats partly restored basal extracellular noradrenaline levels in the hippocampus, leading to retarded seizure development. In these studies, the antiepileptogenic effect correlated well with the extent of graft derived noradrenergic or cholinergic innervation of the stimulated brain structure. However, the clinical relevance of these findings is unclear, because lesions of these neuromodulatory systems are not characteristic features of human epilepsy. In an amygdala kindling model, Kokaia et al. [1994b] showed that rats with GABA releasing matrices bilaterally implanted dorsal to the substantia nigra exhibited only focal limbic seizures in response to electrical stimulation, whereas animals with control matrices devoid of GABA sustained generalized convulsions. However, the anticonvulsant effects observed so far have been transient, either because GABA release from the grafts declined over time, or because the host target neurons downregulate their own GABA receptors following transplantation [Kokaia et al., 1994b; Löscher et al., 1998]. It remains to be shown whether GABA releasing implants can induce increased and long lasting inhibition in an epileptic brain region [Björklund and Lindvall, 2000].

The usefulness of cell transplantation for the treatment of intractable epilepsy in man is not clear. Intracerebral implantation of porcine fetal striatal GABA rich tissue has been performed in a group of epileptic patients in whom surgical removal of the brain region receiving the transplant was planned [A Pilot Short-Term Safety and Feasibility Study of Implanting GABA-Producing Porcine Fetal Neuronal Cells into Epileptogenic Tissue of Patients with Focal Epilepsy with Single or Multiple Epileptogenic Sites in the Temporal and/or Frontal Lobes, Phase I, Sponsor: Diacrin, Inc., Charlestown, MA, http://www.diacrin.com]. However, it is pertinent to note that the technique of xenotransplanted porcine neural cells is relatively new and, consequently, burdened with unknown risks. There is a risk of rejection (rash, fever, hypertension, etc.) in the human using xenografts or of transmission of infectious agents incorporated into the genome of the transplanted porcine cells during the xenotransplantation procedure (for example, the porcine endogenous retrovirus). In this respect, it is interesting to remember that the porcine cell trial transplanted into the brains of stroke patients was put on hold on April 17, 2000 because of adverse events in two patients.

Stereotactic Epilepsy Surgery

Stereotactic lesions have frequently been performed with the aim to prevent seizure spread along preexisting and preferred seizure propagating pathways or to directly destroy diseased areas of the brain that act as a focus of epileptic discharges. Other mechanisms including the reduction of the volume of excitable neurons, or the increase of threshold of irritability have also been proposed. The most common targets were fornical fibers, thalamic nuclei, Forel H field, amygdala and hippocampus. "Combined" lesions in various combinations within the limbic system have also been performed.

Yet, the usefulness of stereotactic epilepsy surgery has been repeatedly challenged, and the placement of irreversible lesions for the treatment of epilepsy has been virtually abandoned for several decades (with the exception maybe of stereotactic amygdalotomy in patients with amygdalar epilepsy [Siegfried and Wieser, 1988]). For now it shall suffice to say that the high expectations placed on stereotactic epilepsy surgery have not been met, irrespective of the target area. Nevertheless, the extensive knowledge deriving from early attempts to suppress seizures by stereotactic epilepsy surgery is relevant to the renewed interest in neurostimulation for the treatment of epilepsy. The therapeutic yield of stereotactic ablation of subcortical and cortical targets will therefore be individually discussed in the following section on potential targets for DBS in epilepsy.

Potential Targets for Deep Brain Stimulation in Epilepsy

The interest in electric stimulation for the treatment of epilepsy was rekindled with the beginning of the modern era of DBS in the late 1980s, when Benabid et al. [1987] had reported the use of high frequency DBS of the nucleus ventralis intermedius (Vim) for the treatment of extrapyramidal tremor, and with the increasing experience of DBS for other indications, including movement disorders other than tremor, and chronic pain and psychiatric disorders. The idea of subcortical electric stimulation for the treatment of epilepsy arose from the recognition of widespread reciprocal subcortico-cortical connections and progressive recruitment of subcortical structures during evolution of seizures [Theodore and Fisher, 2004]. Hence, electric stimulation for the treatment of epilepsy aims to influence key "pacemaker" areas in the brain that are thought to be important in seizure genesis or propagation, thereby decreasing seizure severity and frequency. Based on the findings of animal studies and uncontrolled clinical studies, and taking into consideration the connectivity and close functional relations of subcortical nuclei to the cortex and limbic structures, a number of subcortical and cortical structures have been suggested to be promising targets in this respect. These targets include, amongst others, the cerebellum, thalamic nuclei (such as the CM, AN and DM), STN, caudate nucleus, mamillary bodies, amygdala and hippocampus [Schaltenbrand and Walker, 1982; Lüders, 2004].

Historically, the earliest attempts to suppress seizures with electrical stimulation began with the stimulation of the cerebellum. In 1955, Cooke and Snider demonstrated the arrest of focal cortical seizures following stimulation of the cerebellar cortex in animals. Numerous animal studies in various animal seizure models followed that also reported a decrease of seizures with this target [Dow *et al.*, 1962; Mutani *et al.*, 1969; Babb *et al.*, 1974; Hutton *et al.*, 1972; Hablitz and Rea, 1976]. Others, however, failed to confirm an antiseizure effect with cerebellar stimulation [Grimm *et al.*, 1970; Myers *et al.*, 1975)]. In humans, cerebellar stimulation for the treatment of epilepsy (and other diseases) was pioneered by Cooper and colleagues in the mid 1970s [Cooper, 1973; Cooper *et al.*, 1973, 1976, 1977, 1977-1978]. Davis *et al.* [1984] then reported on cerebellar stimulation in 32 patients with focal and generalized seizures, finding complete seizure control or reduction to occasional seizures in 18 (56.2%), worthwhile improvement in nine (28.1%), and no effect in five patients (15.6%). According to Lüders *et al.* [2004], at least 11 uncontrolled studies including a total of 112 patients were performed between 1977 and 1987, with excellent results (seizure free) in 27%, moderate improvement in 53%, and no change in seizure frequency in 20% of patients. However, these encouraging results could not be not confirmed in two controlled trials including five [Van Buren *et al.* 1978] and 12 patients [Wright *et al.* 1984]. Both these studies failed to demonstrate a significant change in seizure frequency, which has lead to a discontinuation of cerebellar stimulation for the treatment of epilepsy in man (with the exception of Velasco *et al.* [2005], who recently reported on a significant reduction in tonic clonic seizures and tonic seizures in a double blind, randomized controlled pilot study of bilateral cerebellar stimulation for treatment of intractable motor seizures).

The Forel H field

With the advent of improved stereotaxy in the 1960ies, the Forel H field quickly became a target for therapeutically motivated lesions to improve symptoms of Parkinson's disease, hyperkinesias and certain types of epilepsies [Spiegel *et al.*, 1963]. Jinnai *et al.* [1976] reported on 64 epilepsy patients who underwent unilateral and bilateral Forel H-tomy (performed in intervals of weeks to > 6 months) with a follow up of 1 to 12 years. They had used a target located 2 mm posterior to the midpoint of the intercommissural AC-PC-line, 4 mm ventral and 4.5 to 5 mm lateral to the wall of the 3rd ventricle. The results of this study are summarized in *Tables I* and *II*. In patients who underwent bilateral Forel H-tomy, the authors noted substantial side effects such as akinetic type of motor disturbance, disturbances of speech and swallowing.

Table I. Effects of Forel H-tomy on epilepsy type.

Epilepsy type	Forel H-tomy	Outcome		
		Excellent	Good	Poor & no effect
Idiopathic (n = 13)	Bilateral wp (pp) Unilateral wp (pp)	3 (0) 2 (0)	1 (2) 1 (1)	0 (1) 1 (1)
Symptomatic (n = 51)	Bilateral wp (pp) Unilateral wp (pp)	2 (1) 13 (0)	5 (2) 3 (0)	4 (6) 11 (4)
Total		21	15	28

wp, well placed; *pp*, poorly placed (or out of target).
Modified from: Jinnai D, Mukawa J, Kobayashi K. Forel-H-tomy for the treatment of intractable epilepsy. *Acta Neurochir* (Vienna) 1976; 23 (Suppl.): 159-165.

Table II. Effects of Forel H-tomy on seizure type.

Seizure type	Abolished			Diminished			Unchanged		
Grand mal	6	{2}	(14)	1	{1}	(2)		{1}	
Petit mal						(1)			
Myoclonic		{1}			{2}				
Hemiconvulsions			(2)			(1)			
Focal	2		(10)	2		(2)			
Akinetic						(2)			
Lennox	2		(1)	2		(1)			(5)
Reflex	1								
Psychomotor							3		(6)

No brackets, Symptomatic cases with bilateral well placed electrodes; *{ }*, Idiopathic cases with bilateral well placed electrodes; *( )*, Symptomatic cases with unilateral well placed electrode.
Modified from: Jinnai D, Mukawa J, Kobayashi K. Forel-H-tomy for the treatment of intractable epilepsy. *Acta Neurochir* (Vienna) 1976; 23 (Suppl.): 159-165.

Yoshii [1977-1978] reported on a 2 to 7 years follow up in 15 patients who underwent Forel H-tomy (the operation was actually carried out in 20 patients, but only 15 of those were reported in their study), finding the procedure to be "markedly effective" or "effective" in seven (46.7%), worthwhile in five (33.3%), and "ineffective" in three patients (20%). Efficacy was greater in patients with bilateral operation, and in patients with grand mal seizures or patients with minor seizures, if compared to patients with other seizure types. Furthermore, six patients demonstrated an improvement of their personality and emotional skills. Koshino *et al.* [1975] found complete seizure control or worthwhile improvement in three of 13 patients (23.1%), but failure in 10 patients (76.9%) with generalized (n = 7) or hemiconvulsive (n = 6) seizures. In a study including nine patients, Rachkov and Bezukh [1983] noted that early post stereotactic investigations may reveal better efficacy of surgical treatment of generalized epilepsy and may also be helpful for gaining a better insight into Forel H functions. In a study including six adult patients with chronic intractable epilepsy associated with multifocal EEG abnormalities, Ramani *et al.* [1980] found a significant reduction in the frequency of generalized tonic clonic seizures in four patients (66.7%), whereas no effect was seen in three patients (50%) with complex partial seizures and in one patient (16.7%) with akinetic myoclonic seizures (the average follow up was 40 months in this study). Neuropsychological testing revealed a mild to moderate postoperative decline in cognitive functions in four of the six patients. Laitinen [1967] demonstrated a seizure reduction in five of seven patients [71.4%] with generalized seizures, but only little improvement with respect to myoclonic attacks.

In 1987, Ravagnati carried out a careful study of all available data with regard to stereotactic lesions placed in the fields of Forel, summarizing that 31 of 103 patients (30.1%) became seizure free or only had occasional seizures, 31 patients (30.1%) had a worthwhile improvement, and 41 patients (39.8%) showed no effect with Forel H-tomy [Jinnai and Nishimoto, 1963; Jinnai, 1966; Laitinen, 1967; Mullan *et al.*, 1967; Chiorino *et al.*, 1968; Jinnai and Mukawa, 1970; Koshino *et al.*, 1975; Mukawa *et al.*, 1975; Jinnai *et al.*, 1976; Yoshii, 1977-1978; Ramani *et al.*, 1980; Marossero *et al.*, 1980; Bidzinksi and Ostrowski, 1981]. Ravagnati concluded that "in primary generalized seizures as well as in multifocal epilepsies, lesions in the thalamus... have produced disappointing results. For grand mal seizures, whether of primary or secondary generalized type, the fields of Forel can be considered a promising target, but further evaluation of its efficacy and safeness is needed". His conclusions were similar to those of Spencer and Spencer [1985] who in their review article on surgical treatment of epilepsy stated that "the results of stereotactic lesions in various locations are difficult to evaluate with the single exception of field H of Forel, which in many reports has been effective for grand mal seizures". Ojemann and Ward [1975] in their review also concluded that "the fields of Forel seem to be a promising target in the treatment of seizures, particularly grand mal seizures, whether of the primary or secondary generalized type". These authors also noted that "further clinical investigations with this target area in intractable epilepsy of these types would seem to be indicated". Their conclusions were mainly based on previous studies reporting on the effect of lesioning of the Forel H fields in patients with epilepsy (in some of these studies, subventral thalamatomies were performed, which had also included parts of the Forel H fields). Walker [1982] suggested that the finding of a positive effect on generalized but not on myoclonic or psychomotor seizures might be related to differences in primary pathways of seizure propagation, taking into account that the latter seizure types do not travel through striothalamic tracts. Ramani et al. [1980] noted that "fields of Forel surgery, while partially effective in generalized tonic clonic seizures, appears justified only in patients with such severe preexisting cognitive deficits, that the benefits of seizure control definitely outweigh the risk of further cognitive decline".

The Subthalamic Nucleus

The consideration of the STN as a target for stimulation in patients with epilepsy was greatly influenced by the positive experience of STN stimulation in patients with movement disorders. The rationale of stimulation of the STN for the treatment of epilepsy arose from the concept of the nigral control of epilepsy system (NCES) in experimental animal studies [Iadarola and Gale, 1982; Gale, 1985]. There is experimental evidence that the so called dorsal midbrain anticonvulsant zone (DMAZ) in the superior colliculi may be under constant inhibitory control of efferent fibers from the substantia nigra pars reticulata. Inhibition of the STN by high frequency stimulation has been suggested to block the inhibitory effect of the subtantia nigra pars reticulata on the DMAZ, and thus to activate the latter, resulting in an increase of the seizure threshold at cortical sites [Loddenkemper et al., 2001].

In animals, high frequency stimulation of the STN has been demonstrated to suppress seizures in various seizure models including the Genetic Absence Epilepsy Rat of Strasbourg (GAERS) [Vercueil et al., 1998], the kainic acid seizure model [Bressand et al., 1999; Loddenkemper et al., 2001; Pan et al., 2004], kindled seizures [Lado et al., 2003], flurothyl seizures [Lado et al., 2003], and spontaneous absence seizures [Vercueil et al., 1998]. Lado et al. [2003] showed that bilateral high frequency STN stimulation at 130 Hz produced a significant increase in the seizure threshold for clonic flurothyl seizures in rats, whereas no effect was found with stimulation at 260 Hz. Moreover, STN stimulation at 800 Hz significantly lowered seizure threshold for tonic clonic seizures. Unilateral disinhibition of the STN, in contrast, has been shown to be likely proconvulsant in rats [Dybdal and Gale, 2000]. Hence, there is good evidence for the anticonvulsant effect of electrical stimulation of the STN in animals, but this effect obviously depends on the stimulation frequency and the type of seizure.

In humans, several uncontrolled studies including at least nine patients with epilepsy have been performed to date, reporting an up to 80% reduction in seizure frequency with bilateral STN stimulation in six, and no change in the remaining patients [Benazzouz et al., 1995; Tronnier et al., 1999; Benazzouz and Hallett, 2000; Loddenkemper et al., 2001; Benabid et al., 2002; Chabardès et al., 2002; Däuper et al., 2002; Dinner et al., 2002; Benabid et al., 2004; Neme et al., 2004]. More specifically, Benabid et al. [2002] demonstrated that long term high frequency STN stimulation at 130 Hz resulted in an 80% reduction in the number and severity of seizures caused by focal cortical dysplasia in a pediatric patient. In a study by Chabardès et al. [2002] on five patients (including the pediatric patient reported in the study of Benabid et al. [2002]), three patients (60%) showed a good response, one patient (20%) had a < 50% improvement in seizure frequency, and one patient (20%) showed no change in seizure patterns after 6 months of chronic 130 Hz STN stimulation. Overall, the mean reduction of seizure frequency was 62.4% (range 41.5-80.7%) in this study. Loddenkemper *et al.* [2001] reported a seizure reduction of 80% in two of five patients (40%) with intractable partial seizures after 16 months of STN stimutation, but no effect in the remaining two patients. Gonzalez-Martinez and colleagues reported on mixed results with STN stimulation at the AANS meeting in 2002, finding seizure reduction rates of 82%, 61% and 30% in three of four patients, and no effect in one patient.

In an electrophysiological study in man, Hamer *et al.* [2003] reported on EEG recordings simultaneously recording from subdural electrodes placed on the precentral gyrus and bilateral STN depth electrodes in a patient with focal clonic seizures, finding that a) the STN activity was mainly ipsilateral to the cortical activity, b) cortical spikes did not necessarily elicit STN spikes, and c) the cortical EEG waves following the polyspikes generally outlasted the waves recorded in the STN. The authors concluded that STN activation may not reflect an essential component of clonic seizures, though the spread of cortical spikes to the STN may contribute to the continuation of the seizure activity of the cortex in general.

In summary, modulation of the seizure threshold by stimulation of the STN appears to be a promising future treatment option for patients with some forms of pharmacologically intractable epilepsy, though results from controlled studies are not available to date and much has to be done in order to answer the questions as to the efficacy of STN DBS. Several centers are now performing long term protocols for DBS of the STN in patients with intractable epilepsy.

The Fornix

Based on the consideration that the fornix is the major outlet of the hippocampus, section of the fornix (so called fornicotomy) has been performed early by many surgeons. Hassler and Riechert [1957] placed lesions bilaterally in the fornix at the posterior margin of the anterior commissure in a patient with temporal lobe seizures and concluded that the interruption of the fornix and anterior commissure may diminish frequency and spreading of attacks in patients with temporal lobe seizures. Umbach [1966] reported on the effects of fornix lesions (bilateral in 5 cases) combined with lesions of the anterior commissure in 18 patients with TLE, finding that partial seizures were eliminated in four patients (22.2%), and generalized seizures in 11 of 13 patients (84.6%). Orthner and Lohmann [1966; n = 2] and Schaltenbrand *et al.* [1966; n = 5] made similar experiences. Schaltenbrand *et al.* [1966] found improvement in four of five patients (80%) with concomitant lesioning of the anterior commissure and the pallidum. Bouchard and Umbach [1972] found a reduction of 65% for generalized seizures in a study including 50 patients. Barcia-Salorio and Broseta [1976] studied the indications and long term results of stereotactic fornicotomy with concomitant lesioning of the anterior commissure in 42 patients with TLE and behavioral disturbances, finding satisfactory results in 78.6% of their patients, though mainly when aggression was the main clinical feature (the best results were related to a high IQ and a short clinical history). Sonnen *et al.* [1976], in contrast, found no definite improvement in seizure frequency in eight patients that underwent amygdalotomy followed by fornicotomy in some of the cases (however, three of their patients improved with respect to behavior). Mundinger *et al.* [1976] reported on 29 patients with psychomotor seizures who underwent fornicotomy (bilateral in three cases) and lesioning of the anterior commissure and the amygdala, finding a good outcome in six patients (20.7%), a worthwhile improvement in 13 patients (44.8%) and a treatment failure in 10 patients (34.5%). Ganglberger [1984] found complete seizure control in four of 10 patients (40%), and improvement in nine patients (90%) following concomitant lesioning of the amygdala and the DM.

Memory function is considered to be a major concern after bilateral section of the anterior fornix in man. However, in a review comprising 193 patients (of whom 180 patients underwent fornicotomy for the treatment of epilepsy, and 13 patients removal of a third ventricle colloid cyst), Garcia-Bengochea and Friedman [1987] noted persistent postoperative memory loss in no more than four patients. Hassler and Riechert [1957] in their case report stated that unilateral fornicotomy was generally well tolerated, whereas bilateral symmetrical interruption of the fornices caused an excitatory state with disorientation in time and place and amnesia of more than one week's duration. They consequently concluded that bilateral fornicotomy should not be carried out in symmetrical positions in order to prevent memory impairment.

The Mamillary Bodies

The consideration of the MB and MTT as targets for therapeutically motivated lesions in patients with epilepsy was mainly based on the functional and anatomical connectivity of the MB and MTT to other limbic structures (cf. Papez circuit, page 38), and also on the early reports by Jinnai et al. [1969] showing that bilateral lesions in the MB resulted in an almost 2-fold increase in pentylenetretrazol (PTZ) threshold in cats.

In guinea pigs, Mirski and Ferrendelli [1983, 1986b] showed selective metabolic activation of the MB using [^{14}C]-2-deoxyglucose autoradiography during a threshold convulsive stimulus induced by the co-infusion of PTZ and ethosuximide. In subsequent work, the authors then showed that bilateral interruption of the MMT had a substantial protective effect against the convulsant PTZ in guinea pigs [Mirski and Ferrendelli, 1984a, 1984b, 1987]. Lesioning of the fornix and the mamillary peduncles have also been shown to be protective against PTZ seizures, though to a lesser degree than MTT lesions. The composite analysis of lesions in the mid diencephalon revealed that the most protective lesions were those that primarily damaged the MTT, but only small portions of adjacent brain tissue, whereas large lesions additionally involving the MTT were not protective. Mirski and Ferrendelli [1987] argued that this observation, although seemingly paradoxical, may be understood in light of the accumulated evidence demonstrating both facilitatory and inhibitory influences in the diencephalon on the expression of seizures [Andy and Mukawa, 1959; Gellhom et al., 1959; Milhorat et al., 1966; Mullan et al., 1967; Jinnai et al., 1969; Gloor et al., 1977; Quesney et al., 1977]. The protective effect of bilateral MTT or MB lesions (as well as fornix lesions) further implies that the MTT acts as a final common pathway of propagation of paroxysmal activity to the thalamus and cortex from MB associated subcortical structures. This concept is in accordance with the findings of Green and Morin [1953] who found "seizure like activity" in the cerebral cortex only with diencephalic stimulation from within posterior hypothalamic, fornical, MTT or anterior thalamic structures.

The efficacy of stereotactic ablation or DBS of the MB and MTT for the treatment of epilepsy in man is not clear. Sano et al. [1970a] investigated the clinical effects of stereotactic lesioning of the posterior hypothalamus in 22 patients with intractable psychomotor, absence or generalized seizures. The authors demonstrated complete seizure control in one patient (4.5%), a seizure reduction in six patients (27.3%), and no benefit in 15 patients (68.2%). It is noteworthy that in this series two patients (9.1%) died in status epilepticus, and that the EEG recordings in the main remained unchanged postsurgery. More recently, the group around Raftopoulos in Leuven, Belgium, reported on their experience with chronic DBS of the MB and MTT for epilepsy [Duprez et al., 2005; Raftopoulos et al., 2005; van Rijckevorsel et al., 2005]. Raftopoulos et al. [2005] demonstrated the occurrence of epileptiform discharges in MB recordings of a patient with intractable epilepsy. These discharges were commonly restricted to the MB, although spread to the ipsilateral MTT area, and subsequently to the contralateral MB and MTT area, could be found with discharges of a duration of 100 seconds or longer. Van Rijckevorsel et al. [2005] reported MB-MTT EEG findings in three patients with intractable seizures, finding (1) background EEG patterns characterized by low amplitude waves (usually < 25 µV for MB and < 20 µV for MTT) with a variable combination of theta/beta rhythms, (2) diffusion of scalp epileptiform activity to the left MTT and pseudoperiodic slow spikes within the right MTT electrodes after a clinical seizure or a seizure with subtle clinical signs in a patient with a small hypothalamic hamartoma, (3) right MB ictal discharges characterized by an initial low voltage 20 Hz discharge followed by repetitive spikes of progressive higher voltage and low voltage slow waves of a duration of 4 to 108 seconds, occasionally spreading to the right MTT and to the left side in a patient with partial seizures of presumable right temporal onset, and (4) a seizure with rhythmic delta waves in the left MB-MTT electrode during 10 to 15 minutes and occasional pseudoperiodic slow spikes in the right MTT electrode in a patient with partial seizures of frontal or temporal onset. The authors concluded that the theta/beta pattern represents the predominant physiologic profile of MB, and that paroxysmal epileptiform discharges can be readily observed in human MB recordings.

Results from controlled studies on the efficacy of MB or MTT DBS are not available to date. However, taking into consideration the functional and anatomical connectivity of the MB and MTT to other limbic structures, these structures may be regarded as a potential target for the treatment of epilepsy by electrical stimulation.

The Medial Thalamic Nuclei (Anterior and Dorsomedial)

Thalamic DBS as a treatment for intractable epilepsy has been proposed based on previous animal and human observations suggesting involvement of the thalamus in the maintenance and propagation of seizures. Animal studies have demonstrated that lesioning of AN afferents, the application of muscimol to inhibit neuronal firing, or electrical high frequency stimulation of the AN may increase the seizure threshold or reduce frequency of generalized seizures in the pentylenetetrazol seizure model [Mirski and Ferrendelli, 1984a, 1986a, 1987; Mirski and Fisher, 1994; Mirski et al., 1986, 1997, 2003]. Hamani et al. [2004b] showed that bilateral AN lesions or high frequency AN stimulation are protective against pilocarpine induced seizures and status epilepticus in animals.

In humans, AN stimulation for epilepsy was pioneered by Cooper and his colleagues, who reported a > 60% seizure reduction in five of six patients [Cooper et al., 1984; Cooper and Upton, 1985; Upton et al., 1985, 1987]. Exact details of stimulation were not provided in these studies, but overall AN stimulation reduced seizures by more than 60% in five of six patients, allowing for an average 30% decrease in medication requirements. Subsequent unblinded pilot trials confirmed that chronic AN stimulation may result in a significant decrease in seizure frequency in the long term [Sussman et al., 1988; Hodaie et al., 2002; Kerrigan et al., 2004; Andrade et al., 2006]. In an abstract, Sussman et al. [1988] reported on a significant improvement in three of five patients with intractable epilepsy. In 2002, Hodaie et al. reported on the efficacy of anterior thalamic DBS in a pilot study including five patients with intractable seizures of different etiologies. The patients received high frequency stimulation beginning 4 weeks after implantation. The mean follow up was 15 months. No change in medication was done in the first year after implantation. Changes in stimulation parameters were done multiple times in all patients, including a 2-month period of single blinded stimulation OFF. There were no serious adverse effects with AN implantation and stimulation. The authors found a mean seizure reduction of 54%. Two patients showed > 75% reduction. It is interesting to note that in the > 50% good responders group, no change in stimulation parameters (voltages, frequency, bipolar or monopolar stimulation) alone or in combination was as effective in reducing the frequency of seizures as simple implantation of the AN electrodes (that is before activation of stimulation). An excellent response to implantation only (91 and 82% reduction from baseline) was a good outcome indicator, while intermediate reductions (27 to 47%) were associated with variable outcomes after the stimulators were turned ON. There was no significant change in seizure frequency during single blinded stimulation OFF periods in either good or poor responders. The authors left it open whether the sustained long term beneficial response to AN DBS in this small open label trial represented an effect of microthalamotomy caused by electrode insertion or an effect induced by electrical stimulation through the electrodes, or a combination of these or other factors. Kerrigan *et al.* [2004] found a significant improvement regarding the severity of seizures in four of five patients (80%) with medically intractable partial seizures treated with bilateral AN stimulation (in particular with respect to the frequency of secondarily generalized tonic clonic seizures and complex partial seizures associated with falls), but a significant reduction in total seizure frequency was found in only one (20%) of their patients. More recently, Andrade *et al.* [2006] reported the long term follow up (19-81 months, mean 5 years) of six patients with intractable symptomatic generalized or multifocal/partial epilepsy with secondarily generalized tonic clonic seizures implanted with AN thalamic electrodes for therapeutic DBS. Overall, electrode implantation and stimulation in the AN was followed by a > 50% seizure reduction in five of six patients (83.3%), and two patients (33.3%) showed a greater than 75% reduction (however, it is noteworthy that significant benefit was not seen until the addition of further adjuvant antiepileptic drugs at year 5 and 6 in two of the patients included in this study). Nevertheless, these long term findings were in keeping with the results previously reported by the same group [Hodaie *et al.*, 2002], and also with the findings from previous uncontrolled pilot studies of other groups [Cooper *et al.*, 1984; Cooper and Upton, 1985; Sussman *et al.*, 1988; Kerrigan *et al.*, 2004]. No controlled studies have been performed to date, but a multicenter prospective randomized trial of scheduled chronic AN stimulation in persons with medically intractable localization related epilepsy is under way [SANTE trial; Graves *et al.*, 2004].

The Centromedian Nucleus

Based on the hypothesis that destruction of the CM, as a part of the thalamic non specific system, would exert an impact on the process of synchronization in the thalamocortical circuitry, this target has been repeatedly investigated with respect to seizure control in patients with intractable epilepsy. Chkhenkeli *et al.* [2004] demonstrated the active participation of the CM in the spread and maintenance of epileptic activity in 11 patients with partial motor and secondarily generalized seizures. The authors demonstrated a "recruiting reaction" with low frequency 2 to 6 Hz CM stimulation that was accompanied by a synchronization of interictal epileptic activity in 92% of stimulations, whereas high frequency stimulation at 20 to 130 Hz produced desynchronization of background EEG activity accompanied by reduction of interictal epileptic patterns in 78% of stimulations. Both desynchronization and suppression of epileptic activity were mostly observed within the confines of the hemisphere ipsilateral to the side of stimulation, and were more evident on neocortical electrical activity than on the interictal epileptic activity of mesiobasal temporal lobe structures. These results are in good accordance with the findings of Zumsteg *et al.* [2006a] who found a diffuse though mainly ipsilateral and highly significant cortical activation with high intensity stimulation of the CM in a study using SNPM of LORETA (see page 50).

Stereotactic lesioning of the CM for the treatment of epilepsy has been carried out by Ramamurthi *et al.* [1974]. In a study including six patients with intractable myoclonic or salaam seizures, this group found complete seizure control in three patients (50%), a worthwhile improvement in one patient (16.7%), and no benefit in two patients (33.3%). In the same year, Sano [1974] reported on a worthwhile improvement in only two of five patients (40%), and a lack of efficacy in the remaining three patients (60%).

Velasco *et al.* [1987] were the first to employ bilateral CM stimulation in patients with intractable epilepsy, finding a marked seizure reduction in an uncontrolled study including five patients. Chkhenkeli and Šramka [1989] reported that stimulation of the CM resulted in a decrease of cortical epileptiform discharges. One important observation of Velasco *et al.* [1993] was the effects of CM stimulation on generalized tonic clonic seizures, demonstrating that the number of generalized seizures decreased most markedly in their series of patients. The same group of researchers later reported their long term results in 13 patients with bilateral CM stimulation with a mean follow up of 41 months, noting a significant decrease (defined as

> 80% seizure reduction) in the incidence of generalized tonic clonic seizures and atypical absences, but no change in the incidence of complex partial seizures [Velasco et al., 2000a]. The authors concluded that the antiepileptic effect with chronic DBS of the CM may be the result of activation of a nonspecific reticulothalamocortical system responsible for generalized electrocortical responses such as recruiting, desynchronization, negative direct current shifts, and the three per second spike wave complex pattern.

However, notwithstanding this encouraging preliminary data, Fisher et al. [1992] in a double blind controlled cross over study including seven patients with intractable epilepsy found only a modest improvement in the control of generalized tonic clonic seizures, namely a non significant 30% reduction in seizure frequency. In particular, there was no significant difference in the response to periods of stimulation ON or OFF. The negative results of Fisher et al. [1992] were in accordance with the experiences of the Toronto group, who also found that stimulation through the CM was not associated with a beneficial result in the overall control of seizures in the two patients included in their study (in one patient, implantation and stimulation did decrease the number of secondarily generalized tonic clonic seizures (GTC), although the number of complex partial seizures increased. In the other patient with only GTC seizures, no beneficial effects were observed with CM stimulation) [Andrade et al., 2006]. In summary, it is our personal opinion that the usefulness of CM stimulation regarding seizure control is controversial at best.

The Periaqueductal Gray

The idea that generalized convulsions may be related to disordered function in brainstem structures is not new [Temkin, 1970]. Gastaut and Fisher-Williams [1959] demonstrated that generalized convulsions could be elicited by electrical stimulation of the medulla oblongata and noted that generalized convulsions in animals can occur despite ablation of the cerebral cortex, the greater part of the telencephalon, the diencephalon and the mesencephalon. Based on these findings and on the writings of Penfield and Jasper [1946, 1954], the view emerged that primary generalized seizures may originate in midbrain and upper brainstem structures (the "centrencephalic" theory). Conversely, numerous investigators independently showed that chemical or electrical stimulation of the cortex was sufficient to produce generalized convulsions (the "telencephalic" theory) [Gibbs and Gibbs, 1952]. Davidson and Watson [1959] suggested that neuronal aggregates were equally unstable and behave as an unstable system, that is, "go critical" under appropriate environmental circumstances. It was Gloor [1968, 1979] who eventually expanded these opposing ideas by proposing a "corticoreticular" hypothesis, emphasizing the complex interplay between cortical and subcortical structures. Although it is not necessary that any of these possibilities be mutually exclusive [Nashold et al., 1972], it is now acknowledged that the great majority of generalized convulsions in man may originate in cortical structures [Lund, 1952; Williams, 1965; Bancaud, 1971, 1972], but then spread and generalize with prominent participation of the reticular formation and other subcortical structures [Walker et al., 1956; Wada and Cornelius, 1960; Wilder and Schmidt, 1965; Jasper, 1969; Morillo et al., 1982]. Furthermore, there is evidence from pharmacological studies supporting the concept that subcortical structures play an important role in the propagation and generalization of seizures [Fromm, 1987]. The ability to depress the reticular formation actually appears to be an essential characteristic of antiepileptic drugs [Fromm, 1985; Fromm et al., 1984].

Notwithstanding the key role of the cortex in the generation of generalized seizures, the observation that seizures can be experimentally elicited by electrical, mechanical or chemical stimulation of subcortical (even spinal) structures in animals is of great interest with respect to DBS for the treatment of epilepsy. The focus here shall be on the effects of ablation or electrical stimulation of the PAG. Kreindler et al. [1958] demonstrated that high intensity electrical stimulation of the cat and rat PAG (or brainstem reticular formation) produced convulsions that outlasted the duration of the stimulus and that could still be elicited after decerebration by high midbrain transsection. These subcortically triggered "brainstem attacks" differed both in motor pattern and in duration from cortically triggered convulsions and were clearly predominant over simultaneously triggered cortical convulsions. Bergmann et al. [1963] described the occurrence of generalized convulsions during electrical stimulation of the mesodiencephalic "nystagmogenic region" (as defined by Lachmann et al. [1958]) in unanesthetized rabbits. These convulsions were self sustaining (outlasting the stimulation) and independent of the cortical motor region. The authors suggested that these convulsions had been triggered by the spread of the current to the mesencephalic reticular formation and thus were related to the "brainstem attacks" reported by Kreindler et al. [1963]. Burnham et al. [1981] found that self sustained "brainstem triggered convulsions" can be triggered by high intensity electrical stimulation of any level of the rat brainstem reticular core (from the medulla to the mesencephalon, including the PAG), whereas stimulation at sites rostral to the mesencephalon or stimulation of the long descending tracts produced negative results [Burnham et al., 1987]. With respect to chemical stimulation, Ralston and Langer [1965] produced epileptic discharges and convulsions by local application of proconvulsant agents such as tungstic acid gel into the reticular formation of the midbrain, pons and medulla in cats. The systemic administration of chemoconvulsants such as PTZ, bemegride, strychnine or bicucilline has also been shown to elicit paroxysmal discharges and to greatly enhance neuronal firing in the mesecephalic and brainstem reticular formation [Faingold, 1977, Faingold et al., 1983; Velasco et al., 1975, 1976, 1982].

In humans, the PAG has mainly received attention with respect to pain treatment, as outlined on pages 55-56. Studies on the effects of PAG ablation or stimulation in patients with epilepsy are limited. Spiegel and Wycis [1962], Takabayashi et al. [1966] and Niedermeyer et al. [1969] found no evidence as to the involvement of the mesencephalic reticular structures in patients with classic "centrencephalic" epilepsies. In contrast, Nashold et al. [1972] investigated two patients classified as severe intractable "centrencephalic epileptics", finding spontaneous generalized seizures frequently originating in the area of the central tegmentum in one, and evoking seizures by low frequency stimulation of various subcortical structures including the central tegmentum in the other.

Furthermore, Wilson and Nashold [1968] elicited diencephalic seizure discharges that were not accompanied by concomitant cortical discharges. No controlled studies have been performed to date. Nevertheless, it is our opinion that the PAG may be regarded as a potential target for the treatment of epilepsy, considering the vast amount of evidence from animal studies suggesting the role of the brainstem reticular core in major convulsions.

The Caudate Nucleus

Electrical stimulation of the caudate nucleus has been shown to inhibit seizures of rhinencephalic origin and cortical and hippocampal penicillin- and aluminium-hydroxy induced seizure foci in a number of animal studies [Mutani et al., 1969; Wagner et al., 1975; Oakley and Ojemann, 1982; La Grutta et al., 1988]. Psatta [1983] reported on the effects of feedback caudate nucleus stimulations on the interictal spiking activity of epileptic foci automatically detected by a neuroanalyzer in adult cats, finding a spike depression that occurred instantly after the onset of feedback stimulation.

In humans, several uncontrolled studies of the group around Šramka and Chkhenkeli have reported on the antiseizure efficacy of caudate nucleus stimulation. Šramka et al. [1976] found a decrease in seizure frequency in five of six patients with intermittent caudate stimulation, and Chkhenkeli [1978] demonstrated an improvement with low frequency stimulation of the caudate nucleus in a study including 74 patients with epilepsy. Šramka et al. [1980] then reported on the results of therapeutic low frequency electrical stimulation of the caudate nucleus performed in a group of 26 patients, finding good therapeutic effects in two patients, but only mild improvement or no effect in the remaining (16 of the 26 patients had previously undergone destructive stereotactic surgery in various deep brain structures, and stimulation was performed as an additional procedure; additional stimulation of temporal lobe structures was carried out in three patients). Gabašvili *et al.* [1988] reported that low frequency stimulation of the caudate nucleus terminated epileptic activity in six patients who had been in status epilepticus for 4 to 7 days. In a later study including 38 patients, Chkhenkeli and Chkhenkeli [1997] demonstrated that low frequency stimulation of certain points of the ventral part of caudate nucleus reliably led to (1) a decrease of interparoxysmal activity in neocortical and mesial temporal epileptic foci, (2) a decrease of focal discharges in the aforementioned areas, and (3) abrupt cessation of spreading and generalized discharges (clinical data were not assessed in this study). In 2004, Chkhenkeli *et al.* showed that low frequency stimulation at a rate of 4 to 8 Hz of the ventral part of head of the caudate nucleus (a) suppressed subclinical epileptic discharges and reduced the frequency of complex partial and secondary generalized seizures, and (b) decreased the frequency of sharp transients in the interictal epileptic activity and terminated the epileptic discharges in the mesiobasal temporal lobe structures and neocortex in 41 of 57 patients (71.9%) with bilateral interictal epileptiform abnormalities. This suppressive effect did not only occur upon ipsilateral interictal activity and epileptic discharges, but also on contralateral focal discharges and generalized discharges originating from temporal lobe structures contralateral to the side of stimulation.

It is important to note that antiseizure effects with electrical stimulation of the caudate nucleus have generally been achieved by applying low frequency stimulation at rates of 4 to 8 Hz, whereas stimulation with less than 4 Hz did not show a discernible inhibitory effect on interictal neocortical or rhinencephalic epileptic activity. The administration of high frequency stimulation at rates of 30 to 100 Hz caused effects contrary to those achieved with low frequency stimulation, that is an enhancement of epileptiform activity recorded from the caudate nucleus or rhinencephalic brain structures [Chkhenkeli *et al.*, 2004]. The authors therefore suggested that the suppression of neocortical epileptic activity may be the result of inhibitory processes due to activation of the caudate nucleus. This is in accordance with the experimental findings of Klee and Lux [1962], who demonstrated that the activation of the head of the caudate nucleus is correlated with hyperpolarization of cortical neurons.

Moreover, there is evidence for a certain degree of point to point specificity within the caudatocortical circuitry. In the study of Chkhenkeli *et al.* [2004], analysis of the excitatory and inhibitory effects of high and low frequency stimulation of 712 different points within the head of the caudate nucleus indicated that the inhibitory effect was more reliably, that is in 87%, elicited from stimulation of its ventral part. This caudatocortical point to point specificity is in line with the findings of animal studies and with morphological data obtained from the human brain, demonstrating the existence of four intracaudate cytoarchitectonic fields, namely the dorsal, medial, ventrolateral, and ventral field [Namba, 1957]. A number of functional caudatocortical circuits have been proposed to account for these electrophysiological findings. Heuser *et al.* [1961] proposed the existence of a functional entity (which they called the "caudate loop") encompassing the head of the caudate nucleus, the neocortex and the non specific thalamic nuclei. La Grutta *et al.* [1971] suggested the existence of reciprocal connections from the olfactory brain to the head of the caudate nucleus that may be involved in suppressing the spread of rhinencephalic epileptic activity. Sorbera *et al.* [1981] noted that the inhibitory influence of the caudate nucleus is mediated through longer direct striatal-nigro-amygdalar connections, rather than through local olfactory brain-caudate connections. Fariello [1976] postulated that the different effects of caudate nucleus stimulation at various frequencies probably indicate frequency related preferential activation of different neuronal systems within the head of the caudate nucleus.

The Hippocampus

For more than half a century, direct cortical electrical stimulation is used as a standard clinical method of evaluating and localizing eloquent cortical regions as part of invasive presurgical evaluation for epilepsy surgery [Penfield and Jasper, 1954]. Cortical stimulation, when used for localization purposes, frequently gives rise to afterdischarges consisting of runs of epileptiform activity that occurred during or immediately after application of the electrical stimulus. Under some circumstances, afterdischarges can be prolonged and associated with various clinical manifestations of epileptic seizures [Wieser, 1982; Fernandes de Lima et al., 1990]. Conversely, afterdischarges elicited by cortical stimulation have been shown to be significantly decreased or even terminated by application of another brief burst of pulse stimulation to the cortex [Lesser et al., 1999]. Analogously, there is also evidence from animal studies. An increase of seizure threshold with electrical stimulation of cortical structures has been investigated in various animal models [Jennum and Klitgaard, 1996; Barbarosie and Avoli, 1997; Li et al., 1998; Akamatsu et al., 2001; Velíšek et al., 2002; Khosravani et al., 2003]. The best known example is the repetitive stimulation of the amygdala in rats leading to a permanent increase in seizure susceptibility (so called "electrical kindling"). Weiss et al. [1998] have shown that the development of kindling can be blocked by a low intensity and continuous stimulus simultaneously applied through the same electrode used for induction of "kindling".

Based on these considerations, several investigators have reported on the antiseizure effect of direct stimulation of the hippocampus and the amygdala. Velasco et al. [2000b] reported the clinical, EEG and histopathologic effects of subacute electrical stimulation of the hippocampal formation in 10 patients with intractable temporal lobe seizures who underwent presurgical evaluation with bilateral hippocampal depth electrodes or unilateral subdural basotemporal electrodes. Following presurgical investigation, all patients underwent *en bloc* temporal lobectomy and the histopathologic effects of electrical stimulation on the tissue were analyzed using light microscopy. Stimulation parameters were biphasic Lilly wave pulses delivered at a rate of 130 Hz for 23 hours per day for a total duration of about 2 to 3 weeks. The authors found a complete control of seizures and a significant decrease in interictal EEG spiking in the hippocampus in seven of 10 patients (70%) who underwent continuous subacute stimulation of the hippocampal formation or parahippocampal gyrus for a total duration of 5 to 6 days. The most evident and fastest responses were found by stimulation of either the anterior pes hippocampi close to the amygdala or the anterior parahippocampal gyrus (i.e. the entorhinal cortex). No clear antiepileptic responses were found if the stimulation was interrupted or performed outside the hippocampus. Microscopic analysis of the stimulated tissue showed no clear histopathological differences between stimulated and non stimulated hippocampal tissues. The authors concluded that subacute electrical stimulation of the hippocampal formation is a safe procedure capable of suppressing temporal lobe epileptogenesis with no additional damage to the stimulated tissue. Velasco et al. [2000c] then demonstrated that chronic hippocampal stimulation persistently blocked temporal lobe epileptogenesis for 3 to 4 months with no apparent additional undesirable effects on short term memory. The authors concluded that this antiseizure effect was most likely related to physiologic inhibition of the stimulated hippocampus, as evidenced by an increased threshold and decreased duration of afterdischarges induced by hippocampal stimulation, flattening of the hippocampal evoked response recovery cycles, SPECT hypoperfusion of the hippocampal region, and increased hippocampal benzodiazepine receptor binding. A number of uncontrolled studies or anecdotal reports encompassing at least 27 patients subsequently reported favorable clinical effects, namely a reduction in seizure frequency [Yamamoto et al., 2002; Chkhenkeli et al. 2004] or positive electrophysiological effects – i.e. a decrease of interictal epileptiform discharges [Yamamoto et al., 2002; Vonck et al., 2002; Kossoff et al., 2004; Osorio et al., 2005] in patients undergoing hippocampal stimulation.

In a double-blind, multiple cross-over, randomized controlled study including four patients with refractory MTLE whose risk to memory contraindicated temporal lobe resection Tellez-Zenteno et al. [2006] applied continuous subthreshold electrical stimulation at a rate of 190 Hz through a depth electrode implanted along the axis of the left hippocampus. The stimulators were randomly turned ON 1 month and OFF 1 month during each of three treatment cycles, and the outcomes between ON, OFF and baseline periods were compared. There were no adverse effects. Three of four patients (75%) improved with respect to seizure frequency, with a non significant median seizure reduction of 15%. One patient (25%) showed substantial long term seizure improvement with a follow up of 4 years. The findings of this study appear to confirm that there is some form of benefit with hippocampal electrical stimulation in patients with MTLE, although the magnitude of effect was clearly smaller than reported in previous non randomized, unblinded studies. Moreover, the authors stated that an implantation effect cannot be ruled out, considering that the effects seemed to carry over into the OFF period. In this respect, it is interesting to note that seizure improvement following electrode implantation without subsequent stimulation has also been observed in patients undergoing presurgical evaluation [Katariwala et al., 2001].

Two studies also investigated the efficacy of seizure triggered responsive hippocampal stimulation by using a responsive neurostimulator that can automatically analyze electrocortical potentials, detect electrographic seizures, and rapidly deliver targeted electrical stimuli. Kossoff et al. [2004] reported the findings of four out of 40 patients receiving responsive cortical stimulation via subdural electrodes implanted for epilepsy surgery evaluations, finding that electrographic seizures were altered and suppressed in these patients during trials of neurostimulation lasting up to 68 hours, with no major side effects. Furthermore, stimulation appeared to improve the baseline EEG in one of their patients. Osorio et al. [2005] reported on the effects of high frequency electrical hippocampal stimulation triggered by automated seizure detections in four patients, overall finding a mean reduction in seizure rate of 55.5% (– 100 to + 36.8%) and a mean reduction of – 86% (-100 to -58.8%) in those three patients with a > 50% seizure reduction ("responders"). It is of note that these effects on epileptogenic tissue were immediate and also outlasted the stimulation period.

Future studies increasing the number and time of follow up of patients under hippocampal stimulation are necessary before considering chronic hippocampal stimulation a reliable procedure for controlling intractable temporal lobe seizures. Controlled double-blind randomized studies evaluating the efficacy of chronic hippocampal stimulation are under way.

The Amygdala

Studies investigating the use of stereotactic lesioning or stimulation of the amygdala with the aim to suppress seizures in patients with intractable epilepsy date back to the 1960ies. Schwab et al. [1965] reported improvement in seven of 10 patients (70%) with psychomotor seizures following unilateral stereotactic amygdalotomy, whereas complete seizure control (or reduction to occasional seizures) was achieved in three patients (30%). Chitanondh and Laksanavicharn [1969] found a reduction in seizure frequency in 10 (32.2%) and complete seizure control in three of 31 patients (9.7%) with psychomotor seizures following unilateral (n = 26) or bilateral (n = 5) stereotactic amygdalotomy. Vaernet [1972] described improvement in 25 of 45 patients (55.6%) with unilateral and bitemporal TLE. Complete seizure control or occasional seizures was achieved in six of 37 patients (16.2%) with unilateral, and in two of 8 patients (25%) with bilateral lesioning. Ramamurthi et al. [1974] found improvement in 24 of 31 patients (77.4%). Complete seizure control was achieved in 10 of 21 patients (47.6%) with unilateral, and in four of 10 patients (40%) with bilateral lesioning. Sonnen et al. [1976] reported on eight patients with psychomotor and generalized seizures, finding complete seizure control or worthwhile improvement in two (25%), and failure in six patients (75%) following bilateral (n = 7) or unilateral (n = 1) amygdalotomy. In contrast, no improvement was found in three smaller patient series comprising 11 patients [Schaltenbrand et al., 1966; Wycis, 1969; Narabayashi and Mizutani, 1970]. In summary of these studies, 29 of 136 patients (21.3%) with psychomotor seizures showed complete seizure control, while 39 (28.7%) had worthwhile improvement and 68 (50%) had treatment failure [Ravagnati, 1987].

A number of studies also reported on the efficacy of amygdalotomy with respect to generalized seizures (these were mostly secondarily generalized seizures in patients with psychomotor seizures) [Narabayashi and Mizutani, 1970; Diemath, 1972; Heimburger et al., 1978; Narabayashi, 1979]. In summary of these studies, 12 of 94 patients (12.7%) showed complete seizure control, 36 (38.3%) had worthwhile improvement, and 46 patients (48.9%) had treatment failure.

It is pertinent to note that neither unilateral nor bilateral amygdalotomy has been shown to result in major disability. Using psychometric testing, Ramamurthi and Kalyanaraman [1982], found no psychological deficit in 120 patients who underwent bilateral amygdalotomy. In particular, memory functions appeared not to be affected in any of these patients. Moreover, there was no Klüver Bucy syndrome, though transitory hypersexualism and hyperphagia occurred in two of 260 patients (0.8%) with bilateral amygdalotomy (both of which had a previous history of encephalitis). Rather, there was an improvement in psychological performance in those patients who had shown seizure control after operation, and irritability and restlessness has also been shown to improve postsurgery [Ramamurthi et al., 1974; Mempel, 1971].

Conclusions and Outlook

The role of stereotactic ablative surgery for the treatment of epilepsy is not clear. The appropriate interpretation of early studies is mainly limited by the fact that the great majority of these studies were carried out using an uncontrolled outcome assessment, that is, control groups were usually lacking (and much less true surgical sham controls). Moreover, the majority of these studies were unblinded, that is, outcome was frequently assessed by the same group of researchers that have also performed stereotactic ablative surgery. These circumstances clearly hinder the ascertainment of how much of any benefit may have been related to placebo.

Notwithstanding these limitations, modern stereotactic ablative surgery using current image-guided technology offers the opportunity to revisit some of the subcortical and cortical targets investigated in early studies. The basic idea of stereotactic ablation for the treatment of epilepsy is the interruption of seizure propagating pathways or to directly destroy diseased areas of the brain that act as a focus of epileptic discharges (other mechanisms that have been proposed are the reduction of the volume of excitable neurons, or the increase of threshold of irritability). It is fair to say that there is virtually no subcortical structure that has not yet been lesioned with the aim to control seizures in patients with epilepsy, and also that the high expectations placed on stereotactic epilepsy surgery have generally not been met, irrespective of the target area. Nonetheless, it is likely that stereotactic surgery of at least some of these subcortical or cortical targets, or combinations thereof, may indeed provide antiseizure efficacy. Moreover, modern radiosurgery (gamma surgery) may offer a valuable alternative treatment option in this respect [Mori et al., 2000; Chen et al., 2001; Mathieu et al., 2006; Prayson and Yoder, 2007].

The extensive knowledge deriving from the experience with stereotactic epilepsy surgery is relevant to the renewed interest in neurostimulation for the treatment of epilepsy. DBS has theoretical advantages over surgery because it is adaptable if seizures change and is reversible if functional disruption of the epileptogenic cortex causes adverse effects. With the limited data available to date, this technique appears to be safe. From the experience with the treatment of movement disorders and pain we know that complications are primarily associated with the implantation procedure itself, with a 5% risk of infection and a 5 to 7.5% risk of intracerebral hemorrhage leading to clinical symptoms. Moreover, experience with DBS for treatment of PD has shown that tissue damage can be avoided by observing appropriate charge density [Haberler et al., 2000]. Charge densities safely delivered to human cortex for acute intermittent stimulation are in the range of 50-60 $\mu C/cm^2$/phase [Risinger and Gumnit, 1995]. Animal studies suggest that tissue damage is correlated with charge density per phase and total charge per phase, as well as with cumulative exposure of tissue to stimulation [Yuen et al., 1981]. Damage induced by continuous stimulation appears more severe than that induced by intermittent stimulation with equal or even longer total exposure time [Gordon et al., 1990; Risinger and Gumnit, 1995].

DBS can be directed to one or several epileptic foci, to a specific path of seizure propagation, or to a particular structure with more global modulatory effects. Modulation of the seizure threshold by DBS of subcortical or cortical structures appears to be a promising future treatment option for patients with some forms of pharmacologically intractable epilepsy. Continuous, cycling and responsive stimulation applied to the cortex or to deep brain structures may suppress seizures via different mechanisms and pathways and in that way be complementary and even synergistic [Morrell, 2006]. However, much has to be done in order to answer the questions as to the efficacy of DBS. For most targets, controlled DBS studies in patients with epilepsy have not been performed to date, and the optimal location (various deep brain nuclei or cortical) and characteristics of the stimulation are still to be determined. However, several centers are now performing long term protocols for DBS (e.g. STN stimulation) and a multicenter prospective randomized trial of scheduled chronic AN stimulation in persons with medically intractable localization related epilepsy is currently under way [SANTE trial; Graves et al., 2004].

Responsive stimulation may offer additional specificity (treatment may be provided when needed). Penfield and Jasper [1954] probably were the first to apply focal electrical stimulation to humans in order to terminate spontaneous seizures detected by electrocorticography at the time of resective surgery. Subsequent studies have been conducted in patients with intracranial electrodes placed to localize seizure onsets prior to epilepsy surgery, and a number of small pilot trials suggested that this kind of therapy may indeed reduce seizure frequency, at least in some patients with intractable epilepsy. Closed loop responsive stimulation requires systems that detect abnormal electrographic activity (that is, abnormal electrographic discharges are to be detected before there is evolution into a clinical seizure) and provide subsequent brief cortical stimulation in response to abnormal electrographic discharges. Lesser et al. [1999] showed that responsive cortical electrical stimulation can shorten afterdischarges elicited during functional mapping. In this study, 17 patients with subdural electrodes received brief bursts of stimulation (biphasic 0.3 ms, 50 Hz pulse for a duration of 0.3-2 s) in order to abort afterdischarges. The duration of the afterdischarges was significantly shorter in those patients receiving responsive stimulation. Other investigators have also reported that responsive stimulation shortens or terminates electrographic discharges induced by stimulation during brain mapping [Motamedi et al., 2002; Chkhenkeli et al., 2004]. Kossoff et al. [2004] used an external device that automatically analyzes the electrocorticogram and provides targeted cortical stimulation and applied this technique in four patients with subdural electrodes implanted for epilepsy surgery evaluations. Electrographic seizures were altered and suppressed by responsive stimulation in these patients, and there were no significant adverse events. Osorio et al. [2005] in a small pilot study reported that responsive stimulation terminated some spontaneous seizures in eight patients, four with bilateral anterior thalamic stimulation and four with focal cortical stimulation. A multi-institutional clinical study in patients with medically intractable partial onset seizures treated with a cranially implanted responsive neurostimulator (RNS, NeuroPace, Inc., Mountain View, California) is under way. The RNS pulse generator continuously analyzes the patient's electrocorticogram and automatically triggers electrical stimulation when specific electrocorticogram characteristics programmed by the clinician indicative of precursors of seizures are detected. The pulse generator then stores diagnostic information detailing detections and stimulations, including multichannel stored electrocorticograms. In a feasibility study of this device, a 45% decrease in seizures in seven of eight patients was reported with a mean follow up of 9 months without serious device-related adverse events [Fountas et al., 2005].

Sufficiently sensitive and specific seizure detection algorithms play a key role for responsive neurostimulation. Seizure prediction algorithms, which attempt to identify preictal states using a variety of linear and nonlinear methods, are of special interest. However, these prediction methods require significant computing power and are not currently practical for use in an implanted system [Iasemidis et al., 2005]. The ability of responsive stimulation to terminate seizures, in turn, depends on the stimulation parameters, such as the current intensity, stimulus duration, stimulus waveform, pulse frequency, and the timing and spatial location of the stimulation in relation to the spike discharge. In this respect, it is pertinent to note that the results of therapeutic stimulation to terminate seizures in kindled rats are not consistent: Slow 1 Hz stimulation inhibited seizures [Weiss et al., 1998], whereas in other studies stimulation with 3 Hz or 60-100 Hz stimulation facilitated kindled seizures [Dennison et al., 1995; Weiss et al., 1998]. Vercueil et al. [1998] found that epileptiform activity in the STN of rats was terminated most effectively at stimulation frequencies in excess of 130 Hz. Mirski et al. [1997] demonstrated that stimulation with 100 Hz inhibited seizures in rats treated with pentylenetetrazol. In humans, the optimal stimulation frequency to terminate seizures has not been established. In a study by Kinoshita et al. [2005], both high (50 Hz) and low (0.9 Hz) frequency cortical stimulation of the seizure onset zone had a suppressive effect on spike frequency and reduced high frequency activity in four patients with epilepsy implanted with subdural electrodes. Furthermore, the efficacy of DBS in men very likely varies depending on the anatomic region treated and on the selection of anodes and cathodes. Stimulation with an alternating current may have different effects than a direct current. Goodman *et al.* [2005] treated amygdala kindled rats with preemptive low frequency 1 Hz sine wave stimulation and found that the incidence of severe seizures significantly decreased. In addition, low frequency sine wave stimulation inhibited the ability to produce kindled seizures. The safety of sine wave stimulation in men has not been established.

References

Aggleton JP, Desimone R, Mishkin M. The origin, course, and termination of the hippocampothalamic projections in the macaque. *J Comp Neurol* 1986; 243: 409-421.

Akamatsu N, Fueta Y, Endo Y, Matsunaga K, Uozumi T, Tsuji S. Decreased susceptibility to pentylenetetrazole-induced seizures after low frequency transcranial magnetic stimulation in the rat. *Neurosci Lett* 2001; 310: 153-156.

Akert K. August Forel – cofounder of the neuron theory (1848-1931). *Brain Pathol* 1993; 3: 425-430.

Akert K. Comparative anatomy of frontal cortex and thalamofrontal connections. In: Warren JM, Akert K eds. *The Frontal Granular Cortex and Behavior*. New York: McGraw-Hill 1964: 372-396.

Akert K. Limbisches System. In: Drenckhahn D, Zenker W eds. *Benninghoff Anatomie*, Vol. 2/15. Völlig neu bearbeitete Auflage. München Wien, Baltimore: Urban & Schwarzenberg 1994: 603-627.

Albe-Fessard D. Electrophysiological methods for the identification of thalamic nuclei. *Z Neurol* 1973; 205: 15-28.

Albe-Fessard D, Gillett E. Interaction of afferent impulses of somatesthetic origin and of cortical origin at the level of the median center; unitary activities. *J Physiol* (Paris) 1958; 50: 108-111.

Amaral DG, Cowan WM. Subcortical afferents to the hippocampal formation in the monkey. *J Comp Neurol* 1980; 189: 573-591.

Amorapanth P, Nader K, LeDoux JE. Lesions of periaqueductal gray dissociate-conditioned freezing from conditioned suppression behavior in rats. *Learn Mem* 1999; 6: 491-499.

Anderson JL, Leith NJ, Barrett RJ. Tolerance to amphetamine's facilitation of self-stimulation responding: anatomical specificity. *Brain Res* 1978; 145: 37-48.

Andrade DM, Zumsteg D, Hamani C, Hodaie M, Sarkissian S, Lozano AM, Wennberg RA. Long-term follow-up of patients with thalamic deep brain stimulation for epilepsy. *Neurology* 2006; 66: 1571-1573.

Andrews PI, Dichter MA, Berkovic SF, Newton MR, McNamara JO. Plasmapheresis in Rasmussen's encephalitis. *Neurology* 1996; 46: 242-246.

Andy OJ, Mukawa J. Brain stem lesion effects on electrically induced seizures (electroencephalographic and behavioral study). *Electroencephalogr Clin Neurophysiol* 1959; 11: 397.

Andy OJ, Stephan H. Stereotaxic surgery of the limbic system. In: Schaltenbrand G, Walker AE eds. *Stereotaxy of the Human Brain*. Stuttgart, New York: Georg Thieme Verlag 1982: 629-644.

Angevine JB Jr., Locke S, Yakovlev PI. Limbic nuclei of thalamus and connections of limbic cortex. V. Thalamocortical projection of the magnocellular medial dorsal nucleus in man. *Arch Neurol* 1964; 10: 165-180.

Antal A, Nitsche MA, Paulus W. Transcranial direct current stimulation and the visual cortex. *Brain Res Bull* 2006; 68: 459-463.

Babb TL, Mitchell AG Jr, Crandall PH. Fastigiobulbar and dentatothalamic influences on hippocampal cobalt epilepsy in the cat. *Electroencephalogr Clin Neurophysiol* 1974; 36: 141-154.

Bancaud J. Apport de l'exploration fonctionnelle par voie stéréotaxique à la chirurgie de l'épilepsie. *Neurochirurgie* 1959; 5: 55-112.

Bancaud J. Rôle du cortex cérébral dans les épilepsies "géneralisées" d'origine organique. *Presse Med* 1971; 79: 669-673.

Bancaud J. Mechanisms of cortical discharges in "generalized" epilepsies in man: In: Petsche H; Brazier MAB eds. *Synchronization of EEG Activity in Epilepsies*. New York: Springer 1972: 368-380.

Barbarosie M, Avoli M. CA3-driven hippocampalentorhinal loop controls rather than sustains in vitro limbic seizures. *J Neurosci* 1997; 17: 9308-9314.

Barcia-Salorio JL, Broseta J. Stereotactic fornicotomy in temporal epilepsy: indications and long-term results. *Acta Neurochir* (Wien) 1976; 23 (Suppl.): 167-175.

Benabid AL, Pollak P, Louveau A, Henry S, de Rougemont J. Combined (thalamotomy and stimulation) stereotactic surgery of the VIM thalamic nucleus for bilateral Parkinson disease. *Appl Neurophysiol* 1987; 50: 344-346.

Benabid AL, Minotti L, Koudsie A, De Saint MA, Hirsch E. Antiepileptic effect of high-frequency stimulation of the subthalamic nucleus (corpus luysi) in a case of medically intractable epilepsy caused by focal dysplasia: a 30-month follow-up: technical case report. *Neurosurgery* 2002; 50: 1385-1391.

Benabid AL, Koudsie A, Chabardes S, Vercueil L, Benazzouz A, Minotti L, Le Bas JF, Kahane P, de Saint Martin A, Hirsch E. Subthalamic nucleus and substantia nigra pars reticulata stimulation: the Grenoble experience. In: Lüders HO ed. *Deep Brain Stimulation and Epilepsy*. London, New York: Martin Dunitz 2004: 335-348.

Benazzouz A, Hallett M. Mechanism of action of deep brain stimulation. *Neurology* 2000; 55 (Suppl.6): 13-16.

Benazzouz A, Piallat B, Pollak P, Benabid AL. Responses of substantia nigra pars reticulata and globus pallidus complex to high frequency stimulation of the subthalamic nucleus in rats: electrophysiological data. *Neurosci Lett* 1995; 189: 77-80.

Berger H. Ueber das Elektroenkephalogramm des Menschen III. *Arch Psychiatr Nervenheilk* 1931; 94: 16-60.

Berger JR. Memory and the mammillothalamic tract. *Am J Neuroradiol* 2004; 25: 906-907.

Bergman H, Wichmann T, Karmon B, DeLong MR. The primate subthalamic nucleus. 2. Neuronal activity in the MPTP model of parkinsonism. *J Neurophysiol* 1994; 72: 507-520.

Bergmann F, Costin A, Gutman J. A low threshold convulsive area in the rabbit's mesencephalon. *Electroencephalogr Clin Neurophys* 1963; 15: 683-690.

Bernoulli C, Siegfried J, Baumgartner G, Regli F, Rabinowicz T, Gajdusek DC, Gibbs CJ Jr. Danger of accidental person-to-person transmission of Creutzfeldt-Jakob disease by surgery. *Lancet* 1977; 26: 478-479.

Beurrier C, Bezard E, Bioulac B, Gross C. Subthalamic stimulation elicits hemiballismus in normal monkey. *Neuroreport* 1997; 8: 1625-1629.

Bidzinski J, Ostrowski K. Destruction of Forel's field in the surgical treatment of epilepsy. *Neurol Neurochir Pol* 1981; 15: 49-52.

Bindman LJ, Lippold OC, Redfearn JW. Long-lasting changes in the level of the electrical activity of the cerebral cortex produced by polarizing currents. *Nature* 1962; 196,584-585.

Björklund A, Lindvall O. Cell replacement therapies for central nervous system disorders. *Nature Neuroscience* 2000; 3,537-544.

Bouchard G, Umbach W. Indications for the open and stereotactic brain surgery in epilepsy. In: Fusek I, Kunc Z eds. *Present Limits of Neurosurgery.* Amsterdam: Excerpta Medica 1972.

Bressand K, Dematteis M, Kahane P, Benazzouz A, Benabid AL. Involvement of the subthalamic nucleus in the control of temporal lobe epilepsy: study by high frequency stimulation in rats. *Abstr Soc Neurosci* 1999; 25: 1656 (abstract).

Broca P. Anatomie comparée des circonvolutions cérébrales. Le grand lobe limbique et la scissure limbique dans la série des mammifères. *Rev Anthropol* 1878: 1: 385-498.

Bruet N, Windels F, Bertrand A, Feuerstein C, Poupard A, Savasta M. High frequency stimulation of the subthalamic nucleus increases the extracellular contents of striatal dopamine in normal and partially dopaminergic denervated rats. *J Neuropathol Exp Neurol* 2001; 60: 15-24.

Burnham WM, Albright P, Schneiderman J, Chiu P, Ninchoji T. "Centrencephalic" mechanisms in the kindling model. In: Wada JA ed. *Kindling 2.* New York: Raven Press 1981: 161-178.

Burnham WM. Electrical stimulation studies: Generalized convulsions triggered from the brain stem. In: Fromm GH, Faingold CL, Browning RA, Burnham WM eds. *Epilepsy and the Reticular Formation.* Neurology and Neurobiology (Liss AR) 1987: 25-38.

Burzaco JA. Fundus striae terminalis, an optimal target in sedative stereotactic surgery. In: Laitinen L, Livingston K eds. *Surgical Approaches in Psychiatry.* Lancester, England: Medical and Technical Publishing Co 1973: 135-137.

Buser B, Bancaud J. Bases techniques et méthodologiques de l'exploration fonctionelle stéréotaxique du télencéphale. In: Talairach J, Szikla G, Tournoux P, Prossalentis A, Bordas-Ferrer M, Covello L, Iacob M, Mempel E eds. *Atlas d'Anatomie Stéréotaxique du Télencéphale.* Paris: Masson et Cie 1967: 251-323.

Caspers H. Über die Beziehung zwischen Dentritenpotential und Gleichspannung an der Hirnrinde. Pflügers *Arch Ges Physiol* 1959; 269: 157-181.

Caspers H (ed.), Bechtereva NP, Caspars H, Goldring S, Gumnit RJ, Speckmann EJ (collaborators). DC potentials recorded directly from the cortex. *Handbook of Electroencephalography and Clinical Neurophysiology* 1974: 10A: 1-87.

Chabardès S, Kahane P, Minotti L, Koudsie A, Hirsch E, Benabid AL. Deep brain stimulation in epilepsy with particular reference to the subthalamic nucleus. *Epileptic Disord* 2002; 4 (Suppl. 3): 83-93.

Chang HT. The repetitive discharge of corticothalamic reverberating circuit. *J Neurophysiol* 1950; 13: 235-257.

Chen ZF, Kamiryo T, Henson SL, Yamamoto H, Bertram EH, Schottler F, Patel F, Steiner L, Prasad D, Kassell NF, Shareghis S, Lee KS. Anticonvulsant effects of gamma surgery in a model of chronic spontaneous limbic epilepsy in rats. *J Neurosurg* 2001; 94: 270-280.

Chiorino R, Donoso P, Diaz G, Aranda L, Asenjo A, Garcia C. Findings on stereotaxic surgery in the treatment of epilepsy, apropos of a new technic: the campotomy [span]. *Neurocirurgia* 1968; 26: 143-147.

Chitanondh H, Laksanavicharn U. Stereotaxic amygdalotomy in the treatment of temporal automatism. *Excerpta Medica Int Congress Series* 1969; 193: 9.

Chkhenkeli SA. Inhibitory influences of caudate stimulation on the epileptic activity of human amygdala and hippocampus during temporal lobe epilepsy. *Physiol Hum Anim* 1978; 5: 406-411.

Chkhenkeli SA, Chkhenkeli IS. Effects of therapeutic stimulation of nucleus caudatus on epileptic electrical activity of brain in patients with intractable epilepsy. *Stereotact Funct Neurosurg* 1997; 69: 221-224.

Chkhenkeli SA, Šramka M. Therapeutic stimulation of the non-specific thalamic system for the treatment of some forms of epilepsy. Presented at: *IXth Congress of Neurological Surgery*, New Delhi, India, 1989.

Chkhenkeli SA, Sramka M, Lortkipanidze GS, Rakviashvili TN, Bregvadze ESh, Magalashvili GE, Gagoshidze TSh, Chkhenkeli IS. Electrophysiological effects and clinical results of direct brain stimulation for intractable epilepsy. *Clin Neurol Neurosurg* 2004; 106: 318-329.

Chow KL, Blum JS, Blum RA. Cell ratios in the thalamocortical visual system of the Macaca mulatta. *J Comp Neurol* 1950; 92: 227-240.

Clough R, Statnick M, Maring-Smith M, Wang C, Eells J, Browning R, Dailey J, Jobe P. Fetal raphe transplants reduce seizure severity in serotonin-depleted GEPRs. *Neuroreport* 1996; 8: 341-346.

Cohen MW. Glial potentials and their contribution to extracellular recordings. In: Creutzfeldt O ed. Electrical activity from the neuron to the EEG and EMG. Vol.2. In: Rémond A ed.-in-chief. *Handbook of Electroencephalography and Clinical Neurophysiology.* Amsterdam: Elsevier 1976; Vol2B: 43-60.

Cohn R. DC recordings of paroxysmal disorders in man. *Electroencephalogr Clin Neurophysiol* 1964; 17: 17-24.

Comte P, Siegfried J, Wieser HG. Multipolar hollow-core electrode for brain recordings. *Appl Neurophysiol* 1983; 46: 41-46.

Cooke PM, Snider RS. Some cerebellar influences on electrically-induced cerebral seizures. *Epilepsia* 1955; 4: 19-28.

Cooper IS. Effect of thalamic lesions upon torticollis. *N Engl J Med* 1964; 270: 967-972.

Cooper IS. Effect of chronic stimulation of anterior cerebellum on neurological disease. *Lancet* 1973; 1(7796): 206.

Cooper IS, Upton AR. Therapeutic implications of modulation of metabolism and functional activity of cerebral cortex by chronic stimulation of cerebellum and thalamus. *Biol Psychiatry* 1985; 20: 811-813.

Cooper IS, Amin I, Gilman S. The effect of chronic cerebellar stimulation upon epilepsy in man. *Trans Am Neurol Assoc* 1973; 98: 192-196.

Cooper IS, Amin I, Riklan M, Waltz JM, Poon TP. Chronic cerebellar stimulation in epilepsy. Clinical and anatomical studies. *Arch Neurol* 1976; 33: 559-570.

Cooper IS, Amin I, Upton A, Riklan M, Watkins S, McLellan L. Safety and efficacy of chronic stimulation. *Neurosurgery* 1977; 1: 203-205.

Cooper IS, Amin I, Upton A, Riklan M, Watkins S, McLellan L. Safety and efficacy of chronic cerebellar stimulation. *Appl Neurophysiol* 1977-78; 40: 124-34.

Cooper IS, Upton AR, Amin I, Garnett S, Brown GM, Springman M. Evoked metabolic responses in the limbic-striate system produced by stimulation of anterior thalamic nucleus in man. *Int J Neurol* 1984; 18: 179-187.

Cowie RJ, Robinson DL. Subcortical contributions to head movements in macaques. I. Contrasting effects of electrical stimulation of a medial pontomedullary region and the superior colliculus. *J Neurophysiol* 1994; 72: 2648-2664.

Creutzfeldt OD. *Cortex Cerebri.* Berlin: Springer 1983: 484.

Crighel E, Kreindler A. The role of the thalamic pulvinar-LP complex in modulating neocortical reactivity. In: Cooper IS, Riklan M, Rakic P eds. *The Pulvinar-LP Complex.* Springfield Ill, Thomas 1974: 80-94.

Crouch RL. The nuclear configuration of the thalamus of macacus rhesus. *J Comp Neurol* 1934; 59: 451-485.

Cuénod M, Audinat E, Do KQ, Gähwiler BH, Grandes P, Herrling P, Knöpfel T, Perschak H, Streit P, Vollenweider F, Wieser HG. Homocysteic acid as transmitter candidate in the mammalian brain and excitatory amino acids in epilepsy. In: Ben-Ari Y ed. *Excitatory Amino Acids and Neuronal Plasticity.* New York: Plenum Press 1990: 57-63.

Däuper J, Peschel T, Schrader C, Kohlmetz C, Joppich G, Nager W, Dengler R, Rollnik JD. Effects of subthalamic nucleus (STN) stimulation on motor cortex excitability. *Neurology* 2002; 59: 700-706.

Davidson S, Watson CW. Hereditary light sensitive epilepsy. *Neurology* 1956; 6: 235-261.

Davis R, Gray E, Engle H, Dusnak A. The reduction of seizures in cerebral palsy and epileptic patients using chronic cerebellar stimulation. *Acta Neurochir* 1984; 33 (Suppl.): 161-167.

De Oca BM, DeCola JP, Maren S, Fanselow MS. Distinct regions of the periaqueductal gray are involved in the acquisition and expression of defensive responses. *J Neurosci* 1998; 18: 3426-3432.

DeLong MR, Crutcher MD, Georgopoulos AP. Primate globus pallidus and subthalamic nucleus: Functional organization. *J Neurophysiol* 1985; 53: 530-543.

Dempsey EW, Morison RS. The production of rhythmically recurrent cortical potentials after localized thalamic stimulation. *Am J Physiol* 1942; 135: 293-300.

Dennison Z, Teskey GC, Cain DP. Persistence of kindling: effect of partial kindling, retention interval, kindling site, and stimulation parameters. *Epilepsy Res* 1995; 21: 171-182.

Depaulis A, Bandler R eds. *Midbrain Periaqueductal Gray Matter: Functional, Anatomical and Neurochemical Organization.* Kluver Academic Publishers NATO Science Series 21, 1991.

D'Esposito M, Verfaellie M, Alexander MP, Katz DI. Amnesia following traumatic bilateral fornix transection. *Neurology* 1995; 45: 1546-1550.

Diemath H. Discussion. In: Vaernet ed. *Stereotaxic Amgdalotomy in Temporal Lobe Epilepsy. Confin Neurol* 1972; 34: 182.

Dinner DS, Neme S, Nair D, Montgomery EB Jr, Baker KB, Rezai A, Luders HO. EEG and evoked potential recording from the subthalamic nucleus for deep brain stimulation of intractable epilepsy. *Clin Neurophysiol* 2002; 113: 1391-1402.

Do KQ, Klancnik J, Gähwiler B, Perschak H, Wieser HG, Cuènod M. Release of excitatory amino acids: animal studies and epileptic foci studies in humans. In: Meldrum BS, Moroni F, Simon RP, Woods JH eds. *Excitatory Amino Acids.* New York: Raven Press Ltd. 1991: 677-685.

Dow RS, Fernandez-Guardiola A, Manni E. The influence of the cerebellum on experimental epilepsy. *Electroencephalogr Clin Neurophysiol* 1962; 14: 383-398.

Dujardin E, Jurgens U. Afferents of vocalization-controlling periaqueductal regions in the squirrel monkey. *Brain Res* 2005; 1034: 114-131.

Duprez TP, Serieh BA, Raftopoulos C. Absence of memory dysfunction after bilateral mammillary body and mammillothalamic tract electrode implantation: preliminary experience in three patients. *Am J Neuroradiol* 2005; 26: 195-197 (author reply 197-198).

During MJ. In vivo neurochemistry of the conscious human brain: intrahippocampal microdialysis in epilepsy. In: Robnison T, Justice J eds. *Microdialysis in the Neurosciences.* Amsterdam: Elsevier 1991: 425-442.

During MJ, Spencer DD. Extracellular hippocampal glutamate and spontaneous seizure in the conscious human brain. *Lancet* 1993; 340: 1607-1610.

During MJ, Fried I, Leone P, Katz A, Spencer DD. Direct measurement of extracellular lactate in the human hippocampus during spontaneous seizures. *Journal of Neurochemistry* 1994; 62: 2356-2361.

During MJ, Ryder KM, Spencer DD. Hippocampal GABA transporter function in temporal-lobe epilepsy. *Nature* 1995; 376: 174-177.

Duvernoy HM. *The Human Hippocampus. Functional Anatomy, Vascularization and Serial Sections with MRI.* Second completely revised and expanded edition. Berlin, Heidelberg: Springer 1988.

Dybdal D, Gale K. Postural and anticonvulsant effects of inhibition of the rat subthalamic nucleus. *J Neurosci* 2000; 20: 6728-6733.

Faingold CL. Convulsant-induced enhancement of non-primary sensory evoked responses in reticular formation pathways. *Neuropharmacology* 1977; 16: 73-81.

Faingold CL, Hoffman WE, Caspary DM. On the site of pentylenetetrazol-induced enhancement of auditory responses of the reticular formation: Localized cooling and electrical stimulation studies. *Neuropharmacology* 1983; 22: 961-970.

Fariello R. Forebrain influence on an amygdaloid acute epileptic focus in the cat. *Exp Neurol* 1976; 51: 515-528.

Ferencz I, Kokaia M, Elmer E, Keep M, Kokaia Z, Lindvall O. Suppression of kindling epileptogenesis in rats by intrahippocampal cholinergic grafts. *Eur J Neurosci* 1998; 10: 213-220.

Fernandes de Lima VM, Pijn JP, Nunes Filipe C, Lopes da Silva F. The role of hippocampal commissures in the interhemispheric transfer of epileptiform afterdischarges in the rat: a study using linear and non-linear regression analysis. *Electroencephalogr Clin Neurophysiol* 1990; 76: 520-539.

Fernandez-Molina A, Hunsperger RW. Central representation of affective reactions in forebrain and brainstem; electrical stimulation of amygdala, stria terminalis and adjacent structures. *J Physiol* (Lond) 1959; 145: 251-269.

Fisher RS, Uematsu S, Krauss GL, Cysyk BJ, McPherson R, Lesser RP, Gordon B, Schwerdt P, Rise M. Placebo-controlled pilot study of centromedian thalamic stimulation in treatment of intractable seizures. *Epilepsia* 1992; 33: 841-851.

Foerster O, Altenburger H. Elektrobiologische Vorgänge an der menschlichen Hirnrinde. *Verhandlungen der Gesellschaft Deutscher Nervenärzte (22. Jahresversammlung).* Berlin: Von Vogel FCW 1935: 93-102.

Forel A. Untersuchungen über die Haubenregion. *Arch f Psychiatr* 1877; 7: 393-495.

Forel A. *Le Monde Social des Fourmis*, 5 Vols. Geneve: Kündig 1921-1923.

Forel A. *The Sexual Question* (English adaptation from the 2nd German edition, revised and enlarged by Marshall CF) Brooklyn-New York: Physicians and Surgeons Book Company 1926.

Forel A. Ausstellungskatalog 142, siehe auch: http: //www.edimuster.ch/abstinenz/forel.htm

Fountas KN, Smith JR, Murro AM, Politsky J, Park YD, Jenkins PD. Implantation of a closed-loop stimulation in the management of medically refractory focal epilepsy: a technical note. *Stereotact Funct Neurosurg* 2005; 83: 153-158.

Freeman W, Watts JW. Retrograde degeneration of the thalamus following prefrontal lobotomy. *J Comp Neurol* 1947; 86: 65-93.

Fregni F, Pascual-Leone A. Hand motor recovery after stroke: tuning the orchestra to improve hand motor function. *Cogn Behav Neurol* 2006; 19: 21-33.

Fregni F, Boggio PS, Nitsche M, Bermpohl F, Antal A, Feredoes E, Marcolin MA, Rigonatti SP, Silva MTA, Paulus W, Pascual-Leone A. Anodal transcranial direct current stimulation of prefrontal cortex enhancing working memory. *Exp Brain Res* 2005; 166: 23-30.

Fregni F, Boggio PS, Lima MC, Ferreira MJ, Wagner T, Rigonatti SP, Castro AW, Souza DR, Riberto M, Freedman SD, Nitsche MA, Pascual-Leone A. A sham-controlled, phase II trial of transcranial direct current stimulation for the treatment of central pain in traumatic spinal cord injury. *Pain* 2006a; 122: 197-209.

Fregni F, Boggio PS, Nitsche MA, Marcolini MA, Rigonatti SP, Pascual-Leone A. Treatment of major depression with transcranial direct current stimulation (Letter to the Editor). *Bipolar Disorders* 2006b; 8: 203.

Fregni F, Thome-Souza S, Nitsche MA, Freedman SD, Valente KD, Pascual-Leone A. A controlled clinical trial of cathodal DC polarization in patients with refractory epilepsy. *Epilepsia* 2006c; 47: 335-342.

Fromm GH. Effects of different classes of antiepileptic drugs on brain-stem pathways. *Federation Proc* 1985; 4: 2432-2435.

Fromm GH. The brain-stem, and convulsions: Historical overview: In: Fromm GH, Faingold CL, Browning RA, Burnham WM eds. *Epilepsy and the Reticular Formation.* Neurology and Neurobiology (Liss AR) 1987: 1-8.

Fromm GH, Terrence CF, Chattha AS. Differential effect of antiepileptic and non-antiepileptic drugs on the reticular formation. *Life Sci* 1984; 35: 2665-2673.

Fromm GH, Faingold CL, Browning RA, Burnham WM eds. *Epilepsy and the Reticular Formation.* Neurology and Neurobiology (Liss AR) 1987.

Gabavili VM, Chkhenkeli SA, Šramka M. The treatment of status epilepticus by electrostimulation of deep brain structures. Presented at: *First European Congress of Neurology*, Prag 1988.

Gale K. Mechanisms of seizure control mediated by gamma-aminobutyric acid: role of the substantia nigra. *Fed Proc* 1985; 44: 2414-2424.

Ganglberger JA. Cortical Evoked Potentials. In: Schaltenbrand G, Walker EA eds. *Stereotaxy of the Human Brain*. New York: Thieme-Stratton Inc. 1982: 334-347.

Ganglberger JA. Additional new approach treatment of temporal lobe epilepsy. *Acta Neurochir* 1984; 33 (Suppl.): 149-154.

Garcia-Bengochea F, Friedman WA. Persistent memory loss following section of the anterior fornix in humans. A historical review. *Surg Neurol* 1987; 27: 361-364.

Gastaut H, Fisher-Williams M. The physiopathology of epileptic seizures. In: Field J, Magoun HW eds. *Handbook of Physiology*, Section 1: Neurophysiology, Vol. 1. Washington DC: American Physiological Society 1959: 329-363.

Gellhorn EA, Balling AM, Kawakami M. Studies on experimental convulsions with emphasis on the role of the hypothalamus and the reticular formation. *Epilepsia* 1959; 3: 233-254.

Gibbs FA, Gibbs EL. *Atlas of Electroencephalography*. Vol. 2. Massachusetts: Addison-Wesley Publishing company Inc. 1952.

Gloor P. Generalized cortico-reticular epilepsies. Some considerations on the pathophysiology of generalized bilaterally synchronous spike and wave discharge. *Epilepsia* 1968; 9: 249-263.

Gloor P. Generalized epilepsy with spike-and-wave discharge: A reinterpretation of its electrographic and clinical manifestations. *Epilepsia* 1979; 20: 725-732.

Gloor P. EEG characteristics in Creutzfeld-Jakob Disease. *Ann Neurol* 1980; 8: 341.

Gloor P. *The Temporal Lobe and Limbic System*. New York, Oxford: Oxford University Press 1997.

Gloor P, Quesney LF, Zumstein H. Pathophysiology of generalized penicillin epilepsy in the cat: the role of cortical and subcortical structures. II. Topical application of penicillin to the cerebral cortex and to subcortical structures. *Electroencephalogr Clin Neurophysiol* 1977; 43: 79-94.

Goldring S. Negative steady potential shifts which lead to seizure discharge. *UCLA Forum Sci* 1963; 1: 215-236.

Goodman JH, Berger RE, Tcheng TK. Preemptive low frequency stimulation decreases the incidence of amygdala-kindled seizures. *Epilepsia* 2005; 46: 1-7.

Goodman SJ, Holcombe V. Selective and prolonged analgesia in monkey resulting from brain stimulation. Recent advances in Pain Research and Therapy. *Proceedings of the First World Congress on Pain*. New York: Raven Press 1976; 495-502.

Gordon B, Lesser RP, Rance NE, Hart J Jr, Webber R, Uematsu S, Fisher RS. Parameters for direct cortical electrical stimulation in the human: histopathological confirmation. *Electroencephalogr Clin Neurophysiol* 1990; 75: 371-377.

Graves N, Lozano AM, Wennberg RA, Osorio I, Wilkinson S, Baluch G, French JA, Kerrigan JF, Shetter A, Fisher RS. Brain stimulation for epilepsy: pilot patient results and implementation of a controlled clinical trial. *Epilepsia* 2004; 45 (Suppl.7): 148.

Green JD, Morin F. Hypothalamic electrical activity and hypothalamo-cortical relationships. *Am J Physiol* 1953; 172: 175-186.

Grimm RJ, Frazee JG, Bell CC, Kawasaki T, Dow RS. Quantitative studies in cobalt model epilepsy: the effect of cerebellar stimulation. *Int J Neurol* 1970; 7: 126-140.

Gudden B. Beitrag zur Kenntnis der Corpus mammillare und der sogenannten Schenkel des Fornix. *Arch Psychiat Nervenkr* 1881; 11: 428-452.

Haberler C, Alesch F, Mazal PR, Pilz P, Jellinger K, Pinter MM, Hainfellner JA, Budka H. No tissue damage by chronic deep brain stimulation in Parkinson's disease. *Ann Neurol* 2000; 48: 372-376.

Hablitz JJ, Rea G. Cerebellar nuclear stimulation in generalized penicillin epilepsy. *Brain Res Bull* 1976; 1: 599-601.

Hajek M, Valavanis A, Yonekawa Y, Schiess R, Buck A, Wieser HG. Selective amobarbital test for the determination of language function in epileptic patients with frontal and posterior temporal brain lesions. *Epilepsia* 1998; 39: 389-398.

Hamani C, Saint-Cyr JA, Fraser J, Kaplitt M, Lozano AM. The subthalamic nucleus in the context of movement disorders. *Brain* 2004a; 127: 4-20.

Hamani C, Ewerton FI, Bonilha SM, Ballester G, Mello LE, Lozano AM. Bilateral anterior thalamic nucleus lesions and high-frequency stimulation are protective against pilocarpine-induced seizures and status epilepticus. *Neurosurgery* 2004b; 54: 191-195.

Hamer HM, Luders HO, Knake S, Fritsch B, Oertel WH, Rosenow F. Electrophysiology of focal clonic seizures in humans: a study using subdural and depth electrodes. *Brain* 2003; 126: 547-555.

Hammond C, Feger J, Bioulac B, Souteyrand JP. Experimental hemiballism in the monkey produced by unilateral kainic acid lesion in corpus Luysii. *Brain Res* 1979; 171: 577-580.

Handforth A, DeGiorgio CM, Schachter SC, Uthman BM, Naritoku DK, Tecoma ES, et al. Vagus nerve stimulation therapy for partial-onset seizures: a randomized active-control trial. *Neurology* 1998; 51: 48-55.

Hartwig HG, Wahren W. Anatomy of the hypothalamus. In: Schaltenbrand G, Walker AE eds. *Stereotaxy of the Human Brain*. Stuttgart, New York: Georg Thieme Verlag 1982: 87-106.

Hassler R. Über die Thalamus-Stirnhirn-Verbindungen beim Menschen. *Nervenarzt* 1948; 19: 9-12.

Hassler R. Über die afferenten Bahnen und Thalamuskerne des motorischen Systems des Grosshirns I und II. *Arch Psychiatr* 1949a; 182: 786-818.

Hassler R. Über die Rinden- und Stammhirnanteile des menschlichen Thalamus. *Psychiatr Neurol* 1949b; 1: 181-187.

Hassler R. Anatomie des Thalamus. *Arch Psychiatr* 1950; 148: 249-256.

Hassler R. Architectonic organization of the thalamic nuclei. In: Schaltenbrand G, Walker AE eds. *Stereotaxy of the Human Brain*. Stuttgart, New York: Georg Thieme Verlag 1982: 140-180.

Hassler R, Dieckmann G. Stereotactic treatment of different kinds of spasmodic torticollis (in German). *Confin Neurol* 1970; 32: 135-143.

Hassler R, Hess WR. Experimentelle und anatomische Befunde über die Drehbewegungen und ihre nervösen Apparate. *Arch Psychiat* 1954; 192: 488-526.

Hassler R, Riechert T. Klinische Effekte bei Reizung einzelner Thalamuskerne des Menschen. *Nervenarzt* 1955; 26: 35.

Hassler R, Riechert T. Über einen Fall von doppelseitiger Fornicotomie bei sogenannter temporaler Epilepsie. *Acta Neurochir* 1957; 5: 330-340.

Haymaker W, Anderson E, Nauta WJH eds. *The Hypothalamus*. Springfield Ill: Charles C Thomas 1969: 805-807.

Hayne R, Meyers R. An improved model of a human stereotaxic instrument. *J Neurosurg* 1950; 7: 463-475.

Heimburger RF, Small IF, Small JG, Milstein V, Moore D. Stereotactic amygdalotomy for convulsive and behavioral disorders. Long-term follow-up study. *Appl Neurophysiol* 1978; 41: 43-51.

Herkenham M. The connections of the nucleus reuniens thalami: evidence for a direct thalamo-hippocampal pathway in the rat. *J Comp Neurol* 1978; 177: 589-610.

Hess R. *EEG Handbook*, 2nd unchanged edition. Basel: Sandoz Ltd. 1969.

Heuser G, Buchwald NA, Wyers EJ. The "caudate-spindle". II. Facilitatory and inhibitory caudate-cortical pathways. *Electroencephalogr Clin Neurophysiol* 1961; 13: 519-524.

Hodaie M, Hamani C, Zumsteg D, Andrade DM, Wennberg RA, Lozano AM. Deep brain stimulation in a patient with medically intractable generalized seizures. In: Lüders H, Najm I, Bingaman W eds. *Textbook of Epilepsy Surgery*. Abingdon: Taylor & Francis Group 2007 (in press).

Hodaie M, Wennberg RA, Dostrovsky JO, Lozano AM. Chronic anterior thalamus stimulation for intractable epilepsy. *Epilepsia* 2002; 43: 603-608.

Holstege G, Kuypers HG, Dekker JJ. The organization of the bulbar fibre connections to the trigeminal, facial and hypoglossal motor nuclei. II. An autoradiographic tracing study in cat. *Brain* 1977; 100: 264-286.

Hosobuchi Y, Adams JE, Linchitz R. Pain relief by electrical stimulation of the central gray matter in humans and its reversal by naloxone. *Science* 1977; 197: 183-186.

Huber A, Padrun V, Déglon N, Aebischer P, Möhler H, Boison D. Grafts of adenosine-releasing cells suppress seizures in kindling epilepsy. *Proc Natl Acad Sci USA* 2001; 98: 7611-7616.

Hummel F, Celnik P, Giraux P, Floel A, Wu WH, Gerloff C, Cohen LG. Effects of non-invasive cortical stimulation on skilled motor function in chronic stroke. *Brain* 2005; 128: 490-499.

Hunter J, Jasper HH. Effects of thalamic stimulation in unanesthetized animals. The arrest reaction and petit mal like seizure activation patterns and generalized convulsions. *Electroenceph Clin Neurophysiol* 1949; 1: 305-324.

Hutton JT, Frost JD Jr, Foster J. The influence of the cerebellum in cat penicillin epilepsy. *Epilepsia* 1972; 13: 401-408.

Iadarola MJ, Gale K. Substantia nigra: site of anticonvulsant activity mediated by gamma-aminobutyric acid. *Science* 1982; 218: 1237-1240.

Iasemidis LD, Shiau DS, Pardalos PM, Chaovalitwongse W, Narayanan K, Prasad A, Tsakalis K, Carney PR, Sackellares JC. Long-term prospective on-line real-time seizure prediction. *Clin Neurophysiol* 2005; 116: 532-544.

Ikeda A, Nagamine T, Kunieda T, Yazawa S, Ohara S, Taki W, Kimura J, Shibasaki H. Clonic convulsion caused by epileptic discharges arising from the human supplementary motor area as studied by subdural recording. *Epileptic Disord* 1999; 1: 21-26.

Ingram JL, Osorio I, Steven WB. Anterior thalamic nuclei evoked responses: A preliminary study. *Epilepsia* 2001; 42 (Suppl.7): 29.

Ironside JW. The spectrum of safety: variant Creutzfeldt-Jakob disease in the United Kingdom. *Semin Hematol* 2003; 40 (Suppl.3): 16-22.

Iukharev SP. [Individual anatomic variability of Forel's field H] [Article in Russian] *Arkh Anat Gistol Embriol* 1976; 71: 77-81.

Iyer MB, Mattu U, Grafman J, Lomarev M, Sato S, Wasermann EM. Safety and cognitive effect of frontal DC brain polarization in healthy individuals. *Neurology* 2005; 64: 872-875.

Jasper HH. Thalamic reticular system. In: Sheer DE, ed. *Electrical Stimulation of the Brain*. Austin: University of Texas Press 1961: 277-87.

Jasper HH. Mechanisms of propagation: Extracellular studies. In: Jasper HH, Ward AA Jr, Pope A eds. *Basic Mechanisms of Epilepsy*. Boston: Little, Brown 1969: 421-440.

Jasper HH, Droogleever-Fortuyn J. Experimental studies on the functional anatomy of petit mal epilepsy. *Res Publ Assoc Res Nerv Ment Dis* 1947; 26: 272-298.

Jennum P, Klitgaard H. Repetitive transcranial magnetic stimulations of the rat. Effect of acute and chronic stimulations on pentylenetetrazole-induced clonic seizures. *Epilepsy Res* 1996; 23: 115-122.

Jinnai D. Clinical results and the significance of Forel-H-tomy in the treatment of epilepsy. *Confin Neurol* 1966; 27: 129-136.

Jinnai D, Mukawa J. Forel-H-tomy for the treatment of epilepsy. *Confin Neurol* 1970; 32: 307-315.

Jinnai D, Nishimoto A. Stereotaxic destruction of Forel-H for treatment of epilepsy. *Neurochirurgia* (Stuttg.) 1963; 25: 164-176.

Jinnai D, Mogami H, Mukawa J, Iwata Y, Kobayashi K. Effect of brain-stem lesions on metrazol-induced seizures in cats. *Electroencephalogr Clin Neurophysiol* 1969; 27: 404-411.

Jinnai D, Mukawa J, Kobayashi K. Forel-H-tomy for the treatment of intractable epilepsy. *Acta Neurochir* (Vienna) 1976; 23 (Suppl.): 159-165.

Jung R, Riechert T, Heines KD. Zur Technik und Bedeutung der operativen Elektrocorticographie und subcorticalen Hirnpotentialableitung. *Nervenarzt* 1952; 22: 433-436.

Kaitz SS, Robertson RT. Thalamic connections with limbic cortex. II. Corticothalamic projections. *J Comp Neurol* 1981; 195: 527-545.

Kamikawa K, Noda H, Miyagawa S, Mogami H, Jinnai D. Non-specific projection system of the thalamus and bilateral motor control of subcortical nuclei. *Confin Neurol* 1967; 29: 112-116.

Katariwala NM, Bakay RA, Pennell PB, Olson LD, Henry TR, Epstein CM. Remission of intractable partial epilepsy following implantation of intracranial electrodes. *Neurology* 2001; 57: 1505-1507.

Kerrigan JF, Litt B, Fisher RS, Cranstoun S, French JA, Blum DE, Dichter M, Shetter A, Baltuch G, Jaggi J, Krone S, Brodie M, Rise M, Graves N. Electrical stimulation of the anterior nucleus of the thalamus for the treatment of intractable epilepsy. *Epilepsia* 2004; 45: 346-354.

Khosravani H, Carlen PL, Velazquez JL. The control of seizure-like activity in the rat hippocampal slice. *Biophys J* 2003; 84: 687-695.

Kinoshita M, Ikeda A, Matsuhashi M, Matsumoto R, Hitomi T, Begum T, Usui K, Takayama M, Mikuni N, Miyamoto S, Hashimoto N, Shibasaki H. Electric cortical stimulation suppresses epileptic and background activities in neocortical epilepsy and mesial temporal lobe epilepsy. *Clin Neurophysiol* 2005; 116: 1291-1299.

Kirikae T, Wada J. Electrothalamogram of petit mal seizures. *Med Biol* 1951; 20: 253.

Klee MR, Lux HD. Intracellular studies on the influence of inhibiting potentials in the motor cortex. II. The effect of electric stimulation of the nucleus caudatus. *Arch Psychiatr Nervenkr Z Gesamte Neurol Psychiatr* 1962; 203: 667-689.

Kleiner-Fisman G, Fisman DN, Sime E, Saint-Cyr JA, Lozano AM, Lang AE. Long-term follow-up of bilateral deep brain stimulation of the subthalamic nucleus in patients with advanced Parkinson disease. *J Neurosurg* 2003; 99: 489-495.

Kokaia M, Cenci MA, Elmer E, Nilsson OG, Kokaia Z, Bengzon J, Bjorklund A, Lindvall O. Seizure development and noradrenaline release in kindling epilepsy after noradrenergic reinnervation of the subcortically deafferented hippocampus by superior cervical ganglion or fetal locus coeruleus grafts. *Exp Neurol* 1994a; 130: 351-361.

Kokaia M, Aebischer P, Elmer E, Bengzon J, Kalen P, Kokaia Z, Lindvall O. Seizure suppression in kindling epilepsy by intracerebral implants of GABA - but not by noradrenalin-releasing polymer matrices. *Exp Brain Res* 1994b; 100: 385-394.

Koshino K, Nakano M, Miki M, Matsumura H. Stereotaxic operation for the control of infantile epilepsy and associated behavioral disorder. *Confin Neurol* 1975; 37: 223-231.

Kossoff EH, Ritzl EK, Politsky JM, Murro AM, Smith JR, Duckrow RB, Spencer DD, Bergey GK. Effect of an external responsive neurostimulator on seizures and electrographic discharges during subdural electrode monitoring. *Epilepsia* 2004; 45: 1560-1567.

Krack P, Batir A, Van Blercom N, Chabardes S, Fraix V, Ardouin C, Koudsie A, Limousin PD, Benazzouz A, LeBas JF, Benabid AL, Pollak P. Five-year follow-up of bilateral stimulation of the subthalamic nucleus in advanced Parkinson's disease. *N Engl J Med* 2003; 349: 1925-1934.

Kreindler A, Zuckermann E, Steriade M, Chimion D. Electroclinical features of convulsions induced by stimulation of brain stem. *J Neurophysiol* 1958; 21: 430-436.

Künzle H. Aufbau und Verbindungen der Basalganglien. In: Drenckhahn D, Zenker W eds. *Benninghoff Anatomie*. Volume 2 15. Völlig neu bearbeitete Auflage. München, Wien, Baltimore: Urban & Schwarzenberg 1994: 572-582.

La Grutta V, Amato G, Zacami MT. The importance of the caudate nucleus in the control of convulsive activity in the amygdaloid complex and the temporal cortex of the cat. *Electroencephalogr Clin Neurophysiol* 1971; 31: 57-69.

La Grutta V, Sabatino M, Gravante G, Morici G, Ferraro G, La Grutta G. A study of caudate inhibition on an epileptic focus in the cat hippocampus. *Arch Int Physiol Biochim* 1988; 96: 113-120.

Labar D, Murphy J, Tecoma E. Vagus nerve stimulation for medication-resistant generalized epilepsy. E04 VNS Study Group. *Neurology* 1999; 52: 1510-1512.

Lachmann J, Bergmann F, Monnier M. Central nystagmus elicited by stimulation of the meso-diencephalon in the rabbit. *Am J Physiol* 1958; 193: 328-334.

Lado FA, Velisek L, Moshe SL. The effect of electrical stimulation of the subthalamic nucleus on seizures is frequency dependent. *Epilepsia* 2003; 44: 157-164.

Laitinen LV. Thalamatomy in progressive myclonus epilepsy. *Acta Neurol Scand* 1967; Suppl. 31: 170-171.

Le Gros Clark WE. The structure and connection of the thalamus. *Brain* 1932; 55: 406-470.

Leith NJ, Barrett RJ. Self-stimulation and amphetamine: tolerance to d and l isomers and cross tolerance to cocaine and methylphenidate. *Psychopharmacology* (Berl.) 1981; 74: 23-28.

Leksell L. A stereotaxic apparatus for intracranial neurosurgery. *Acta Chir Scand* 1949; 99: 229-253.

Lesser RP, Kim SH, Beyderman L, Miglioretti DL, Webber WR, Bare M, Cysyk B, Krauss G, Gordon B. Brief bursts of pulse stimulation terminate after discharges caused by cortical stimulation. *Neurology* 1999; 53: 2073-2081.

Levy SR, Chiappa KH, Burke CJ, Young RR. Early evolution of incidence of electroencephalographic abnormalities in Creutzfeldt-Jakob disease. *J Clin Neurophysiol* 1986; 3: 1-21.

Li H, Weiss SR, Chuang DM, Post RM, Rogawski MA. Bidirectional synaptic plasticity in the rat basolateral amygdala: characterization of an activity-dependent switch sensitive to the presynaptic metabotropic glutamate receptor antagonist 2S-alpha-ethylglutamic acid. *J Neurosci* 1998; 18: 1662-1670.

Liebeskind JC, Guilbaud G, Besson JH, Oliveras JL. Analgesia from electrical stimulation of the periaqueductal grey matter in the cat: behavioural observations and inhibitory effects on spinal cord interneurons. *Brain Res* 1973; 50: 444-446.

Lindvall O, Bengzon J, Elmer E, Kokaia M, Kokaia Z. Grafts in models of epilepsy. In: Dunnett SB, Bjorklund A eds. *Functional Neural Transplantation*. New York: Raven Press 1994: 387-413.

Loddenkemper T, Pan A, Neme S, Baker KB, Rezai AR, Dinner DS, Montgomery EB Jr, Luders HO. Deep brain stimulation in epilepsy. *J Clin Neurophysiol* 2001; 18: 514-532.

Loher TJ, Pohle T, Krauss JK. Functional stereotactic surgery for treatment of cervical dystonia: Review of the experience from the lesional era. *Stereotact Funct Neurosurg* 2004; 82: 1-13.

Löscher W, Ebert U, Lehmann H, Rosenthal C, Nikkhah G. Seizure suppression in kindling epilepsy by grafts of fetal GABAergic neurons in rat substantia nigra. *J Neurosci Res* 1998; 15: 196-209.

Lozano AM. The subthalamic nucleus: myth and opportunities. *Mov Disord* 2001; 16: 183-184.

Lüders HO. *Deep brain stimulation and epilepsy*. London, New York: Martin Dunitz, Taylor & Francis Group 2004.

Lüders J, Najm I, Lüders HO. Brain stimulation and epilepsy: basic overview and novel approaches. In: Lüders HO ed. *Deep Brain Stimulation and Epilepsy*. London, New York: Martin Dunitz 2004: 3-17.

Lüders HO, Najm I, Bingaman W eds. *Textbook of Epilepsy Surgery*. Abingdon UK: Taylor & Francis Group (in press).

Lund M. Epilepsy in association with intracranial tumor. *Acta Psychiat Neurol Scand* 1952; Suppl. 81: 3-149.

MacLean PD. The triune brain, emotion of scientific bias. In: Schmitt FO ed. *The Neurosciences, Second Study Program*. New York: Rockefeller University Press 1970: 336-349.

Marossero F, Ravagnati L, Sironi VA, Miserocci G, Franzini A, Ettore G, Cabrini GP. Late results of stereotactic radiofrequency lesions in epilepsy. *Acta Neurochir* 1980; 30 (Suppl.): 145-149.

Mathieu D, Kondziolka D, Niranjan A, Flickinger J, Lunsford LD. Gamma knife radiosurgery for refractory epilepsy caused by hypothalamic hamartomas. *Stereotact Funct Neurosurg* 2006; 84: 82-87.

Matsumura M, Kojima J, Gardiner TW, Hikosaka O. Visual and oculomotor functions of monkey subthalamic nucleus. *J Neurophysiol* 1992; 67: 1615-1632.

Mayanagi Y, Walker AE. DC potentials of temporal lobe seizures in the monkey. *J Neurol* 1975; 209: 199-215.

Mayer DJ, Wolfle TL, Akil H, Carder B, Liebeskind JC. Analgesia from electrical stimulation in the brain stem of the rat. *Science* 1971; 174: 1351-1354.

McCallister LW, Connelly JC, Kaufman MP. Stimulation of H fields of Forel decreases total lung resistance in dogs. *J Appl Physiol* 1988; 65: 2156-2163.

McDonnell G, Burke P. The challenge of prion decontamination. *Clin Infect Dis* 2003; 36: 1152-1154.

Mempel E. The effect of partial amygdalectomy on emotional disturbances and epileptic seizures. *Pol Med J* 1971; 10: 968-974.

Milhorat TH, Baldwin M, Hantman DA. Experimental epilepsy after rostral reticular formation excision. *J Neurosurg* 1966; 24: 595-611.

Mirski MA, Ferrendelli JA. Individual and combined effects of convulsant and anticonvulsant drugs on regional brain metabolism. *Soc Neurosci* 1983; 9: 627.

Mirski MA, Ferrendelli JA. Interruption of the mammillothalamic tract prevents seizures in guinea pigs. *Science* 1984a; 226: 72-74.

Mirski MA, Ferrendelli JA. Interruption of the connections of the mammillary bodies protects against experimental generalized seizures. *Epilepsia* 1984b; 25: 661.

Mirski MA, Ferrendelli JA. Anterior thalamic mediation of generalized pentylenetetrazol seizures. *Brain Res* 1986a; 399: 212-23.

Mirski MA, Ferrendelli JA. Selective metabolic activation of the mammillary bodies and their connections during ethosuximide-induced suppression of pentylenetetrazol seizures. *Epilepsia* 1986b; 27: 194-203.

Mirski MA, Ferrendelli JA. Interruption of the connections of the mammillary bodies protects against generalized pentylenetetrazol seizures in guinea pigs. *J Neurosci* 1987; 7: 662-670.

Mirski MA, Fisher RS. Electrical stimulation of the mammillary nuclei increases seizure threshold to pentylenetetrazol in rats. *Epilepsia* 1994; 35: 1309-1316.

Mirski MA, McKeon AC, Ferrendelli JA. Anterior thalamus and substantia nigra: two distinct structures mediating experimental generalized seizures. *Brain Res* 1986; 397: 377-380.

Mirski MA, Rossell LA, Terry JB, Fisher RS. Anticonvulsant effect of anterior thalamic high frequency electrical stimulation in the rat. *Epilepsy Res* 1997; 28: 89-100.

Mirski MA, Tsai YC, Rossell LA, Thakor NV, Sherman DL. Anterior thalamic mediation of experimental seizures: selective EEG spectral coherence. *Epilepsia* 2003; 44: 355-365.

Monnier M, Fischer R. Stimulation électrique et coagulation thérapeutique du thalamus chez l'homme. *Confinia Neurol* (Basel) 1951; 11: 282-286.

Monnier M, Fischer R. *La stimulation électrique du thalamus chez l'homme. Résultats somatotopiques. Livre jubilaire du Dr. André Thomas.* Paris: Mather 1955.

Mori Y, Kondziolka D, Balzer J, Fellows W, Flickinger JC, Lunsford LD, Thulborn KR. Effects of stereotactic radiosurgery on an animal model of hippocampal epilepsy. *Neurosurgery* 2000; 46: 157-165 (discussion 165-168).

Morillo LE, Ebner TJ, Bloedel JR. The early involvement of subcortical structures during the development of a cortical seizure focus. *Epilepsia* 1982; 23: 571-585.

Morison RS, Dempsey EW. A study of thalamocortical relations. *Am J Physiol* 1942; 135: 280-292.

Morison RS, Dempsey EW. Mechanism of thalamo-cortical augmentation and repetition. *Am J Physiol* 1943; 138: 297-308.

Morrell M. Brain stimulation for epilepsy: can scheduled or responsive neurostimulation stop seizures? *Curr Opin Neurol* 2006; 19: 164-168.

Morris GL 3rd, Mueller WM. Long-term treatment with vagus nerve stimulation in patients with refractory epilepsy. The Vagus Nerve Stimulation Study Group E01-E05. *Neurology* 1999; 53: 1731-1735.

Moruzzi G, Magoun HW. Brain stem reticular formation and activation of the EEG. *Electroencephalogr Clin Neurophysiol* 1949; 1: 455-473.

Motamedi GK, Lesser RP, Miglioretti DL, Mizuno-Matsumoto Y, Gordon B, Webber WR, Jackson DC, Sepkuty JP, Crone NE. Optimizing parameters for terminating cortical afterdischarges with pulse stimulation. *Epilepsia* 2002; 43: 836-846.

Mountcastle VB, Henneman E. The representation of tactile sensibility in the thalamus of the monkey. *J Comp Neurol* 1952; 97: 409-440.

Mouton LJ. *Spinal efferents and afferents of the periaqueductal gray: Possible role in pain, sex and micturation.* Thesis (Proefschrift, Rijksuniversiteit Groningen) 1999 [http://irs.ub.rug.nl/ppn/188049061]

Mukawa J. Fiber connections of the Forel H-field as seen in Marchi preparations. *Acta Med Okayama* 1964a; 18: 207-220.

Mukawa J. Effects of brainstem and subcortical lesions on corticogenic epileptic convulsion with special reference to Forel H-field. *Acta Med Okayama* 1964b; 18: 153-171.

Mukawa J, Dimura T, Nagao I, Kobayashi K, Iwata Y. Forel-H-tomy for the treatment of intractable epilepsy. Special reference to postoperative electroencephalographic changes. *Confin Neurol* 1975; 37: 302-307.

Mullan S, Vailati G, Karasick J, Mailis M. Thalamic lesions for the control of epilepsy. *Arch Neurol* 1967; 16: 277-285.

Mundinger F, Becker P, Groebner E, Bachschmid G. Late results of stereotactic surgery of epilepsy predominantly temporal lobe type. *Acta Neurochir* 1976; 23 (Suppl.): 177-182.

Münkle MC, Waldvogel HJ, Faull RL. The distribution of calbindin, calretinin and parvalbumin immunoreactivity in the human thalamus. *J Chem Neuroanat* 2000; 19: 155-173.

Mutani R, Bergamini L, Doriguzzi T. Experimental evidence for the existence of an extrarhinencephalic control of the activity of the cobalt rhinencephalic epileptogenic focus. Part 2. Effects of the paleocerebellar stimulation. *Epilepsia* 1969; 10: 351-362.

Myers RR, Burchiel KJ, Stockard JJ, Bickford RG. Effects of acute and chronic paleocerebellar stimulation on experimental models of epilepsy in the cat: studies with enflurane, pentylenetetrazol, penicillin, and chloralose. *Epilepsia* 1975; 16: 257-267.

Namba M. Cytoarchitectonische Untersuchungen am Striatum. *Z Hirnforsch* 1957; 3: 247-271.

Narabayashi H. Functional differentiation in and around the ventrolateral nucleus of the thalamus based on experience in human stereoencephalotomy. *Johns Hopk Med J* 1968; 122: 295-300.

Narabayashi H. Long range results of medial amygdalotomy on epileptic traits in adult patients. In: Rasmussen T, Marino R eds. *Functional Neurosurgery.* New York: Raven 1979: 243-252.

Narabayashi H, Mizutani T. Epileptic seizures and the stereotaxic amygdalotomy. *Confin Neurol* 1970; 32: 289-297.

Narabayashi H, Ushimura Y. *Stereoencephalotomy.* 47th Japan Neuro Psych Conf Kyoto 1950.

Nashold BS, Stewart B; Wilson WP. Depth electrode studies in centrencephalic epilepsy. *Confin Neurol* 1972; 34: 252-263.

Nauta WJH. An experimental study of the fornix system in the rat. *J Comp Neurol* 1956; 104: 247-271.

Nauta WJH. Hippocampal projections and related neural pathways to the midbrain in the cat. *Brain* 1958: 319-340.

Nauta WJH, Haymaker W. Hypothalamic nuclei and fiber connections. In: Haymaker W, Anderson E, Nauta WJH eds. *The Hypothalamus.* Springfield Ill: Charles C. Thomas 1969: 136-209.

Neme S, Montgomery EB Jr., Rezai A, Wilson K, Lüders HO. Subthalamic nucleus stimulation in patients with intractable epilepsy: the Cleveland experience. In: Lüders HO ed. *Deep Brain Stimulation and Epilepsy.* London, New York: Martin Dunitz 2004: 349-355.

Netter FH. *Atlas of Human Anatomy.* Ardsley USA: CIBA-GEIGY Corp. 1989 (distributed and printed by CIBA-GEIGY Limited, Basel, 1991).

Nichols TE, Holmes AP. Nonparametric permutation tests for functional neuroimaging: a primer with examples. *Hum Brain Mapp* 2002; 15: 1-25.

Niedermeyer E, Laws ER Jr., Walker AE. Depth EEG findings in epileptics with generalized spike-wave complexes. *Arch Neurol* 1969; 21: 51-58.

Nitsche MA, Paulus W. Excitability changes induced in the human motor cortex by weak transcranial direct current stimulation. *J Physiol* 2000; 527: 633-639.

Oakley JC, Ojemann GA. Effects of chronic stimulation of the caudate nucleus on a preexisting alumina seizure focus. *Exp Neurol* 1982; 75: 360-367.

Ohye C. Use of selective thalamotomy for various kinds of movement disorder, based on basic studies *Stereotact Funct Neurosurg* 2000; 75: 54-65.

Ojemann GA. Speech and short-term verbal memory. Alterations evoked from stimulation in pulvinar. In: Cooper IS, Riklan M, Rakic P eds. *The Pulvinar-LP Complex.* Springfield Ill, Thomas 1974: 173-184.

Ojemann GA, Ward AA Jr. Stereotactic and other procedures for epilepsy. In: Purpura DP, Penry JK, Walter RD eds. *Advances in Neurology*, Vol. 8. New York: Raven Press 1975: 241-263.

Ordway GA, Waldrop TG, Iwamoto GA, Gentile BJ. Hypothalamic influences on cardiovascular response of beagles to dynamic exercise. *Am J Physiol* 1989; 257: 1247-1253.

Orthner H, Lohmann R. Erfahrungen mit stereotaktischen Eingriffen bei Epilepsie. *Dtsch med Wschr* 1966; 91: 984-991.

Osorio I, Frei MG, Sunderam S, Giftakis J, Bhavaraju NC, Schaffner SF, Wilkinson SB. Automated seizure abatement in humans using electrical stimulation. *Ann Neurol* 2005; 57: 258-268.

Pan A, Boongird A, Kunieda T, Naim I, Lüders HO. Focal limbic seizures induced by kainic acid: effects of bilateral subthalamic nucleus stimulation. In: Lüders HO ed. *Deep Brain Stimulation and Epilepsy.* London, New York: Martin Dunitz, Taylor&Francis Group 2004: 199-208.

Pant SS, Benton JW, Dodge PR. Unilateral pupillary dilation during and immediately following seizures. *Neurology* 1966; 16: 837-840.

Papez JW. A proposed mechanism of emotion. *Arch Neurol Psychiatry* 1937; 38: 725-743.

Papez JW. Visceral brain, its component parts and their connections. *J Nerv Ment Dis* 1958; 126: 40-56.

Parent A. Auguste Forel on ants and neurology. *Can J Neurol Sci* 2003; 30: 284-291.

Pascual-Marqui RD. Review of methods solving the EEG inverse problem. *Int J Bioelectromagnetism* 1999; 1: 75-86.

Pascual-Marqui RD, Michel CM, Lehmann D. Low resolution electromagnetic tomography: a new method for localizing electrical activity in the brain. *Int J Psychophysiol* 1994; 18: 49-65.

Paulus W. Outlasting excitability shifts induced by direct current stimulation of the human brain. *Clin Neurophysiol* 2004; 57 (Suppl.): 708-714.

Penfield WG, Jasper HH. Highest level seizures. *Res Publ Assn Nerv Ment Dis* 1946; 26: 252-271.

Penfield WG, Jasper HH. *Epilepsy and the Functional Anatomy of the Human Brain.* Boston: Little Brown & Co 1954.

Poletti CE, Creswell G. Fornix system efferent projections in the squirrel monkey: an experimental degeneration study. *J Comp Neurol* 1977; 175: 101-128.

Powell EW. Limbic projections to the thalamus. *Exp Brain Res* 1973; 17: 394-401.

Prayson RA, Yoder BJ. Clinicopathologic findings in mesial temporal sclerosis treated with gamma knife radiotherapy. *Ann Diagn Pathol* 2007; 11: 22-26.

Priori A. Brain polarization in humans: a reappraisal of an old tool for prolonged non-invasive modulation of brain excitability. *Clin Neurophysiol* 2003; 114, 589-595.

Psatta DM. Control of chronic experimental focal epilepsy by feedback caudatum stimulations. *Epilepsia* 1983; 24: 444-454.

Purpura DP, McMurtry JG. Intracellular activities and evoked potential changes during polarization of motor cortex. *J Neurophysiol* 1965: 166-185.

Quesney LF, Gloor P, Kratzenberg E, Zumstein H. Pathophysiology of generalized penicillin epilepsy in the cat: The role of cortical and subcortical structures. I. Systemic application of penicillin. *Electroencephalogr Clin Neurophysiol* 1977; 42: 640-655.

Rachkov BM, Bezukh SM. Effect of single-stage stereotaxic destruction of Forel's field H on neurologic functions and the structure of paroxysms in patients with generalized epilepsy] [article in Bulgarian]. *Zh Nevropatol Psikhiatr Im S S Korsakova* 1983; 83: 824-827.

Raftopoulos C, van Rijckevorsel K, Abu Serieh B, de Tourtchaninoff M, Ivanoiu A, Mary G, Grandin C, Duprez T. Epileptic discharges in a mammillary body of a patient with refractory epilepsy. *Neuromodulation* 2005; 8: 236-240.

Ralston RL, Langer H. Experimental epilepsy of brain-stem origin. *Electroencephalogr Clin Neurophysiol* 1965; 18: 325-333.

Ramamurthi B, Kalyanaraman S. Stereotaxic targets for epilepsy. In: Schaltenbrand G, Walker AE eds. *Stereotaxy of the Human Brain.* Stuttgart, New York: Georg Thieme Verlag 1982: 653-660.

Ramamurthi B, Kalyanaraman S, Sayeed ZA, Dharmapal N. Surgical Treatment of epilepsy. In: Harris P, Mawdsley C eds. *Epilepsy: Proceedings of the Hans Berger Centenary Symposium.* Edinburgh: Churchill Livingston 1974: 203-208.

Ramani SV, Yap JC, Gumnit RJ. Stereotactic fields of Forel interruption for intractable epilepsy. *Appl Neurophysiol* 1980; 43: 104-108.

Ravagnati L. Stereotactic surgery for epilepsy. In: Wieser HG, Elger CE eds. *Presurgical Evaluation of Epileptics.* Heidelberg: Springer 1987: 361-371.

Reynolds DV. Surgery in the rat during electrical analgesia induced by focal brain stimulation. *Science* 1969; 164: 444-445.

Ribstein M. Exploration du cerveau humain par electrodes profundes. *Electroencephalogr Clin Neurophysiol* 1960; Suppl.16: 1-129.

Richardson DE, Akil H. Pain reduction by electrical brain stimulation in man. Part 1: Acute administration in periaqueductal and periventricular sites. *J Neurosurg* 1977; 47: 178-183.

Richardson DE, Akil H. Pain reduction by electrical brain stimulation in man. Part 2: Chronic self-administration in the periventricular gray matter. *J Neurosurg* 1977; 47: 184-194.

Riechert T, Mundinger F. Beschreibung und Anwendung eines Zielgerätes für stereotaktische Hirnoperationen: II Modell. *Acta Neurochir* 1955; Suppl.3: 308-337.

Riechert T, Umbach W. Cortical and subcortical EEG patterns during stereotaxic operations in subcortical structures of the human brain. *Electroenceph Clin Neurophysiol* 1955; 7: 663-664.

Rieck RW, Huerta MF, Harting JK, Weber JT. Hypothalamic and ventral thalamic projections to the superior colliculus in the cat. *J Comp Neurol* 1986; 243: 249-265.

Risinger M, Gumnit R. Intracranial electrophysiologic studies. *Neuroimaging Clin N Am* 1995; 5: 559-573.

Rogers SW, Andrews PI, Gahring LC, Whisenand T, Cauley K, Crain B, Hughes TE, Heinemann SF, McNamara JO. Autoantibodies to glutamate receptor GluR3 in Rasmussen's encephalitis. *Science* 1994; 265: 648-651.

Romanelli P, Heit G, Hill B, Kraus A, Hastie T, Bronte-Stewart HM. Microelectrode recording revealing a somatotopic body map in the subthalamic nucleus in humans with Parkinson disease. *J Neurosurg* 2004; 100: 611-618.

Rush AJ, George MS, Sackeim HA, Marangell LB, Husain MM, Giller C, Nahas Z, Haines S, Simpson RK, Goodman R. Vagus nerve stimulation (VNS) for treatment-resistant depressions: a multicenter study. *Biol Psychiatry* 2000; 47: 276-286.

Russchen FT, Amaral DG, Price JL. The afferent input to the magnocellular division of the mediodorsal thalamic nucleus in the monkey, Macaca fascicularis. *J Comp Neurol* 1987; 256: 175-210.

Sano K. Indications for and results of making central lesions in the brain for epileptic patients. In: Harris P, Mawdsley C eds. *Epilepsy.* London: Churchill 1974: 215-221.

Sano K, Yoshioka M, Mayanagi Y, Sekino H, Yoshimasu N: Stimulation and destruction of and around the interstitial nucleus of Cajal in man. *Confin Neurol* 1970a; 32: 118-125.

Sano K, Yoshioka M, Sekino H, Mayanagi Y, Yoshimasu N. Functional organization of the internal medullary lamina in man. *Confin Neurol* 1970b; 32: 374-380.

Saper CB. Organization of cerebral cortical afferent systems in the rat. II. Hypothalamocortical projections. *J Comp Neurol* 1985; 237: 21-46.

Sasaki K, Staunton HP, Dieckmann G. Characteristic features of augmenting and recruiting responses in the cerebral cortex. *Exp Neurol* 1970; 26: 369-392.

Schaltenbrand G, Wahren W. *Atlas for Stereotaxy of the Human Brain (Architectonic Organization of the Thalamic Nuclei by Rolf Hassler)* - 2nd, revised and enlarged Edition. Stuttgart: Georg Thieme Publishers 1977 (including Guide to this atlas).

Schaltenbrand G, Wahren W. Electroanatomical observations. In: Schaltenbrand G, Walker AE eds. *Stereotaxy of the Human Brain.* Stuttgart, New York: Georg Thieme Verlag 1982: 390-409.

Schaltenbrand G, Walker AE eds. *Stereotaxy of the Human Brain.* Stuttgart, New York: Georg Thieme Verlag 1982.

Schaltenbrand G, Spuler H, Nadjmi M, Hopf HC, Wahren W. The stereotaxic treatment of epilepsy. *Confin Neurol* 1966; 27: 111-113.

Schlag J, Villablanca J. Cortical incremental responses to thalamic stimulation. *Brain Res* 1967; 6: 119-142.

Schulman E, Auer J. Caudate efferents to the thalamus. *Anat Rec* 1957; 127: 363.

Schwab RS, Sweet WH, Mark VH, Kjellberg RN, Ervin FR. Treatment of intractable temporal lobe epilepsy by stereotactic amygdala lesions. *Trans Am Neurol Assoc* 1965; 90: 12-19.

Scoville WB, Milner B. Loss of recent memory after bilateral hippocampal lesions. *J Neurol Neurosurg Psychiatry* 1957; 20: 11-21.

Shetty AK, Turner DA. Fetal hippocampal grafts containing CA3 cells restore host hippocampal glutamate decarboxylase-positive interneuron numbers in a rat model of temporal lobe epilepsy. *J Neurosci* 2000; 20: 8788-8801.

Shuchman M. Approving the vagus-nerve stimulator for depression. *N Engl J Med* 2007; 356: 1604-1607.

Siegfried J, Wieser HG. Effets de la stimulation de la substance grise periaqueductale chez l'homme sur l'activité spontanée et évoquée. *Neurochir* 1978; 24: 407-414.

Siegfried J, Wieser HG. The actual role of stereotactic operations on deep brain structures in the treatment of medically refractory epilepsies. In: Broggi G ed. *The Rational Basis of the Surgical Treatment of Epilepsies.* London: Libbey 1988: 113-119.

Sikes RW, Chronister RB, White LE, Jr. Origin of the direct hippocampus--anterior thalamic bundle in the rat: a combined horseradish peroxidase--Golgi analysis. *Exp Neurol* 1977; 57: 379-395.

Sillanpaa M, Jalava M, Kaleva O, Shinnar S. Long-term prognosis of seizures with onset in childhood. *N Engl J Med* 1998; 338: 1715-1722.

Simma K. Zur Projektion des Centrum medianum und Nucleus parafascicularis thalami beim Menschen. *Monatsschr Psychiatr Neurol* 1951; 122: 32-46.

Simonyan K, Jürgens U. Afferent subcortical connections into the motor cortical larynx area in the rhesus monkey. *Neuroscience* 2005; 130: 119-131.

Sonnen AE, Manen JV, van Dijk B. Results of amygdalotomy and fornicotomy in temporal lobe epilepsy and behaviour disorders. *Acta Neurochir* (Wien) 1976; 23 (Suppl.): 215-220.

Sorbera F, Crescimanno G, Amato G, La Grutta V. Effetti della stimulazione condizionante della substantia nigra sullättivita epileptica amigdaloidae nel gatto. *Bull Soc Ital Biol Sper* 1981; 57: 1901-1904.

Speckmann EJ. Experimentelle Epilepsieforschung - Grundlagen, Modelle, Ergebnisse nach: E.J. Speckmann, Experimentelle Epilepsieforschung, Wissenschaftliche Buchgesellschaft, Darmstadt 1986; Konzept und Realisation: AMV AV-Kommunikation und Medizin-Verlag, München Produktion: Bayerl & Partner Film, München Desitin Videothek, Hamburg 1989.

Speckmann EJ, Caspers H eds. *Origin of Cerebral Field Potentials*. Stuttgart: Thieme 1979.

Spencer DD, Spencer SS. Surgery for epilepsy. *Neurol Clin* 1985; 3: 313-330.

Spiegel EA, Wycis HT. Thalamic recordings in man with special reference to seizure discharges. *Electroenceph Clin Neurophysiol* 1950; 2: 23-29.

Spiegel EA, Wycis HT. Diencephalic mechanisms in petit-mal epilepsy. *Electroenceph Clin Neurophysiol* 1951; 3: 473-475.

Spiegel EA, Wycis HT. *Stereoencephalotomy*. Part I. New York: Grune and Stratton 1952.

Spiegel EA, Wycis HT. Chronic implantation of intracerebral electrodes in humans. In: Sheer DE ed., *Electrical Stimulation of the Brain*. Austin: University of Texas Press 1961: 37-44.

Spiegel EA, Wycis HT. *Stereoencephalotomy*. Part II. Clinical and physiological applications. New York: Grune and Stratton 1962: 453-480.

Spiegel EA, Wycis HT, Marks M, Lee AJ. Stereotaxic apparatus for operations on the human brain. *Science* 1947; 196: 349-350.

Spiegel EA, Wycis HT, Szekely EG, Adams I, Flanagan M, Baird HN. Campotomy in various extrapyramidal disorders. *J Neurosurg* 1963; 20: 871-884.

Squire LR, Moore RY. Dorsal thalamic lesion in a noted case of human memory dysfunction. *Ann Neurol* 1979; 6: 503-506.

Sramka M, Fritz G, Galanda M, Nadvornik P. Some observations in treatment stimulation of epilepsy. *Acta Neurochir* (Wien) 1976; 23 (Suppl.): 257-262.

Sramka M, Fritz G, Gajdosova D, Nadvornik P. Central stimulation treatment of epilepsy. *Acta Neurochir Suppl* (Wien) 1980; 30: 183-187.

Steinhoff BJ, Racker S, Herrendorf G, Poser S, Grosche S, Zerr I, Kretzschmar H, Weber T. Accuracy and reliability of periodic sharp wave complexes (PSWC) in Creutzfeldt-Jakob disease. *Arch Neurol* 1996; 53: 162-166.

Steinhoff BJ, Zerr I, Glatting M, Schulz-Schaeffer W, Poser S, Kretzschmar HA. Diagnostic value of periodic complexes in Creutzfeldt-Jakob disease. *Ann Neurol* 2004; 56: 702-708.

Steriade M. *The Thalamus*. Amsterdam: Elsevier Science Publishing 1997.

Stodieck SRG, Wieser HG. Autonomic phenomena in temporal lobe epilepsy. *J Autonom Nerv Syst* 1986; Suppl.: 611-621.

Stodieck SRG, Wieser HG. Epicortical DC changes in epileptic patients. In: Wolf P, Dam M, Janz D, Dreifuss FE eds. *Advances in Epileptology*. New York: Raven Press 1987; 16: 123-127.

Stodieck SRG, Wieser HG. The effects of polarization on human epileptic foci. In: Thoma H ed. *Proc. 1st Vienna International Workshop on Functional Electrostimulation*. Vienna 1983 (Abstract in *Artif Organs* 1984; 8/3: 392).

Sugita K, Doi T, Mutsaga N, Takaoka Y. Clinical study of fornicotomy for psychomotor epilepsy and behavior disorder. In: Umbach W ed. *Special Topics in Stereotaxis*. Stuttgart: Hippokrates 1971: 42-52.

Sugita K, Kobayashi S. General considerations of pain. In: Schaltenbrand G, Walker AE eds. *Stereotaxy of the Human Brain*. Stuttgart, New York: Thieme 1982: 462-468.

Sussman NM, Goldman HW, Jackel RA, Kaplan L, Callanan M, Bergen J, Harner RN. Anterior thalamic stimulation in medically intractable epilepsy. Part II. Preliminary clinical results. *Epilepsia* 1988; 29: 677.

Takebayashi H, Komai N, Imamura H. Depth EEG, analysis of the epilepsies. *Confin Neurol* 1966; 27: 144-148.

Talairach J, De Ajuriaguerra J, David M. Études stéréotaxiques et structures encéphaliques profondes chez l'homme. *Presse Méd* 1952; 28: 605-609.

Talairach J, David M, Tournoux P, Corredor H, Kvasina T. *Atlas d'Anatomie Stéréotaxique des Noyaux Gris Centraux*. Paris: Masson 1957.

Talairach J, David M, Tournoux P. *L'Exploration Chirurgicale Stéréotaxique du Lobe Temporal dans l'Épilepsie Temporale: repérage anatomique stéréotaxique et technique chirurgicale*. Paris: Masson 1958.

Talairach J, Szikla G, Tournoux P, Prossalentis A, Bordas-Ferrer M, Covello L, Jacob M, Mempel E, Buser P, Bancaud J. *Atlas d'Anatomie Stéréotaxique du Télencéphale.* Paris: Masson 1967.

Talairach J, Bancaud J, Szikla G, Bonis A, Geier S, Vedrenne C. New approach to the neurosurgery of epilepsy. Stereotaxic methodology and therapeutic results. 1. Introduction and history. *Neurochirurgie* 1974; 20: 1-240.

Talairach J, Tournoux P. *Co-Planar Stereotactic Atlas of the Human Brain.* Stuttgart: Thieme, 1988.

Tasker RR, Emmers R. Patterns of somesthetic projection in SI and SII of the human thalamus. *Confin Neurol* 1967; 29: 160-162.

Tasker RR, Emmers R. Double somatotopic representation in the human thalamus, its application in localisation during thalamotomy for Parkinson's disease. *Third Symposium on Parkinson's Disease.* Livingstone, Edinburgh, London 1969: 100.

Tellez-Zenteno JF, McLachlan RS, Parrent A, Kubu CS, Wiebe S. Hippocampal electrical stimulation in mesial temporal lobe epilepsy. *Neurology* 2006; 66: 1490-1494.

Temkin O. *The Falling Sickness. A History of Epilepsy from the Greeks to the Beginnings of Modern Neurology.* 2nd edition. Baltimore: Johns Hopkins Press 1971: 467

Terzuolo CA, Bullock TH. The measurement of imposed voltage gradient adequate to modulate neuronal firing. *Proc Natl Acad Sci USA* 1956; 42: 687-693.

The Vagus Nerve Stimulation Study Group. A randomized controlled trial of chronic vagus nerve stimulation for treatment of medically intractable seizures. *Neurology* 1995; 45: 224-230.

Theodore WH, Chen R, Vega-Bermudez F, Boroojerdi B, Werhahn K, Cohen L. Transcranial magnetic stimulation for the treatment of seizures: a controlled study. *Neurology* 2002; 52: 560-562.

Theodore WH, Fisher RS. Brain stimulation for epilepsy. *Lancet Neurol* 2004; 3: 111-118.

Tönnes J, Hajek M, Mirkovic N, Stierli B, Behrmann JT, Wieser HG, Streit P. Acute Rasmussen's encephalitis: are there patients without autoantibodies to glutamate receptor GluR3? *Society for Neuroscience.* Los Angeles 1998.

Traub RD, Pedley TA. Virus-induced electrotonic coupling: hypothesis on the mechanism of periodic EEG discharges in Creutzfeldt-Jakob disease. *Ann Neurol* 1981; 10: 405-410.

Tronnier VM, Krause M, Heck A, Kronenbürger M, Bonsanto MM, Fogel W. Deep brain stimulation for the treatment of movement disorders. *Neurol Psychiat Brain Res* 1999; 6: 199-212.

Turner BH. The convolutions of the brain. A study in comparative anatomy. *J Anat Physiol* 1981a; 25: 105-153.

Turner BH. The cortical sequence and terminal distribution of sensory related afferents to the amygdaloid complex of the rat and monkey. In: Ben Ari Y ed. *The Amygdaloid Complex.* INSERM Symposium no. 20. Amsterdam: Elsevier North Holland Biomedical Press 1981b: 51-62.

Twyman RE, Gahring LC, Spiess J, Rogers SW. Glutamate receptor antibodies activate a subset of receptors and reveal an agonist binding site. *Neuron* 1995; 14: 755-762.

Uemura H: Pathologisch anatomische Untersuchung über die Verbindungsbahnen zwischen dem Kleinhirn und dem Hirnstamm. *Schweiz Arch Neurol* 1917; 1: 131-226.

Umbach W. Vegetative Reaktionen bei elektrischen Reizungen und Ausschaltungen in subcorticalen Hirnstrukturen des Menschen. *Acta Neuroveg* (Wien) 1961: 23: 225-245.

Umbach W. Long-term results of fornicotomy for temporal epilepsy. *Confin Neurol* 1966; 27: 121-123.

Umbach W, Riechert T. Elektrophysiologische und klinische Ergebnisse stereotaktischer Eingriffe im limbischen System bei temporaler Epilepsie. *Nervenarzt* 1964; 35: 482-488.

Ungerleider LG, Christensen CA. Pulvinar lesions in monkeys produce abnormal eye movements during visual discrimination training. *Brain Res* 1977; 136: 189-196.

Upton AR, Cooper IS, Springman M, Amin I. Suppression of seizures and psychosis of limbic system origin by chronic stimulation of anterior nucleus of the thalamus. *Int J Neurol* 1985-86; 19-20: 223-230.

Upton AR, Amin I, Garnett S, Springman M, Nahmias C, Cooper IS. Evoked metabolic responses in the limbic-striate system produced by stimulation of anterior thalamic nucleus in man. *Pacing Clin Electrophysiol* 1987; 10: 217-225.

Uthman BM, Reichl AM, Dean JC, Eisenschenk S, Gilmore R, Reid S, Roper SN, Wilder BJ. Effectiveness of vagus nerve stimulation in epilepsy patients: a 12-year observation. *Neurology* 2004; 63: 1124-1126.

Vaernet K. Stereotaxic amygdalotomy in temporal lobe epilepsy. *Confin Neurol* 1972; 34: 176-180.

Valenstein ES, Nauta WJ. A comparison of the distribution of the fornix system in the rat, guinea pig, cat, and monkey. *J Comp Neurol* 1959; 113: 337-363.

Van Buren JM, Borke RC. *Variations and connections of the human thalamus.* Vol. 1, The nuclei and cerebral connections of the human thalamus Vol. 2, *Variations of the Human Diencephalon.* Heidelberg: Springer 1972.

Van Buren JM, Wood JH, Oakley J, Hambrecht F. Preliminary evaluation of cerebellar stimulation by double-blind stimulation and biological criteria in the treatment of epilepsy. *J Neurosurg* 1978; 48: 407-416.

Van der Kooy D. The reticular core of the brain-stem and its descending pathways: anatomy and function. In: Fromm GH, Faingold CL, Browning RA, Burnham WM eds. *Epilepsy and the Reticular Formation. Neurology and Neurobiology* (Liss AR) 1987; 27: 9-23.

Van Groen T, Wyss JM. Extrinsic projections from area CA1 of the rat hippocampus: olfactory, cortical, subcortical, and bilateral hippocampal formation projections. *J Comp Neurol* 1990a; 302: 515-528.

Van Groen T, Wyss JM. The connections of presubiculum and parasubiculum in the rat. *Brain Res* 1990b; 518: 227-243.

Van Rijckevorsel K, Abu Serieh B, de Tourtchaninoff M, Raftopoulos C. Deep EEG recordings of the mammillary body in epilepsy patients. *Epilepsia* 2005; 46: 781-785.

Vanhatalo S, Holmes MD, Tallgren P, Voipio J, Kaila K, Miller JW. Very slow EEG responses lateralize temporal lobe seizures: an evaluation of non-invasive DC-EEG technique. *Neurology* 2003; 60: 1098-1104.

Vann SD, Aggleton JP. The mammillary bodies: two memory systems in one? *Nat Rev Neurosci* 2004; 5: 35-44.

Velasco AL, Velasco M, Velasco F, Menes D, Gordon F, Rocha L, Briones M, Marquez I. Subacute and chronic electrical stimulation of the hippocampus on intractable temporal lobe seizures: preliminary report. *Arch Med Res* 2000b; 31: 316-28.

Velasco F, Velasco M, Estrada-Villanueva F, Machado JP. Specific and non-specific multiple unit activities during the onset of pentylenetetrazol seizures. I. Intact animals. *Epilepsia* 1975; 16: 207-214.

Velasco F, Velasco M, Maldonaldo H, Estrada-Villanueva F. Specific and non-specific multiple unit activities during the onset of pentylenetetrazol seizures. II. Acute lesions interrupting nonspecific system connections. *Epilepsia* 1976; 17: 461-475.

Velasco F, Velasco M, Romo R. Specific and non-specific multiple unit activities during pentylenetetrazol seizures in animals with mesencephalic transsections. *Electroencephalogr* Clin Neurophysiol 1982; 53: 289-297.

Velasco F, Velasco M, Ogarrio C, Fanghanel G. Electrical stimulation of the centromedian thalamic nucleus in the treatment of convulsive seizures: a preliminary report. *Epilepsia* 1987; 28: 421-430.

Velasco F, Velasco M, Velasco AL, Jimenez F. Effect of chronic electrical stimulation of the centromedian thalamic nuclei on various intractable seizure patterns: I. Clinical seizures and paroxysmal EEG activity. *Epilepsia* 1993; 34: 1052-1064.

Velasco F, Velasco M, Jimenez F, Velasco AL, Brito F, Rise M, Carrillo-Ruiz JD. Predictors in the treatment of difficult-to-control seizures by electrical stimulation of the centromedian thalamic nucleus. *Neurosurgery* 2000a; 47: 295-304 (discussion 304-305).

Velasco F, Carrillo-Ruiz JD, Brito F, Velasco M, Velasco AL, Marquez I, Davis R. Double-blind, randomized controlled pilot study of bilateral cerebellar stimulation for treatment of intractable motor seizures. *Epilepsia* 2005; 46: 1071-1081.

Velasco M, Velasco F, Velasco AL, Boleaga B, Jimenez F, Brito F, Marquez I. Subacute electrical stimulation of the hippocampus blocks intractable temporal lobe seizures and paroxysmal EEG activities. *Epilepsia* 2000c; 41: 158-169.

Velasco M, Velasco F, Velasco AL. Centromedian-thalamic and hippocampal electrical stimulation for the control of intractable epileptic seizures. *J Clin Neurophysiol* 2001; 18: 495-513.

Velíček L, Velískova J, Stanton PK. Low-frequency stimulation of the kindling focus delays basolateral amygdala kindling in immature rats. *Neurosci Lett* 2002; 326: 61-63.

Vercueil L, Benazzouz A, Deransart C, Bressand K, Marescaux C, Depaulis A, Benabid AL. High frequency stimulation of the subthalamic nucleus suppresses absence seizures in the rat: comparison with neurotoxic lesions. *Epilepsy Res* 1998; 31: 39-46.

Victor M. The irrelevance of mammillary body lesions in the causation of the Korsakoff amnesic state. *Int J Neurol* 1987-88; 21-22: 51-57.

Vogt C, Vogt O. Thalamus-Studien I-III. *Psychol* 1941; 50: 33-154.

Vogt C. La myéloarchitecture du thalamus du cerebropithèque. *Psychol Neurol* 1909; 12: 285-324.

Vonck K, Boon P, Achten E, De Reuck J, Caemaert J. Long-term amygdalohippocampal stimulation for refractory temporal lobe epilepsy. *Ann Neurol* 2002; 52: 556-565.

Wada JA, Cornelius LR. Functional alteration of deep structures in cats with chronic focal cortical irritative lesions. *Arch Neurol* 1960; 3: 425-447.

Wagner R 2nd, Feeney DM, Gullotta FP, Cote IL. Suppression of cortical epileptiform activity by generalized and localized ECoG desynchronization. *Electroencephalogr Clin Neurophysiol* 1975; 39: 499-506.

Walker AE. The projection of the medial geniculate body to the cerebral cortex in the macaque monkey. *J Anat* 1937; 71: 319-331.

Walker AE. *The Primate Thalamus.* Chicago: University Chicago Press 1938a.

Walker AE. The thalamus of the chimpanzee II. Its nuclear structure, normal and following hemidecortication. *J Comp Neurol* 1938b; 69: 487-507.

Walker AE. Normal and pathophysiological physiology of the thalamus: In: Schaltenbrand G, Walker AE eds. *Stereotaxy of the Human Brain.* Stuttgart, New York: Georg Thieme Verlag 1982: 181-217.

Walker AE, Poggio GF, Andy OJ. Structural spread of cortically-induced epileptic discharges. *Neurology* 1956; 616-626.

Wallenberg A. Sekundäre, sensible Bahnen im Gehirnstamm des Kaninchens, ihre gegenseitige Lage und ihre Bedeutung für den Aufbau des Thalamus. *Anat Anz* 1900: 18: 81.

Waltz JM, Riklan M, Stellar S, Cooper IS. Cryothalamotomy for Parkinson's disease. A statistical analysis. *Neurology* 1966; 16: 994-1102.

Warwick R, Williams PL eds. *Gray's Anatomy,* 35th ed. Edinburgh: Longman Group Ltd 1973: 902.

Wasserman EM, Jordan Grafman J. Recharging cognition with DC brain polarization. *Trends Cogn Sci* 2005; 9: 503-505.

Weiss SR, Eidsath A, Li XL, Heynen T, Post RM. Quenching revisited: low level direct current inhibits amygdala-kindled seizures. *Exp Neurol* 1998; 154: 185-192.

Wennberg R. Short term benefit of battery depletion in vagus nerve stimulation for epilepsy. *J Neurol Neurosurg Psychiatry* 2004; 75: 939.

Wichmann T, Bergman H, DeLong MR. The primate subthalamic nucleus. 1. Functional properties in intact animals. *J Neurophysiol* 1994a; 72: 494-506.

Wieser HG. *Electroclinical Features of the Psychomotor Seizure. A Stereo-electroencephalographic Study of Ictal Symptoms and Chrono-topographical Seizure Patterns Including Clinical Effects of Intracerebral Stimulation.* Stuttgart, London: G. Fischer-Butterworths 1983a: 242.

Wieser HG. Stereoelectroencephalographic correlates of focal motor seizures. In: Speckmann EJ, Elger CE eds. *Epilepsy and Motor System.* Baltimore: Urban-Schwarzenberg 1983b: 287-309.

Wieser HG. Selective amygdalohippocampectomy: Indications, investigative technique and results. In: Symon L, Brihaye J, Guidetti B, Loew F, Niller JD, Nornes H, Pasztor E, Pertuiset B, Yasargil MG eds. *Advances and Technical Standards in Neurosurgery* 1986a; 13: 39-133.

Wieser HG. Psychomotor seizures of hippocampal-amygdalar origin. In: Pedley TA, Meldrum BS eds. *Recent Advances in Epilepsy*, Number 3. Edinburg, London: Churchill Livingstone 1986b: 57-79.

Wieser HG. Stereo-electroencephalography. In: Wieser HG, Elger CE eds. *Presurgical Evaluation of Epileptics.* Heidelberg: Springer 1987a: 192-204.

Wieser HG. Stereo-EEG, intraoperative monitoring and anaesthesia. In: Halliday M, Butler SR, Paul R eds. *A Textbook of Clinical Neurophysiology.* London: John Wiley & Sons Ltd. 1987b: 269-304.

Wieser HG. The phenomenology of limbic seizures. In: Wieser HG, Speckmann EJ, Engel J Jr eds. *The Epileptic Focus. Current Problems in Epilepsy* 3. London, Paris: John Libbey 1987c: 113-136.

Wieser HG. Temporal lobe epilepsy, sleep and arousal: Stereo-EEG findings. In: Degen R, Rodin EA eds. *Epilepsy, Sleep and Sleep Deprivation.* Amsterdam: Elsevier 1991: 137-167.

Wieser HG: Rasmussen's encephalitis: New treatment strategies. *The Third YONSEI Epilepsy Symposium, Seoul*, June 6, 1996 (Abstr. Book, p.145).

Wieser HG. Electrophysiological aspects of forced normalization. In: Trimble MR and Schmitz B eds. *Forced Normalization and Alternative Psychoses of Epilepsy.* Petersfield UK: Wrightson Biomedical Publ 1998: 95-119.

Wieser HG. Temporal lobe epilepsies. In: Meinardi H ed. *Handbook of Clinical Neurology.* Vol. 73 (29): *The Epilepsies*, Part II. Amsterdam: Elsevier Science BV 2000: 53-96.

Wieser HG. Stereoelectroencephalography and Foramen ovale electrode recording. In: Niedermeyer E, Lopes da Silva F eds. *Electroencephalography: Basic Principles, Clinical Applications, and Related Fields.* Fourth Edition. Baltimore: Williams & Wilkins 1999: 725-740.

Wieser HG, Creutzfeldt O. Physiology of the frontal cortex. In: Wieser HG, Elger CE eds. *Presurgical Evaluation of Epileptics.* Berlin, Heidelberg: Springer-Verlag 1987: 23-27.

Wieser HG, Elger CE eds. *Presurgical Evaluation of Epileptics.* Heidelberg: Springer 1987.

Wieser HG, Kausel W. Limbic seizures. In: Wieser HG, Elger CE eds. *Presurgical Evaluation of Epileptics.* Heidelberg: Springer 1987: 227-248.

Wieser HG, Schindler K. Foramen ovale and epidural electrodes in the definition of the seizure onset zone. In: Lüders HO, Najm I. Bingaman W eds. *Textbook of Epilepsy Surgery.* Abingdon UK: Taylor & Francis Group (in press).

Wieser HG, Siegel AM. Relations between the EEG of the cortex, thalamus and periaqueductal gray in patients suffering from epilepsy and pain syndromes. In: Zschocke S, Speckmann E-J eds. *Basic Mechanisms of the EEG.* Boston: Birkhäuser 1993: 145-182.

Wieser HG, Siegfried J. Hirnstamm-Ableitungen (Makroelektroden) beim Menschen. l. Elektrische Befunde im Wachzustand und Ganznachtschlaf. *Z EEG-EMG* 1979a; 10: 8-19.

Wieser HG, Siegfried J. Hirnstamm-Ableitungen (Makroelektroden) beim Menschen. 2. Klinische und elektrische Effekte bei Stimulation im periaquäduktalen Grau (PGM); Augenbewegungsabhängige Aktivität; visuelle und somatosensorische Reizantworten im PGM. *Z EEG-EMG* 1979b; 10: 62-69.

Wieser HG, Graf HP, Bernoulli C, Siegfried J. Quantitative analysis of intracerebral recordings in epilepsia partialis continua. *Electroenceph Clin Neurophysiol* 1978; 44: 14-22.

Wieser HG, Elger CE, Stodieck SRG. The 'Foramen Ovale Electrode': A new recording method for the preoperative evaluation of patients suffering from mesio-basal temporal lobe epilepsy. *Electroenceph Clin Neurophysiol* 1985a; 61: 314-322.

Wieser HG, Hailemariam S, Regard M, Landis T. Unilateral limbic epileptic status activity: Stereo-EEG, behavioural, and cognitive data. *Epilepsia* 1985b; 26: 19-29.

Wieser HG, Valavanis A, Roos A, Isler P, Renella RR. "Selective" and "superselective" temporal lobe memory tests. I. Neuroradiological, neuroanatomical and electrical data. In: *Advances in Epileptology.* New York: Raven Press 1989a; 17: 20-27.

Wieser HG, Do KQ, Perschak H, Cuénod M. Modulation of extracellular aspartate level during epileptiform events in primary epileptogenic area of patients (Abstract). *Satellite Symp on Physiology, Pharmacology and Development of Epileptogenic Phenomena.* Frankfurt July 4-8, 1989b.

Wieser HG, Swartz BE, Delgado-Escueta AV, Bancaud J, Walsh GO, Maldonado H, Saint-Hilaire JM. Differentiating frontal lobe seizures from temporal lobe seizures. *Adv Neurol* 1992; 57: 267-285.

Wieser HG, Bjeljac M, Khan N, Müller S, Siegel AM, Yonekawa Y. Interplay of interictal discharges and seizures: some clinical and EEG findings. In: Wolf P ed. *Epileptic Seizures and Syndromes*. London: John Libbey 1994: 563-578.

Wieser HG, Müller S, Schiess R, Khan N, Regard M, Landis T, Bjeljac M, Buck A, Valavanis A, Yasargil G, Yonekawa Y. The anterior and posterior selective temporal lobe amobarbital tests: angiographical, clinical, electroencephalographical PET and SPECT findings, and memory performance. *Brain and Cognition* 1997; 33: 71-97.

Wieser HG, Henke K, Zumsteg D, Taub E, Yonekawa Y, Buck A. Activation of the left motor cortex during left leg movements after right central resection. *J Neurol Neurosurg Psychiatry* 1999; 67: 487-491.

Wieser HG, Ortega M, Friedman A, Yonekawa Y. Long-term seizure outcomes following amygdalohippocampectomy. *J Neurosurg* 2003; 98: 751-763.

Wieser HG, Schwarz U, Blättler T, Bernoulli C, Sitzler M, Stoeck K, Glatzel M. Serial EEG findings in sporadic and iatrogenic Creutzfeldt-Jakob disease. *Clin Neurophysiol* 2004; 115: 2467-2478.

Wieser HG, Schindler K, Zumsteg D. EEG in Creutzfeld-Jakob disease. *Clin Neurophysiol* 2006; 117: 935-951.

Wieser HG, Jones-Gotman M, Smith ML, Zumsteg D, Mueller S, Buck A, Regard M, Yonekawa Y, Valavanis A. Selective temporal lobe amobarbital memory test. *Epileptologia* 2007; 15: 85-106.

Wilder BJ, Schmidt RP. Propagation of epileptic discharge from chronic neocortical foci in monkey. *Epilepsia* 1965: 6: 297-309.

Williams D. The thalamus and epilepsy. *Brain* 1968; 88: 539-556.

Williams D, Parsons Smith G. The spontaneous electrical activity of the human thalamus. *Brain* 1949; 72: 450-482.

Wilson WP, Nashold BS. Epileptic discharges occurring in the mesencephalon and thalamus. *Epilepsia* 1968; 9: 265-273.

Windels F, Bruet N, Poupard A, Urbain N, Chouvet G, Feuerstein C, Savasta M. Effects of high frequency stimulation of subthalamic nucleus on extracellular glutamate and GABA in substantia nigra and globus pallidus in the normal rat. *Eur J Neurosci* 2000; 12: 4141-4146.

Winkelmann A. Wilhelm von Waldeyer-Hartz (1836-1921): an anatomist who left his mark. *Clin Anat* 2007; 20: 231-234.

Witter MP, Groenewegen HJ. The subiculum: cytoarchitectonically a simple structure, but hodologically complex. *Prog Brain* Res 1990; 83: 47-58.

Witter MP, Ostendorf RH, Groenewegen HJ. Heterogeneity in the dorsal subiculum of the rat. Distinct neuronal zones project to different cortical and subcortical targets. *Eur J Neurosci* 1990; 2: 718-725.

World Health Organisation. Consensus on criteria for diagnosis of sporadic CJD. *Wkly Epidemiol Rec* 1998; 73: 361-365.

Wright GD, McLellan DL, Brice JG. A double-blind trial of chronic cerebellar stimulation in twelve patients with severe epilepsy. *J Neurol Neurosurg Psychiatry* 1984; 47: 769-774.

Wycis HT. Discussion. In: Adams J, Rutkin B eds. Treatment of temporal lobe epilepsy by stereotaxic surgery. *Confin Neurol* 1969; 31: 80-85.

Yakovlev PI, Locke S, Angevine JB. The limbus of the cerebral hemisphere, limbic nuclei of the thalamus and the cingulus bundle. In: Purpura DP, Yahr MD eds. *The Thalamus.* New York, London: Columbia University Press 1966: 77-97.

Yakovlev PI, Locke S, Koskoff DY, Patton RA. Limbic nuclei of the thalamus and connections of limbic cortex. I. Organization of the projections of the anterior group of nuclei and of the midline nuclei of the thalamus to the anterior cingulate gyrus and hippocampal rudiment in the monkey. *Arch Neurol* 1960; 3: 620-641.

Yakovlev PI. Motility, behavior and the brain. Stereodynamic organization and neural coordinates of behavior. *J Nerv Ment Dis* 1948; 107: 313-335.

Yamamoto J, Ikeda A, Satow T, Takeshita K, Takayama M, Matsuhashi M, Matsumoto R, Ohara S, Mikuni N, Takahashi J, Miyamoto S, Taki W, Hashimoto N, Rothwell JC, Shibasaki H. Low-frequency electric cortical stimulation has an inhibitory effect on epileptic focus in mesial temporal lobe epilepsy. *Epilepsia* 2002; 43: 491-495.

Yeterian EH, Pandya DN. Corticothalamic connections of paralimbic regions in the rhesus monkey. *J Comp Neurol* 1988; 269: 130-146.

Yoneoka Y, Takeda N, Inoue A, Ibuchi Y, Kumagai T, Sugai T, Takeda K, Ueda K. Acute Korsakoff syndrome following mammillothalamic tract infarction. *R Am J Neuroradiol* 2004; 25: 964-968.

Yoshii N. Follow-up study of epileptic patients following Forel-H-tomy. *Appl Neurophysiol* 1977-1978; 40: 1-12.

Yoshii N, Adachi K, Kudo T, Schmizu S, Nishioka S, Nakahama H. Further studies on the stereotaxis for pain relief. *Tohuku J Exp Med* 1970; 102: 225-232.

Yuen TG, Agnew WF, Bullara LA, Jacques S, McCreery DB. Histological evaluation of neural damage from electrical stimulation: considerations for the selection of parameters for clinical application. *Neurosurgery* 1981; 9: 292-299.

Zumsteg D, Jenny D, Wieser HG. Vocal cord adduction during vagus nerve stimulation for treatment of epilepsy. *Neurology* 2000; 54: 1388-1389.

Zumsteg D, Friedman A, Wennberg RA, Wieser HG. Source localization of mesial temporal interictal epileptiform discharges: Correlation with intracranial foramen ovale electrode recordings. *Clin Neurophysiol* 2005; 116: 2810-2818.

Zumsteg D, Lozano AM, Wieser HG, Wennberg RA. Cortical activation with deep brain stimulation of the anterior thalamus for epilepsy. *Clin Neurophysiol* 2006a: 117: 192-207.

Zumsteg D, Lozano AM, Wennberg RA. Depth electrode recorded cerebral responses with deep brain stimulation of the anterior thalamus for epilepsy. *Clin Neurophysiol* 2006b; 117: 1602-1609.

Zumsteg D, Lozano AM, Wennberg RA. Rhythmic cortical EEG synchronization with low frequency stimulation of the anterior and medial thalamus for epilepsy. *Clin Neurophysiol* 2006c; 117: 2272-2278.

Zumsteg D, Lozano AM, Wennberg RA. Mesial temporal inhibition in a patient with deep brain stimulation of the anterior thalamus for epilepsy. *Epilepsia* 2006d; 47: 1958-1962.

Index

[^{14}C]-2-deoxyglucose autoradiography 141

10-20 electrode system, international 7

3rd ventricle 137, 141

6-hydroxydopamine 135

A

Abducens, nucleus 34

Absence seizure 3, 88, 92-93, 100-103, 111-112, 127, 138-139, 141, 144

Absence status epilepticus 92-93, 100

AC, alternating current 17, 153

Accelerometer 90, 129

Acetazolamide 81

Acetylcholine 135

Acoustic stimulation 129, 132

Activation, see Arousal

AD, afterdischarge 9, 11, 16, 23-25, 69-71, 79, 135, 147, 153

Adenosine 135

AED, antiepileptic drug 134, 143-144

Afferent fibers 30, 32-35, 45-56, 142

Afterdischarges (AD) 9, 11, 16, 23-25, 69-71, 79, 135, 147, 153

Ag/AgCl electrodes 7, 14

Aggression 30, 39, 50, 56, 140

AHE, amygdalohippocampectomy 20, 23, 60, 66, 71, 76, 79, 85, 121

Akinesia 52, 137

Akinetic seizure 138

ALA, alanine 25-26

Alanine (ALA) 25-26

Alcohol 40, appendix

Alexander table 5

Allocortex 45

Alpha rhythm 54, 128, 131-132

Altered thinking, ictal 84-85

Alternating current (AC) 17, 153

Aluminium-hydroxy, seizure model 145

Ambient cistern 122

Amnesia, ictal 11, 66

Amnesia, side effect 141

Amnestic syndrome (Korsakoff syndrome) 40

Amplitude quotient (Q) 97-98

Amygdala 4, 11, 13, 17-20, 23-25, 27, 34, 38, 47-49, 54, 61-69, 71, 74, 77, 78, 79, 81, 85-86, 116, 118-122, 124, 135, 136-137, 140, 146-149, 154

Amygdalohippocampectomy (AHE) 20, 23, 60, 66, 71, 76, 79, 85, 121

Amygdalotomy, stereotactic 136, 140, 148-149

AN, anterior nucleus of the thalamus 2, 44-47, 136, 141-143, 152

Analgesia 56

Ancestral projection route 45

Anesthesia dolorosa 127, 129

Angiography 4-5, 105

Anisocoria, ictal 65

Anodic stimulation 14-18, 153

Anomic errors, ictal 53

Anoxic injury 40

Ansa lenticularis, ansa lentiformis 30-31

Anterior commissure 4, 32, 42, 45, 53, 140

Anterior main nucleus, of the anterior thalamic region 44

Anterior nucleus of the thalamus (AN) 2, 44-47, 136, 141-143, 152

Anterior thalamic head direction signal 40

Anterograde cell degeneration 47

Anteroventral nucleus, of the anterior thalamic region 44

Antidromic activation 46, 49

Antiepileptic drug (AED) 134, 143-144

Anxiety, with stereotactic stimulation/lesioning 48, 50, 56

Aphasia, see Speech disturbance

Appetite, with stereotactic stimulation/lesioning 48

Apraxia, with stereotactic stimulation/lesioning 53

ARAS, ascending reticular activation system 32, 50, 56-57, 122

Arousal 43, 56-57, 122, 129, 132,

Ascending head sensation, ictal 73

Ascending reticular activating system (ARAS) 32, 50, 56-57, 122

ASN, asparagine 26

ASP, aspartate 20, 24-27

Asparagine (ASN) 26

Aspartate (ASP) 20, 24-27

Asphyxia, perinatal 66, 71

Ataxia, with stereotactic stimulation/lesioning 35

Athetoid movements, with stereotactic stimulation/lesioning 36

Atonic falls, ictal 80, 82

Atonic generalized seizures 121

Atypical cortical lamination 85

Auditory aura 60, 80

Auditory system 54

Augmenting EEG response 46

Auguste Forel 30, 191

Aura, epileptic 11, 16, 23, 60, 66, 74, 77, 79-80, 84

Automatic spike detection algorithms 9, 21, 24, 27, 145, 148, 153

Automatisms, ictal 66, 71, 73, 116, 121

Autonomic signs, with stereotactic lesioning/stimulation 34, 43, 48, 53, 56, 61-62, 72

B

BA, Brodmann area 6, 45, 47-50, 54

Ballism, with stereotactic stimulation/lesioning 36-37

Basal forebrain 45, 135

Basal ganglia 30-31, 33-37, 43, 48-49, 51-52, 54-55, 136, 140, 146

Basal nucleus of Meynert 34, 43, 191

Base plane 42

Battery depletion, in VNS 134

Behavior 16, 19, 37, 39-40, 50, 56, 80, 104, 116, 134, 140

Bemegride, seizure model 145

Benzodiazepine receptor binding 147

Beta activity, ictal 141-142

Beta activity, coherence 115-116

Beta spindles 116, 120

Bicucilline, seizure model 145

Bipolar stimulation 9, 44, 49, 142

Bisynchrony 94

Bladder tone, with stereotactic stimulation/lesioning 56

Blink, see Eye blink

Blood pressure, with stereotactic stimulation/lesioning 56

Botulinum toxin 35

Brachium conjunctivum 30, 49, 51

Bradycardia, ictal 61-62

Brain biopsy, 121, 126

Brainstem 2, 30, 34-35, 38, 40-41, 45, 49-51, 55-57, 121-124, 128-130, 132, 139, 141, 144-145

Brainstem attacks, brainstem triggered convulsions 144-145

Broca, Paul 37

Brodmann area (BA) 6, 45, 47-50, 54

Bronchodilation, with stereotactic stimulation/lesioning 34

Burr hole 4-7

C

CA, cornu ammonis 32

CA3 cells 135

Calbindin 47

Calciumbinding proteins 47

Callosotomy 88-89, 102

Calretinin 47

Campotomy 34, 36-37

Capsula externa 43

Capsula interna 43, 105, 114, 127, 130

Carbamazepine 66, 104

Cardiotachymeter 67, 124

Cardiovascular control, with stereotactic stimulation/lesioning 34, 56

Cathodic stimulation 14, 16-20, 49, 153

Caudate loop 146

Caudate nucleus, see Nucleus caudatus

CD, cervical dystonia, see Dystonia

Cell transplantation 134-136

Central lateral complex (of the thalamus, CLC) 31, 49-51

Centré median de Luys, see Centromedian nucleus

Centrencephalic theory, of epilepsy 3, 144-145

Centromedian nucleus, of the thalamus (CM) 35-36, 41, 49-50, 127, 136, 143-144

Cephalic aura, ictal 60, 84-85

Cerebellar peduncle 57

Cerebellar stimulation 2, 137

Cerebellothalamic fibers 30-31, 49, 51-52

Cerebellum 30-31, 49, 52. 136-137

Cerebral peduncle 31-33,

Cerebrospinal fluid 14, 88, 104

Cerebrovascular lesion 17, 40, 136,

Cervical dystonia (CD), see Dystonia

Charge densities 149

Chemical stimulation 34, 144-145

Cholecystokinin 54

Cholinergic neurons 34, 135

Choreiform movements, with stereotactic stimulation/lesioning 36

Cingulate cortex 4, 6, 11, 15, 27, 32, 40, 45-46, 54-55, 60-63, 66-68, 72, 74-75, 77-78, 81-82, 85, 89-90, 94-95, 97-100, 102-104, 107, 112, 115, 117-120,

Circuminsular cortex 62-63, 65

Circumstantiality 116

CJD, Creutzfeldt-Jakob disease 2-3, 14, 123-127

Claustrum 34, 43

CLC, central lateral complex of the thalamus 31, 49

Clonazepam 121

Closed loop stimulation, see Feedback stimulation

CM, centromedian nucleus, of the thalamus 35-36, 41, 49-50, 127, 136, 143-144

Coagulation 4, 35, 106, 110, 112, 115, 126-127

Cochlear implants 2

Coding 40, 51

Cognitive evoked potentials 2, 11, 84-87

Cognitive impairment, with stereotactic stimulation/lesioning 39-41, 48, 50, 53, 138-141

Coherence analysis 7, 9, 115-116

Cold, feeling of, with stereotactic stimulation/lesioning 43, 56

Collicular afferents 33

Colloid cyst 141

Coma 112

Commissures, anterior, posterior 4, 30, 32, 42, 45, 53, 140

Complex partial seizure (CPS) 21, 23, 60-61, 66, 68-69, 71, 73-74, 78, 83, 115-116, 121, 138-141, 143-144, 146, 148

Compressed spectral array (CSA) 7, 24, 27

Conduction velocity 123, 125

Confusion, postictal 121

Confusion, with stereotactic stimulation/lesioning 50

Consciousness, clouding of, ictal 116

Cornu ammonis (CA) 32

Corona radiata 114

Corpus callosum 36, 43, 45, 88-89, 102, 127

Corpus Luysii, see Forel H field

Cortical activation 16, 46, 49-50, 122, 143-144

Cortical dysplasia 85, 139,

Cortical sources, see Cortical activation

Corticoreticular hypothesis, of epilepsy 144

Corticothalamic connections 38, 45-46, 48-49, 53, 91

Cough, with VNS 134

Coupling, electrotonic 127

CPS, complex partial seizure 21, 23, 60-61, 66, 68-69, 71, 73-74, 78, 83, 115-116, 121, 138-141, 143-144, 146, 148

Crawling, feeling of, with stereotactic stimulation/lesioning 74, 79

Creutzfeldt-Jakob Disease (CJD) 2-3, 14, 123-127

Cross power spectral density (CPSD) 47

CSA, compressed spectral array 7, 24, 27

Cycling stimulation 2, 152

D

DBS, deep brain stimulation 2, 30, 37, 47, 49, 134, 136-154

DC, see Direct Current

Deafferentation of the cortex 49

Débilité motrice 88

Decerebration 144

Decortication 49

Deep brain stimulation (DBS) 2, 30, 37, 47, 49, 134, 136-154

Déjerine-Roussy, thalamic syndrome 127, 130

Delta activity, ictal 63, 89, 103, 142

Dendritic membranes 127

Dendritic potentials 14

Depolarization 14, 17

Depression, major 17

Depression, with stereotactic stimulation/lesioning 16, 43, 145

Depth electrode, see Electrode

Destructiveness, with stereotactic stimulation/lesioning 50

Desynchronization 17, 143-144

Diagonal band, see Septal diagonal band

Diazepam 101, 104, 116, 120

Dichotomous concept 46

Diencephalic structures 30, 40-41, 45, 50, 141, 144-145

Digitization 7

Dipole, equivalent 65, 102-103

Direct current (DC) shift 144

Direct Current (DC) stimulation, recording 2, 14-20, 154

Discomfort in the throat, with VNS 134

Disorientation, with stereotactic stimulation/lesioning 141

Divergence, of thalamocortical pathways 46

Dizziness, with stereotactic stimulation/lesioning 48

DL-homocysteic acid 34

DM, dorsomedial nucleus of the thalamus 36, 43, 45, 47-49, 54, 84, 88-92, 95-104, 136, 140, 142-143

DMAZ, dorsal midbrain anticonvulsant zone 139

Dopa-induced dyskinesia 51

Dopamine 37, 51

Dorsal horn 56

Dorsal midbrain anticonvulsant zone (DMAZ) 139

Dorsomedial nucleus, of the thalamus (DM) 36, 43, 45, 47-49, 54, 84, 88-92, 95-104, 136, 140, 142-143

Dysarthria 106

Dyskinesia, with stereotactic stimulation/lesioning 36-37, 51, 53

Dysnomia 106

Dyssynergia, with stereotactic stimulation/lesioning 35

Dystonia 2, 34-35

E

ECG, electrocardiogram 7, 61-62

EDA, electrodermal activity 61-64

Edinger-Westphal nucleus, of oculomotor nucleus 57, 129-130, 132

EEG attenuation, ictal 17, 121-122, 124

Electrical sensation, with stereotactic stimulation/lesioning 53

Electrocardiogram (ECG) 7, 61-62

Electroconvulsive therapy 17

Electrocorticography 150

Electrode implantation 4-6, 123, 142-143, 148-149

Electrodermal activity (EDA) 61-64

Electrodes de type aigu 6, 124

Electromyographic recording (EMG) 90, 107-108, 110, 112-114

Electrooculogram (EOG) 7, 90, 130-132

Emboliform nucleus 49

EMG, electromyographic recording 90, 107-108, 110, 112-114

Emotion 37-39, 48, 56, 138

Encephalitis, Rasmussen's 104-115, 120-123

Enkephalin 54

Entopeduncular nucleus 30

Entorhinal cortex 40, 45, 48-49, 147

EOG electrooculogram 7, 90, 130-132

EPC, epilepsia partialis continua 104-115, 120-123

Epigastric aura, ictal 11

Epilepsia partialis continua (EPC) 104-115, 120-123

Epilepsy-prone rats, seizure model 135

Epileptogenic zone 2, 17-21, 103, 120, 149

Episodic information 40

Epithalamus 43

ER, evoked response 11-13, 19-20, 46, 49, 50, 72, 75, 82, 96-100, 105, 109-110, 116, 119, 129-131

Ethosuximide 111

Ethosuximide, seizure model 141

Euphoria, with stereotactic stimulation/lesioning 43

Evoked potentials 11, 46, 54, 79, 84, 86-87, 125, 131

Evoked response (ER) 11-13, 19-20, 46, 49, 50, 72, 75, 82, 96-100, 105, 109-110, 116, 119, 129-131

Excitatory amino acids 2, 20, 24-27

Excitatory interneurons 17

Excitatory state, with stereotactic stimulation/lesioning 141

Excitotoxic lesions 37

Extracellular fluid examination 6, 20, 24-27, 135

Extracellular glia potentials 14

Extrapyramidal tremor 136

Eye movement, ictal 121, 129

Eye movement, with stereotactic stimulation/lesioning 34, 37, 43, 54

Eye movement related potentials, 129-132

Eyelid movement, ictal 114, 129

Eyelid movement, with stereotactic stimulation/lesioning 75

F

Face twitching, ictal 114

Facilitation 14

Facilitatory inputs 51, 141

Fall, ictal 80-82, 115, 121, 143

Faraday cage 8

Fasciculus retroflexus Meynertii 43

Fasciculus thalamicus, see Forel H field

Fasciculus Vicq d'Azyrii, see Mamillothalamic tract

Fatigue, with stereotactic stimulation/lesioning 39, 43

Fear, ictal 66, 71-72, 73-74, 77-79, 84-85

Fear, with stereotactic stimulation/lesioning 48, 56, 72

Fearful behavior 88, 104

Febrile seizure 83-84, 101

Feedback stimulation 2, 145, 148, 153

Feeling of paralysis, ictal 80

Fetal hippocampal grafts, cell transplantation 135-136

Filtering 7

Fimbria fornicis 43, 135

Floating, feeling of, with stereotactic stimulation/lesioning 48

Flurothyl seizures, seizure model 139

Flushing, ictal 23, 73, 121

FO electrode, foramen ovale electrode 14-16, 121-122, 124

Focal seizure, see Simple partial seizure (SPS)

Foramen of Monro 39

Foramen ovale (FO) electrode 14-16, 121-122, 124

Forced normalization 20

Forceps delivery 101, 115

Foreboding, feeling of, with stereotactic stimulation/lesioning 56

Forel H field 30-35, 36, 51, 60-87, 120-123, 136, 137-139

Forel H-tomy 88, 137-138

Formaldehyde 123

Fornicotomy 39, 140-141

Fornix 30, 34, 36, 37-39, 40-41, 43, 65-66, 136, 140-141

Freezing, feeling of, with stereotactic stimulation/lesioning 43, 56

Frontal lobe 4, 6, 17, 21-24, 32, 37, 45, 47-49, 54-55, 71, 79, 81-82, 88-100, 101-104, 111, 115, 116, 121-122, 126-127, 142

Fronto-orbital 4, 22-23, 47-49, 89, 96-99, 102-104

Fundus striae terminalis 39

Funiculus, of the spinal cord 56

G

GABA, gamma aminobutyric acid 20, 36-37, 54, 135-136

GAD interneurons, hippocampal 135

GAERS, genetic absence epilepsy rat of strasbourg, seizure model 139

Galvanic skin response (GSR) 7

Gamma-aminobutyric acid (GABA) 20, 36-37, 54, 135-136

Gamma surgery 134, 149

Ganglion habenulae 38, 43

Gene therapy 135

Generalized seizure 14-16, 21, 23, 47, 66, 73, 79, 83-85, 88, 95, 100, 104, 111-112, 121, 127, 134, 135, 137-139, 140, 141, 142, 143, 144, 145, 146, 148

Generalized status epilepticus 85, 92-93, 100

Genetic Absence Epilepsy Rat of Strasbourg (GAERS), seizure model 39

Genetically epilepsy prone rats, seizure model 135

Gerstmann-like syndrome, postictal 116

Gestual automatism, ictal 73, 121

Gey's solution 21

Gigantocellular head movement region 34

Glia potentials 14, 17

Gliosis 40, 66, 76, 116, 117, 121

Globus pallidus (GP), pars externa (Gpe), pars interna (Gpi) 30-37, 48, 51-55, 140

GLU, Glutamate 20, 24-26, 35, 37, 54

GluR3 autoantibodies 121

Glutamate (GLU) 20, 24-26, 35, 37, 54

GLY, glycine 25, 54

Glycine (GLY) 25, 54

Goose skin, with stereotactic stimulation/lesioning 43

GP, globus pallidus 30-37, 48, 51-55, 140

Graft, see Cell transplantation

Griseum septi 43

GSR, galvanic skin response 7

Gudden's tegmental nuclei 40, 191

Gut tone, with stereotactic stimulation/lesioning 56

H

H1 field, see Forel H field

Habenula 38, 43

Hallucination, ictal 80

Hallucination, with stereotactic stimulation/lesioning 39, 43, 54

Haubenfelder (Forel H field), see Forel H field

Head movement, with stereotactic stimulation/lesioning 34-35, 40, 43, 56

Head sensation, with stereotactic stimulation/lesioning 43, 50, 73

Head trauma 23, 40, 88

Head version, ictal 23, 80, 82, 95, 116

Heart frequency, ictal 61-62, 72, 84-85, 121, 124

Heart rate, monitoring of 7

Hemianopsia 66, 71, 106, 116

Hemiballism, with stereotactic stimulation/lesioning 36-37

Hemiparesis 104, 106, 111, 121, 127, 130

Hemispherectomy 106, 112, 121-122

Hemorrhage 127, 130, 149,

Herpes zoster 127

Hess electrode system 7, 81, 102, 106

Hess, Walter Rudolf 35

High frequency discharge, ictal 15, 22, 62, 80, 82, 84-85, 90

High frequency stimulation 2, 35, 37, 46-47, 131, 136, 139-140, 142-143, 146, 148, 153

High pressure liquid chromatography (HPLC) 21

Hippocampus 2, 4, 11, 13-14, 16-27, 37-41, 45-46, 49, 61-63, 65-71, 74, 77-79, 81-82, 84-85, 107, 118, 121-122, 135-137, 140, 145, 146-148

Histology 35, 66, 76, 85, 116-117, 121

Hoarseness, with VNS 134

Hodgkin lymphoma 127

Hodology, thalamocortical circuitry 45-49, 56, 143

Hollow core electrodes 6-7, 20-23, 26

Homunculus 51-52

HPLC, high pressure liquid chromatography 21

Hypacusis 116

Hyperextension, of the trunk, ictal 80, 82

Hyperkinesia 34, 52, 137

Hyperphagia, with stereotactic stimulation/lesioning 149

Hyperpolarization 17, 146

Hypersexualism, with stereotactic stimulation/lesioning 149

Hypertension, with cell transplantation 136

Hyperventilation, ictal 84-85, 121

Hypotension, with stereotactic stimulation/lesioning 48

Hypothalamic hamartoma 142

Hypothalamus 3, 30-41, 48, 54-57, 78, 136-142

Hypothermia, with cell transplantation 135

I

i.LA, nucleus intralaminaris 49, 52, 55-56, 62

ICP, intercommissural plane, line 30, 42, 53, 137

IED, interictal epileptiform discharge 17-18, 23, 67-68, 71, 100, 105, 111, 143, 145-147

IgG-saporin 135

Immunolesioning 135

Immunoreactivity 47

Immunosuppressive therapy 121, 127

Impedance 15

Implantation, see Electrode implantation

Incontinence of urine, with stereotactic stimulation/lesioning 48

Inferior colliculus 54, 57

Inferior frontal gyrus 61, 63, 67, 71, 77, 81, 85, 102, 107, 112

Inferior temporal gyrus 48, 61, 63, 67, 77, 81, 85, 107

Inferior thalamic peduncle 48

Infralimbic cortex 32

Infraorbital nerve 131

Inhibition, with stereotactic stimulation/lesioning 11, 37, 46-47, 145-147, 153

Inhibitory connections 17, 51, 55, 139, 141, 146

Inhibitory motor areas 42, 109

Inhibitory transmitters 2, 54, 135

Insular cortex 32, 43, 46, 48, 54, 61-63, 65, 67, 72, 75, 77, 81, 107

Integration nuclei 49-50, 54

Intelligence, with stereotactic stimulation/lesioning 48, 86-87

Intercommissural AC-PC-line 42, 53, 137

Intercommissural plane (ICP) 30, 42

Intercontact spacing 6, 101

Interference 46

Interhemispheric seizure onset 88, 90-92, 95

Interictal epileptiform discharge (IED) 15, 17-18, 20, 23, 27, 61-63, 65, 67-68, 71, 74, 77, 79, 81-82, 86, 89-92, 94-95, 100-108, 110-114, 118, 121-122, 124, 127-128, 132, 140-147, 153

Intermediate dorsal nuclei, of the thalamus 53

Internal capsule 30-32, 35, 45, 52

International 10-20 electrode system 7

Interneurons 17, 135

Interstitial nucleus of Cajal (INC) 34-35, 51

Intestinal activity, with stereotactic stimulation/lesioning 56

Intralaminar nuclei 49-50, 52, 55-56

Ion sensitive microelectrodes 20

Itching, feeling of, with stereotactic stimulation/lesioning 74, 79

J

Jacksonian seizure 104

Joint sensibility, with stereotactic stimulation/lesioning 37, 51, 53

K

Kainic acid, seizure model 135, 139

K complex 101, 103-104, 129, 132

Ketogenic diet 134

Kindling, seizure model 135, 136, 139, 147, 153

Kinesthetic neurons 53

Klüver Bucy syndrome, with stereotactic stimulation/lesioning 149

Korsakoff syndrome (amnestic syndrome) 40

Kreuzschiene 8

L

L.po., nucleus lateropolaris 43, 50-52

Lamella lateralis thalami 50

Lamella medialis thalami 43, 50

Lamella meduallaris medialis 43

Language dominance 88

Larynx, innervation of 34, 55-56

Lateral dorsal nucleus of the thalamus (LD) 41

Lateral frontal areas 6, 32, 49, 54, 91-92, 95, 97, 100

Lateral geniculate body 54

Lateral hypothalamic zone 30, 32-34, 54

Lateral nuclear region, of the thalamus 31, 33-34, 50-53

Lateral posterior nucleus of the thalamus (LP) 41, 54

Laughing, ictal 70

LD, lateral dorsal nucleus of the thalamus 41

Lennox-Gastaut syndrome 138

Lenticular fasciculus, see Forel H field

Lentiform fasciculus, see Forel H field

Levopropylhexedrine 101

Lilly wave pulse, see Biphasic waves

Limbic system 32, 37-49, 56, 65, 136, 141-143

Lingual gyrus 85-87, 116, 118-119

Locus coeruleus 34, 55-56, 135

LORETA low resolution electromagnetic tomography 46, 49-50, 143

Low frequency stimulation 37, 46, 143, 145-146, 153

Low resolution electromagnetic tomography (LORETA) 46, 49-50, 143

LP, lateral posterior nucleus of the thalamus 41, 54

M

Magnocellular 47-49

Mamillary bodies (MB) 30, 38-39, 40-41, 45, 137, 141-142

Mamillothalamic tract (MTT) 32, 40-41, 43, 45, 141-142

Manual automatism, ictal 66, 71

Marchi preparations 32

Massa intermedia 44

MB, mamillary bodies 30, 38-39, 40-41, 45, 137, 141-142

MCP, midcommissural plane 42

Mechanical stimulation 144

Mechanism, of cell transplantation 135

Mechanism, of VNS 134

Mechanisms, of stimulation/lesioning 136, 149

Medial forebrain bundle (MFB) 34, 38

Medial lemniscal system 32, 50, 57, 123, 125

Medial longitudinal fasciculus 57

Medial nuclear group, of the thalamus 41-50, 142-144

Medial pallium 45

Medial parabrachial nucleus 34

Medial pulvinar complex 54

Median nerve stimulation, see Somatosensory evoked potentials

Medioventral nucleus (of the medial nuclear region) 47

Medulla oblongata 34, 55-56, 144-145

Memory function, with stereotactic stimulation/lesioning 39-41, 48, 50, 140-141, 147, 149

Mesencephalon 30, 34, 38-39, 45, 49-50, 54-57, 120-132, 139, 144-145

Mesial frontal lobe 4, 47-49, 90-92, 95, 97, 104

Mesial temporal lobe 11, 16-20, 22-23, 27, 47-48, 65, 66-68, 81, 85, 116, 121, 143, 146

Mesial temporal lobe epilepsy (MTLE) 66, 71, 79, 147-148

Mesocortex 45, 47

Mesolimbic system 38

Metabolism, with stereotactic stimulation/lesioning 37, 141

MFB, medial forebrain bundle 34, 38

Microdialysis 20

Microelectrode recordings 20, 37

Micropsia, ictal 116

Microthalamotomy 142

Micturation, with stereotactic stimulation/lesioning 48, 56

Midbrain, see Mesencephalon

Midcommissural plane (MCP) 42

Middle cerebral artery 105

Middle frontal gyrus 89, 97-98, 112

Middle temporal gyrus 15, 27, 32, 54, 61-63, 67-70, 72-75, 77, 81, 85, 118

Migraine 17, 83-85

Mild head injury 88

Monopolar stimulation 49, 142

Mood change, with VNS 134

Motor arrest, ictal 66, 71, 73, 116, 121

Motor cortex 16, 30, 35, 37, 51, 54, 105, 107-116, 145

Motor face area 107-108, 110, 112-116

Motor function 16-17, 34, 37, 42-44, 50, 52, 55-57, 74, 79-80, 104-106, 109, 120-121, 135, 137, 143, 145

Motor hand area 105, 107, 109-110, 112-114

Motor weakness, with stereotactic stimulation/lesioning 74, 79, 109

Movement disorder 30, 35-36, 52, 136, 139, 149

MTLE, mesial temporal lobe epilepsy 66, 71, 79, 147-148

MTT, mamillothalamic tract 32, 40-41, 43, 45, 141-142

Multifocal epilepsy 134, 138, 143

Muscimol, application of 47, 142

Muscle sensations, with stereotactic stimulation/lesioning 51

Mydriasis, ictal 63-64, 121

Myelinated fibers 30, 38, 48-49

Myoclonic seizure 138-139, 143

Myoclonus 60, 73-74, 79-80, 82-83, 104, 106-108, 110-115, 120, 123, 126, 140

N

N18 component, SEP component 125

N20 component, SEP component 125

Naming, impairment of, ictal 84-85

Naming, impairment of, with stereotactic stimulation/lesioning 53-54

Nausea, ictal 23, 73-74, 78

NCES, nigral control of epilepsy system 139

Near field potential 65, 114, 118

Negative motor phenomena, with stereotactic stimulation/lesioning 109

Neuropeptides 54

Neurotransmitter 20-27, 34-37, 54-56, 135-136

Nigral control of epilepsy system (NCES) 139

Nonpolarizable electrodes (Ag/AgCl) 14

Nonlinear algorithm 153

Nonspecific system, of the thalamus 45, 49-50, 143-144, 146

Noradrenaline 56, 135

NR, nucleus ruber 30, 33, 36, 121-123

NRM, nuclei raphe magnus 55-56

NRP, nuclei raphe pallidus 55-56

Nuclei raphe magnus (NRM) 55-56

Nuclei raphe pallidus (NRP) 55-56

Nuclei zentrolaterales 49-50

Nucleus accumbens 54

Nucleus anterio-inferior, of the anterior thalamic region 44-45

Nucleus anterior hypothalami 30

Nucleus anterior principalis, of the anterior thalamic region 44-45

Nucleus anterodorsalis, of the anterior thalamic region 44-45

Nucleus anteromedialis, of the anterior thalamic region 44-45

Nucleus antero-reuniens, of the anterior thalamic region 44-45

Nucleus arcuatus 30

Nucleus caudatus 31, 36-37, 43, 49, 67, 102-103, 112-113, 136-137, 145-146

Nucleus centralis magnocellularis 43, 49

Nucleus centralis parvocellularis 43, 49

Nucleus commissuralis thalami 43

Nucleus dorsalis superficialis 45

Nucleus dorsomedialis (DM) 36, 43, 45, 47-49, 54, 84, 88-92, 95-104, 136, 140, 142-143

Nucleus dorsomedialis hypothalami 30, 79

Nucleus fasciculosus thalami 43

Nucleus gracilis 55

Nucleus habenularis 43

Nucleus intermediodorsalis 34

Nucleus interstitialis 51

Nucleus intralamellaris (medialis) 43

Nucleus intralaminaris (i.La) 49, 52, 55-56, 62

Nucleus lateralis posterior 54

Nucleus lateralis septi 79

Nucleus lateropolaris (L.po) 43, 50-52

Nucleus limitans thalami 43

Nucleus medialis caudalis (also medioventral nucleus) 47

Nucleus medialis caudalis externus, of the medioventral nucleus 47

Nucleus medialis caudalis internus, of the medioventral nucleus 47

Nucleus medialis dorsalis, see Nucleus dorsomedialis

Nucleus paracentralis 34

Nucleus parafascicularis 34

Nucleus paraventricularis 30

Nucleus posterior hypothalami 30

Nucleus praeopticus medialis 30

Nucleus pulvinaris 36, 43, 53-54, 116-120

Nucleus pulvinaris anterior 34

Nucleus pulvinaris intergeniculatus 54

Nucleus pulvinaris oroventralis 43

Nucleus pulvinaris reticularis 43

Nucleus pulvinaris superficialis 53

Nucleus pulvinaris suprabrachialis 54

Nucleus reticularis polaris 43

Nucleus reticularis pulvinaris 43

Nucleus retroambiguus 55-56

Nucleus ruber (NR) 30, 33, 36, 121-123

Nucleus subcoeruleus 34

Nucleus subthalamicus (STN) 2, 30-37, 60-87, 136, 139-140, 153

Nucleus suprachiasmaticus 30

Nucleus supraopticus 30

Nucleus ventralis anterior (VA) 31, 34, 36, 41, 51

Nucleus ventralis posterolateralis (VPL) 34-35, 41

Nucleus ventralis posteromedialis (VPM) 34-35, 41

Nucleus ventrocaudalis anterior (V.c.a.) 43, 51

Nucleus ventrocaudalis parvocellularis externus (V.c.pc.e) 43, 51

Nucleus ventrocaudalis parvocellularis internus (V.c.pc.i) 43, 51

Nucleus ventrocaudalis portae 43

Nucleus ventrocaudalis posterior (V.c.p.) 43

Nucleus ventrointermedius 35, 41, 43, 51, 136

Nucleus ventrointermedius externus (V.im.e) 43, 51

Nucleus ventrointermedius internus (V.im.i) 43, 51

Nucleus ventrolateralis (VL) 34, 36, 41, 50-53, 105-106, 108-115, 126-127

Nucleus ventromedialis hypothalami 30, 79

Nucleus ventro-oralis (V.o.) 35, 43, 51-52

Nucleus ventro-oralis anterior (V.o.a.) 43, 51-52

Nucleus ventro-oralis internus (V.o.i.) 35, 43, 51-52

Nucleus ventro-oralis posterior (V.o.p) 35, 43, 51-52

Nucleus zentrolateralis caudalis 50

Nucleus zentrolateralis intermedius 50

Nucleus zentrolateralis oralis 50

O

Obesity, with stereotactic stimulation/lesioning 48

Object naming, with stereotactic stimulation/lesioning 54

Obsessive compulsive disorder, with stereotactic stimulation/lesioning 50

Occipital lobe 54, 66, 71, 84-86, 115-121, 129, 132

Ocular orbicular muscle 107-108, 110, 112-114

Oculogram (EOG) 7, 129-132

Oculomotor nerve 129-132

Oculomotor nucleus 57, 129

Olfactory brain 37, 146

Oligophrenia 111

OPA (o-pthalaldehyde) precolumn derivatization 21

Opiate 56

Optokinetic nystagmus 129-132

Oral automatism, ictal 66, 71, 73

Oral orbicular muscle 108, 110, 112-113

Orbitofrontal, see Frontal orbital

Oroalimentary automatism, ictal 66, 71, 73

Oropharynx, myoclonus of, ictal 104, 111

Oscillatory activity 36, 132

Overfulness, feeling of, with stereotactic stimulation/lesioning 56

P

P15 component, SEP component 79

PAG, periaqueductal gray matter 2, 39, 54-57, 127-132, 144-145

Pain 2, 30, 48, 50-51, 54-56, 127-132, 136, 145, 152

Paired pulse stimulation 11, 13

Palliative, surgery 20, 23, 60, 85, 88, 121

Pallidotomy 36, 51

Pallidum 30-37, 48, 51-55, 140

Papez circuit 37-38, 40, 45, 141

Parahippocampal gyrus 4, 15, 23, 27, 45-46, 60, 147

Parietal lobe 15, 54, 61-62, 77, 79, 85, 101-103, 107, 118, 121

Parinaud syndrome, with stereotactic stimulation/lesioning 129-130, 132

Parkinson's disease (PD) 2, 34-37, 51, 53, 137, 149

Pars ventralis diencephali 30

Partial seizure, see Focal seizure

Parvocellular 34, 47, 49-51

PC, posterior commissure 4, 30, 32, 42, 53

pCO_2 14

PD, Parkinson's disease 2, 34-37, 51, 53, 137, 149

Pedunculopontine nucleus (PPN) 31, 35

Penicillin, seizure model 145

Pentylenetetrazol (PTZ), seizure model 47, 141-142, 145, 153

Perfusate 21, 23-27

Periamygdaloid cortex 63

Periaqueductal gray matter (PAG) 2, 39, 54-57, 127-132, 144-145

Perifornical cortex 32, 38

Perigenual cortex 47

Periodic sharp wave complexes (PSWC) 126-127

Perirhinal cortex 32, 48

Perivascular lymphocytic cuffs 121

Perseveration, with stereotactic stimulation/lesioning 53

Petit mal seizure 3, 88, 92-93, 100-103, 111-112, 127, 138-139, 141, 144

Petit mal status 92-93, 100

PGM, see Periaqueductal gray matter

PGO, ponto-geniculo-occipital waves 132

Pharynx, with stereotactic stimulation/lesioning 56

Phase reversal 65, 114, 126-127

Phase spectral analysis 7, 9

Phenobarbital 81, 101, 121

Phenytoin 104, 111, 121

Phosphenes, with stereotactic stimulation/lesioning 54

Photic stimulation 131

Pilocarpine, seizure model 47, 135, 142

Placebo 134, 149

Plasmapheresis 121

Pneumencephalogram 4-5, 104

Point-to-point specificity (thalamocortical) 37, 46-47, 146

Pons 31, 34-35, 55-56, 132, 145

Ponto-geniculo-occipital (PGO) waves 132

Porcine endogenous retrovirus 136

Porcine neural cells 136

Porencephalic cyst 66, 71

Posterior commissure (PC) 4, 30, 32, 42, 53

Posterior lateral hypothalamic (LHAp) neurons 32-33

Posteroventral pallidotomy (PVP) 51

Postherpetic trigeminal neuralgia 129

PPN, pedunculopontine nucleus 31, 35

Precommissural fornix 38

Precommissural nuclei 35

Precommissural septum 38

Preeclampsia 83

Prefrontal cortex 17, 47-49, 54-55, 126-127

Prelimbic cortex 32

Premammalian hippocampal homologue 45

Premotor cortex 51, 54, 114

Premotor potentials, of eye movement 129-130, 132

Preoptic area 38, 54, 79

Prerubral area or nucleus 30, 36

Prestitial nuclei 35

Presubiculum 40, 45

Pretectal area 54

Preterm delivery 115

Primidone 104, 111

Prion protein 123-124

Pro-isocortex 47

Projection 30, 32-33, 35, 40, 45-49, 51, 54-57, 118, 120

Propagation, of seizure activity 2-3, 9, 22-23, 46, 60-63, 65-66, 68, 72-74, 78-79, 85-86, 92, 100, 111, 114, 116, 119-120, 136, 139, 140-146, 149, 152

PSWC, periodic sharp wave complexes 126-127

Psychological deficit, with stereotactic stimulation/lesioning 149

Psychomotor seizure 21, 23, 60-61, 66, 68-69, 71, 73-74, 78, 83, 115-116, 121, 138-141, 143-144, 146, 148

Psychosis, with stereotactic stimulation/lesioning 19-20

PTZ, pentylenetetrazol, seizure model 47, 141-142, 145, 151 (151 to be checked)

Pulsating sensation, ictal 84

Pulse width, of stimulus 153

Pulvinar 36, 43, 53-54, 116-120

Pupillary dilatation, with stereotactic stimulation/lesioning 43, 65

Push-pull cannula 6, 20-27

Putamen 30, 43, 49

PVP, posteroventral pallidotomy 51

Pyramidal fibers 52

Q

Quantitative EEG analysis 7

R

Radiosurgery 134, 149

Rage 48

Raphe nuclei 34, 54-57

Rapid eye movements, ictal 121

Rasmussen's encephalitis 104-110, 111-115, 120-123

Reaction time. with stereotactic stimulation/lesioning 53

Reclination, ictal 80, 82

Recruiting 14, 46, 143-144

Red nucleus, see Nucleus ruber

Reflex epilepsy 138

Refractory period 13

Regio preoptica 79

Regio septalis 79

Rejection, of neuronal grafts 136

REM sleep 114, 128-129, 131-132

Repérage 4-5, 101, 105

Repetitive transcranial magnetic stimulation (rTMS) 2, 134

Resection, surgical 17, 22-23, 41, 66, 71, 76, 116, 120, 147,

Respiration, ictal 61, 63, 67, 84-85, 90

Respiration, with stereotactic stimulation/lesioning 43, 56

Responsive stimulation, see Feedback stimulation
Reticular formation 34, 50, 55-57, 122, 144-145

Reticular nucleus of the thalamus (RTh) 30-31, 33, 144

Retroambiguus 55-56

Retrograde cell degeneration 32-34, 47, 49

Rexed's layer V-VIII 56

Rhinencephalon 37, 145-146

Rigidity, with stereotactic stimulation/lesioning 51-52

RNS, Responsive NeuroStimualtion, see Feedback stimulation

rTMS repetitive transcranial magnetic stimulation 2, 134

S

Saccade 37, 121, 128-129, 132

Sadness, with stereotactic stimulation/lesioning B23

Safety 36, 136, 147, 150, 152 (150 and 152 to be checked)

sAHE, selective amygdalohippocampectomy 20, 23, 60, 66, 71, 76, 79, 85, 121

Salaam seizure 143

Secondary generalization, of seizures 16, 21, 23, 66, 73, 79, 83-85, 88, 95, 100, 104, 111-112, 121, 138-139, 143-144, 146, 148

Secondary sensory area 107-108, 110,

Sedation, side effect of cell transplantation 135

SEEG stereo-electroencephalography 3-27, 60, 74, 80, 84, 88, 101, 105, 111, 116, 121, 126

SEF, spectral edge frequency 9, 24

Seizure detection algorithm 9, 21, 24, 27, 148, 153

Seizure propagation, see Propagation

Selection board 8

Selective amygdalohippocampectomy (sAHE) 20, 23, 60, 66, 71, 76, 79, 85, 121

Selective temporal lobe amytal memory test (STLAMT) 23

Self stimulation 34

Semipermeable polymers 135

Sensory cortex 50-51, 105, 107-110, 112-114

Sensory face area 107-110, 112-113

Sensory hand area 50, 105, 107-110

Sensory sensations, with stereotactic stimulation/lesioning 50, 54, 56, 74, 79

SEP, somatosensory evoked potentials 2, 11, 79, 123, 125

Septal diagonal band 79, 135

Septum 38, 48, 54, 79, 135

SER, serotonine 25-26, 55-56, 135

Serotonine (SER) 25-26, 55-56, 135

Sexual behavior, with stereotactic stimulation/lesioning 48, 56, 149

Sham control 17, 134, 149

Sharp wave, see Interictal epileptiform discharge

Sine wave stimulation 153

Single neuron recording 16

Single pulse stimulation 9, 11-13, 16, 19, 23-25, 46-47, 49-50, 64-65, 72, 74-75, 79-80, 82-83, 85-86, 96-100, 116, 147

Skin incision 4

Sleep induction, ictal 121-122, 124

Sleep regulation 52, 56-57, 122

Slow Wave Sleep (SWS) 9, 12-14, 21, 52, 56-57, 90, 100-101, 103-104, 114, 116, 128-129, 131-132

Smelling, with stereotactic stimulation/lesioning 43

SNPM, statistical nonparametric mapping 46, 48, 50, 143

SNr, substantia nigra pars reticulate, see Substantia nigra

Solitary tract nucleus 55

Somatosensory evoked potentials (SEP) 2, 11, 79, 123, 125

Somatostatin 54

Somatotopic organization 35, 50-51

Spatial sampling 3, 153

Spatiotemporal summation 46

SPECT hypoperfusion 147

Spectral edge frequency (SEF) 9, 24

Speech disturbance, with stereotactic stimulation/lesioning 53-54, 137

Spike, see Interictal epileptiform discharge

Spike detection algorithm 9, 21, 24, 27, 148, 153

Spinal cord 34, 51, 55-56, 127, 144

Spinal cord stimulation 127

Spindle-like activity 101, 103-104

Spinning, feeling of, with stereotactic stimulation/lesioning 48

Spinoperiaqueductal gray pathway 55

Spinothalamic tract 55, 57

Spontaneous absence seizures, seizure model 139

Spreading, see Propagation

Sprinter homunculus 52

SSMA, supplementary sensorimotor area 4, 85, 88-92, 95-100, 107, 112

Staring, ictal 73, 121

Statistical nonparametric mapping (SNPM) 46, 48, 50, 143

Status epilepticus 47, 60, 83, 85, 92-93, 100, 106, 121, 141-142, 146

Steam autoclaving 124

Stereo-electroencephalography SEEG 3-27, 60, 74, 80, 84, 88, 101, 105, 111, 116, 121, 126

Sterilization 21, 123

Stimulation frequency 37, 44, 46, 139, 142-143, 145-146, 153

Stimulation parameters, of DBS 2, 9-13, 44, 142, 153

STN, subthalamic nucleus 2, 30-37, 60-87, 136, 139-141, 153

Strange feeling, ictal 84-85

Strangeness, feeling of, with stereotactic stimulation/lesioning 39, 43

Stratum lacunosum moleculare (of the hippocampus) 45

Stria habenularis 43

Stria medullaris thalami 43

Stria terminalis 43, 54, 79

Striatal-nigro-amygdalar connections 146

Striate cortex 119-120

Striatum 30-31, 35-37, 43, 49, 67, 102-103, 112-113, 136-137, 145-146

Striothalamic tracts 139

Stroke 17, 40, 136

Strychnine, seizure model 145

Stuporous states, ictal 88, 92

Subcallosal cortex 47

Subdural electrode (strip/grid) 4, 140, 147-148

Subiculum 40, 45, 48

Substance P 54

Substantia grisea centralis, see Periaqueductal gray matter

Substantia innominata 34

Substantia nigra, pars reticulata (SNr) 30-31, 33-37, 55, 57, 135, 139

Substantia periventricularis, midline nuclei (Walker) 43

Subthalamic fasciculus 31

Subthalamic nucleus (STN) 2, 30-37, 60-87, 136, 139-140, 153

Subthalamotomy 36-37, 137-140

Sulthiame 111

Superior colliculus 33-34, 37, 54, 57, 128-130, 132, 139

Superior frontal gyrus 112

Superior temporal gyrus 32, 48, 54, 60-63, 67, 77, 81, 84-86, 118

Supplementary sensorimotor area (SSMA) 4, 85, 88-92, 95-100, 107, 112

Supramamillary nucleus 33

Supramarginal gyrus 27

Supranucleus pulvinaris intergeniculatus 54

Supranucleus pulvinaris lateralis 53-54

Supranucleus pulvinaris medialis 54

Supranucleus pulvinaris oralis 54

Supranucleus pulvinaris ventralis 54

Swallowing difficulties, with VNS 134

Swallowing disturbance, with stereotactic stimulation/lesioning 43, 56, 137

Sweating, with stereotactic stimulation/lesioning 43

SWS, slow wave sleep 9, 12-14, 21, 52, 56-57, 90, 100-101, 103-104, 114, 116, 128-129, 131-132

Sylvian region 62-63, 112

Synapse 16

Synaptic depolarization 14

Synchronization 46, 84, 86, 127, 132, 143

T

Tachistoscopy 84, 86-87

Tachycardia, ictal 72, 84-85, 121, 124

Taenia thalami 43

Talairach system 3-7, 32, 36, 42

tDCS, transcranial direct current stimulation 16-18

Tegmentum 30, 33-34, 39-40, 45, 50, 54-57, 124, 145, 191

Telencephalic theory, of epilepsy 144

Teleopsia, ictal 116

Temperature regulation, with stereotactic stimulation/lesioning 43, 56

Temporal lobe 4, 11, 15-18, 21-23, 27, 32, 39, 41, 46-49, 54, 60-63, 65-70, 72-75, 77-78, 80-81, 84-86, 88, 107, 116-119, 121-122, 140, 142-143, 146-148

Temporal lobe epilepsy (TLE) 39, 60, 66, 71, 79-80, 83, 85, 140, 147-148

Temporal lobe resection 17, 41, 85, 147

Temporo-occipital cortex 84-86, 117-118, 120, 129

Tentorial herniation 122

Teta/beta rhythms, of the mamillary bodies 141-142

Thalamic fasciculus, see Forel H field

Thalamic syndrome (Déjerine-Roussy) 127, 130

Thalamocortical circuitry 37-54, 65, 141-144

Thalamotomy, see Thalamus, stereotactic surgery

Thalamus 41-54, 83-120, 123-127, 141-144

Thermocoagulation 35, 106, 110, 112, 114-115, 126-127

Thermorhizotomy 127, 129

Theta activity, ictal 62, 88

Theta related cells 40

Thiamine deficiency 40

Tingling sensation, with stereotactic stimulation/lesioning 84

Tiredness, with stereotactic stimulation/lesioning 43

Tissue damage, with DBS 147, 149

TLE, temporal lobe epilepsy 39, 60, 66, 71, 79-80, 83, 85, 140, 147-148

TMN, tuberomamillary neurons 33

TMS, transcranial magnetic stimulation 2, 16, 134

Tolerance 34

Tonic posturing, ictal 80-82, 95, 100, 137

Tonic posturing, with stereotactic stimulation/lesioning 35

Tonic-clonic seizure, see Generalized seizure

Torsion, with stereotactic stimulation/lesioning 43

Torticollis, rotational, horizontal 35

Tractus mamillothalamicus, see Mamillothalamic tract

Train stimulation 9, 11, 23-25, 63, 65, 67-74, 79, 84, 105, 109-110, 119, 129-130, 132

Transcranial direct current stimulation (tDCS) 16-20

Transcranial magnetic stimulation (TMS) 2, 16, 134

Tremor 2, 36, 51-53, 136

Trigeminal neuralgia, postherpetic 127, 129

Trigeminal nucleus 50, 54-55

Trigonum, of the lateral ventricle 53, 116

Truncothalamic nuclei 49

Tuberal lateral hypothalamic (LHAt) neurons 32

Tuberomamillary (TMN) neurons 33

Tungstic acid gel, seizure model 145

Type aigu electrodes 6, 124

U

Uncertainty, feeling of, with stereotactic stimulation/lesioning 48

Unmyelinated fibers 48-49

V

V.c.a., nucleus ventrocaudalis anterior 43, 51

V.c.p., nucleus ventrocaudalis posterior 43

V.c.pc.e, nucleus ventrocaudalis parvocellularis externus 51

V.c.pc.i nucleus ventrocaudalis parvocellularis internus 51

V.im., nucleus ventrointermedius 35, 41, 43, 51, 136

V.im.e., nucleus ventrointermedius externus 43, 51

V.im.i., nucleus ventrointermedius internus 43, 51

V.o., nucleus ventro-oralis 35, 43, 51-52

V.o.a., nucleus ventro-oralis anterior 43, 51-52

V.o.i., nucleus ventro-oralis internus 35, 43, 51-52

V.o.p., nucleus ventro-oralis posterior 43, 51-52

VA, nucleus ventralis anterior 31, 34, 36, 41, 51

Vagus Nerve Stimulating (VNS) 2, 85, 134

Valproic acid 81, 101, 121

Vasoactive intestinal peptide (VIP) 54

Vca, anterior vertical line perpendicular to the AC-PC line 32, 42

Vcp, posterior vertical line perpendicular to AC-PC line 32, 42

Vegetative, see Autonomic

Ventral anterior nucleus of the thalamus (VA) 31, 34, 36, 41, 51

Ventral intermedial nucleus of the thalamus (Vim) 35, 41, 43, 51, 136

Ventral lateral nucleus of the thalamus (VL) 34, 36, 41, 50-53, 105-106, 108-115, 126-127

Ventral posteromedial nucleus of the thalamus (VPM) 34-35, 41

Ventral posterolateral nucleus of the thalamus (VPL) 34-35, 41

Ventral tegmental area 33

Ventral thalamic nuclei 31, 33-34, 41, 50-53

Ventralis-anterior complex of the thalamus (VA) 31, 34, 36, 41, 51

Ventricular enlargement 104, 116

Ventriculography 4-5, 105

Ventrobasal complex 50

Ventrofugal bundle 79

Ventromedial basal nucleus 32

VEP, visual evoked potentials 11, 46, 54

Verbal automatisms, ictal 121

Verbal learning, impairment, with stereotactic stimulation/lesioning 50

Vestibular nuclei 34-35, 51, 54

Vigabatrin 81

Vim, nucleus ventralis intermedius 35, 41, 43, 51, 136

VIP, vasoactive intestinal peptide 54

Visual evoked potentials (VEP) 11, 46, 54

Visual field restriction, ictal 116

Visual hallucinations, with stereotactic stimulation/lesioning 39, 43, 54

VL, nucleus ventrolateralis 34, 36, 41, 50-53, 105-106, 108-115, 126-127

VNS, vagus nerve stimulation 2, 85, 134

Vocalization, with stereotactic stimulation/lesioning 52, 56

Volume conduction 65-66, 114

Vomiting, with stereotactic stimulation/lesioning 43

VPL, ventral posterolateral nucleus of the thalamus 34-35, 41

VPM, ventral posteromedial nucleus of the thalamus 34-35, 41

W

Waking state 12-14, 89-91, 100, 116, 128, 131-132

Warmth, feeling of, with stereotactic stimulation/lesioning 43, 56

Water drinking, ictal 84-85

Waxman-Geschwind syndrome 116

WGA-HRP, wheat germ-agglutinin-conjugated horseradish peroxidase 33-34

Wheat germ-agglutinin-conjugated horseradish peroxidase (WGA-HRP) 33-34

Wing electrode ("Seitenelektrode") 6, 105-106, 108-110

Wyss stimulator 44

X

Xenotransplantation 136

Y

Yakovlev circuit 38, 45, 47-49

Z

Zentrales (Höhlen-)Grau, see Periaqueductal gray matter

Zentrolateral nuclei 50

Zona incerta 30-33, 36, 56

Zonal lamina of fibers 53

Appendix: Historical Note on Auguste Forel

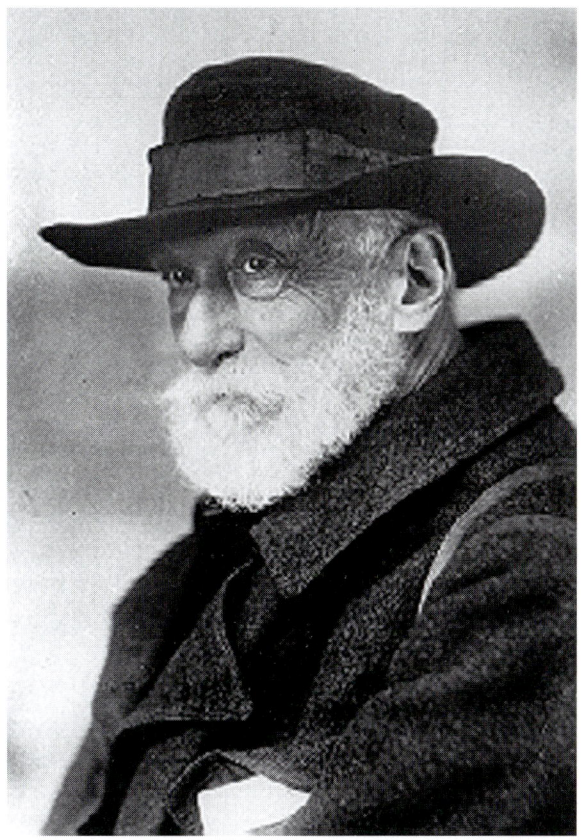

Auguste Forel was born in 1848 in the French part of Switzerland (Morges, Vaud, near Lake Geneva). He developed a lifelong passion for myrmecology (the scientific study of ants) in his childhood, but later chose medicine and neuropsychiatry to earn his living. He attended medical school at the University of Zurich from 1866 to 1871. He wrote his medical thesis – a comparative study of the thalamus – under Theodor Meynert in Vienna from 1871 to 1872. In the following years (1872 to 1879) he worked as an Assistant Physician to Bernhard von Gudden in Munich, leading to his seminal work on the organization of the tegmental region in 1877. In this work, he provided the first description of the zona incerta and the so called H fields (Haubenfeld); an anatomical structure that still bears his name. In 1877, he became "Privatdozent" (Lecturer) at the University of Munich. In 1879, he was appointed Professor of Psychiatry and Director of the Burghölzli Psychiatric Hospital in Zurich. While there, he became interested in the therapeutic value of hypnotism, also continuing his work on brain anatomy and ants. In 1887, his neuroanatomical studies with Gudden's method led him to formulate the neuron theory, four years before Wilhelm von Waldeyer, who received most of the credit for it [Winkelmann, 2007]. Forel then definitively turned his back on neuroscience. After his retirement from the Burghölzli asylum in 1898, and despite a stroke in 1912 that left him hemiplegic, Forel started to write extensively on various social issues such as alcohol abstinence and sexual problems [Forel, 1926]. Before his death in 1931 in Yvorne (Vaud, near Lake Geneva) at the age of 83, Forel published his myrmecological five volume magnum opus on the social world of the ants [Forel, 1921-1923], in which he made insightful observations on the neural control of sensory and instinctive behavior common to both humans and insects. The autopsy of his brain was performed by his former pupil, friend and colleague the well known neuropathologist Oscar Vogt [Akert, 1993; Parent, 2003].

Achevé d'imprimer par Corlet, Imprimeur, S.A.
14110 Condé-sur-Noireau
N° d'Imprimeur : 107104 - Dépôt légal : février 2008

Imprimé en France